THE HYPERACTIVE CHILD IN THE CLASSROOM

The Hyperactive Child In The Classroom

By

FRANK P. ALABISO, Ph.D.
Psychologist, Milton Robinson and Associates
Springville, New York

and

JAMES C. HANSEN, Ph.D.
Department of Counselor Education
State University of New York, Buffalo

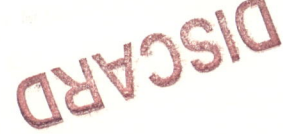

CHARLES C THOMAS • PUBLISHER
Springfield • Illinois • U.S.A.

Andrew S. Thomas Memorial Library
MORRIS HARVEY COLLEGE, CHARLESTON, W. VA.

Published and Distributed Throughout the World by
CHARLES C THOMAS • PUBLISHER
Bannerstone House
301-327 East Lawrence Avenue, Springfield, Illinois, U.S.A.

This book is protected by copyright. No part of it may be reproduced in any manner without written permission from the publisher.

© 1977, by CHARLES C THOMAS • PUBLISHER
ISBN 0-398-03550-4
Library of Congress Catalog Card Number: 76-2590

With THOMAS BOOKS *careful attention is given to all details of manufacturing and design. It is the Publisher's desire to present books that are satisfactory as to their physical qualities and artistic possibilities and appropriate for their particular use.* THOMAS BOOKS *will be true to those laws of quality that assure a good name and good will.*

Printed in the United States of America
A-2

Library of Congress Cataloging in Publication Data

Alabiso, Frank P
    The hyperactive child in the classroom.

    Includes index.
    1. Hyperactive children—Education. 2. Hyperactive children. I. Hansen, James C., joint author.
II. Title.
LC4711.A42   371.9'3   76-2590
ISBN 0-398-03550-4

This part of my life has been for my sons,
Jacob and Jamin.　　　　　　F.A.

My children, Paige, Dana and Scott, make
life and work worthwhile.　　　J.H.

PREFACE

Long before the recent changes in technology facilitated our present level of understanding of hyperactivity, we were frustrated in attempts to help the hyperactive child. Many of our beliefs about hyperactivity have changed radically over the past several years. Within the past decade, research in this area of child development has proliferated. Medical technology and recent advances in our understanding of learning theory have allowed us to view the hyperactive child from a different perspective. We no longer think of him as being mentally retarded or emotionally disturbed, but rather we have come to view him as a youngster who experiences a cluster of dysfunctions in the areas of learning, maturation and emotional development. These dysfunctions act to make the hyperactive child an inefficient learner. His inefficiency in acquiring knowledge, whether it be academic or psychological, seems to be at the crux of his problems in adjustment.

Our concept of hyperactivity must become more complex since we view it as a series of related dysfunctions. While overactivity is the distinguishing characteristic between hyperactivity and other forms of learning and maturational dysfunctions, overactivity alone is not a sufficient description of hyperactive behavior. Indeed, deficits in attention, with associated distractibility, impulsivity and cognitive dysfunction, are additional primary characteristics of hyperactivity.

Regardless of who has identified the child as hyperactive, the one individual who plays a central role in treating the condition is the classroom teacher. Other than the child's parents, no other single individual maintains the potential for a therapeutic effect on the hyperactive child. The classroom experiences are the fulcrum of his learning experiences. His attitudes about adults, his experiences with life, indeed, his very self-image, are shaped to a large extent by his accumulation of classroom experiences.

In this text we have attempted to integrate medical, psychological and educational knowledge about hyperactivity for use by the classroom teacher. This book is designed to help the teacher understand the characteristics of the hyperactive child and then serve as a guide to the classroom management of the child. The book begins with discussion of the characteristics which rightfully constitute a diagnosis of hyperactivity. Hyperactivity is defined as a subcategory of minimal cerebral dysfunction with a cluster of four basic symptoms: high activity level, deficits in attention-distractibility, cognitive dysfunctions and impulsivity. The second chapter presents a more complete description of the hyperactive child, theories of the causes of hyperactivity and several treatment modes. The four remaining chapters are structured to provide the reader with a thorough theoretical understanding of each of the four basic characteristics. We have attempted to bring research findings together with current knowledge of learning theory to provide the classroom teacher with a theoretical orientation and a set of treatment strategies.

We would like to acknowledge Laura Ireland, Christopher Lahey and Bonnie Himes for their technical assistance in preparation of the manuscript. We are also indebted to R. Timothy Rush and Joseph Robins for their comments on the chapter on cognitive dysfunctions.

F.P.A.
J.C.H.

CONTENTS

	Page
Preface	vii

Chapter
1. HYPERACTIVITY 3
   - Evaluation 5
   - Basic Characteristics 6
   - Case Histories 8
2. THE HYPERACTIVE CHILD 33
   - Characteristics of the Syndrome 33
   - Etiology of Hyperactivity 39
   - Modes of Treatment 46
3. ACTIVITY LEVEL IN HYPERACTIVE CHILDREN 73
   - Etiology of Activity Level 75
   - Measurement of Activity Level 83
   - Variables Affecting Activity Level 87
   - Behavioral Control of Activity Level 93
4. ATTENTION-DISTRACTIBILITY IN HYPERACTIVE CHILDREN 119
   - Concepts of Attention 122
   - Concepts of Distractibility 144
   - Modification of Attention Behaviors 153
   - Reinforcement Strategies 162
5. COGNITIVE DYSFUNCTION IN HYPERACTIVE CHILDREN 181
   - Cognitive Abilities 184
   - Memory Abilities 193
   - Learning Set 211
   - Cognitive Styles 213
6. IMPULSIVITY IN HYPERACTIVE CHILDREN 245
   - The Nature of Impulsivity 249
   - Relationship to Other Characteristics of Hyperactivity ... 262
   - Population Characteristics 266

Chapter	Page
Treatment Approaches	279
Strategies for Change	294
Author Index	313
Subject Index	321

THE HYPERACTIVE CHILD
IN THE CLASSROOM

CHAPTER 1

HYPERACTIVITY

THE TERM *hyperactivity* is used so frequently by such a wide variety of individuals responsible for facilitating the growth and development of children that one may have the impression that hyperactivity is commonly understood. Actually this is quite far from the truth. At times it seems as if our prejudices and stereotypes of hyperactive children outdistance our factual understanding of them.

There have always been hyperactive children, yet the written history of the disorder is relatively short. Indeed, prior to 1941, hyperactivity was thought to be either a form of schizophrenia or a type of mental retardation. The work of Werner and Strauss (1941) represented the turning point in our understanding of the hyperactive child. Their research with hyperactive children indicated that the types of errors they made in learning differed from those exhibited by mentally retarded children. Hyperactive children were characterized as experiencing difficulty in visual figures and backgrounds. They were also found to experience deficits in tactile recognition and in organizing incoming receptive stimuli. This differentiation between hyperactivity and mental retardation acted as a catalyst for future research. However, it also opened the gates for a flood of theoretical disagreement as to the nature and parameters of the condition. The terms that we use to label a condition often predetermine how others think about the child who suffers from it. This factor has represented a major problem for the hyperactive child who has been variously labeled as being organically driven (Kahn and Cohen, 1955), neurophrenic (Doll, 1954), and postencephalitic behavior disordered (Levy, 1959), to name a few.

Schrager and his colleagues (1966) closely scrutinized the volumes of research articles describing the condition in an attempt to define the nature of hyperactivity. A close analysis of this data narrowed the description of the hyperactive child as being socially immature, having a short attention span, being highly distractible, impulsive and uninhibited. Several years later, Schrager, et al. (1970) moved towards a social model to describe the hyperactive child. This model viewed the hyperactive child in terms of his proneness to failure in completing the educational tasks during elementary and high school years. Hyperactive children were viewed as members of "a population-at-risk" because they lacked the necessary skills to flow through the educational system. They were viewed as lacking the skills to achieve academic success at the kindergarten and first grade levels. They were observed to lack the skills needed to obtain a positive response from their teachers. Their skill in performing on standardized tests of readiness was described as limited. Finally, they lacked the motivation necessary for high attendance in school.

From a learning point of view, hyperactive children have been identified as suffering from a multiplicity of learning deficits (Gofman, 1970). Their learning styles have been characterized by disorders of language development as well as auditory discrimination and auditory sequencing abilities. They have been reported to suffer from visual-motor and visual-memory deficits along with gross motor incoordination. They are commonly described as suffering from an inability to recognize tactile stimuli and from an inability to correctly formulate right-left discriminations.

In the classroom they have been characterized as presenting a serious management problem to the classroom teacher (Minde et al., 1971). They were described as exhibiting many behavior problems which serve to be distracting to other children in the classroom. They maintain a high rate of academic failure in spite of the fact that their level of intelligence is usually average. Probably the first and foremost challenge they pose for the teacher concerns their difficulties in learning.

The rapidly growing research on hyperactivity, along with the numerous disagreements among investigators as to the characteristics and the nature of the condition, brought into existence a national task force to study hyperactivity and the other conditions classified under the title of minimal brain dysfunction (Clements, 1966). This task force sought to define the various forms of minimal brain dysfunction, to establish criteria for diagnosis, to identify the frequency of such conditions in the general population and to enumerate the variety of treatment modalities. The task force identified hyperactivity as one of the most frequent and most apparent subcategories of learning, physiological and psychological disturbances which come under the title of minimal brain dysfunction. In its overview of the causes of the condition, the task force cited a wide spectrum of biological and social variables (genetic variations, biochemical irregularities, perinatal brain trauma, illnesses and injuries, lag in maturation of a central nervous system, environmental trauma and the effects of socioeconomic cultural milieus). The condition was generally described as one in which children suffered from one or more disturbances in four major areas of functioning. The minimally brain dysfunctioned child was one who was described as suffering from a disturbance in motor functioning along with disturbances of sensory functioning, thinking abilities and learning abilities. Of thirty-seven different terms used to describe minimal cerebral dysfunction, five of them identify the condition known as hyperactivity. This is not surprising in view of the fact that of the one hundred research articles on the characteristics of minimal brain dysfunction surveyed, hyperactivity was at the head of the list of the ten most commonly cited characteristics.

Evaluation

A thorough evaluation of the child is recommended before a diagnosis is made. Evaluation procedures call for the gathering of detailed information on the various areas of the child's functioning. The medical history should include any history of illnesses pertinent to minimal cerebral dysfunction. This history includes prenatal, parinatal and postnatal information. The developmental history describes the child's developmental milestones including details of his motor and language development and the development of the adaptive behavioral social and personality skills. Finally, a family history should include a description of the lineage of both parents and the child's current family constellation. The physical examination is used to rule out systemic disease. Neurological examination is included to evaluate the developmental level of the neurological integration and to rule out specific disorders of the nervous system. Special examinations are recommended including opthalmolgic exams to evaluate both visual acuity, the child's visual processes, and audiometric examinations to rule out disorders of audition. Routine laboratory tests, such as an electroencephalogram (EEG), as well as special Xrays are included in a diagnostic evaluation. A rather extensive educational evaluation is also recommended. The academic history includes a detailed account of the child's school behavior and a history of academic success. This evaluation also includes a psychological evaluation composed of tests to measure the level of intellectual functioning, measures of perceptual functioning and behavioral observations. The academic history involves an assessment of speech and the development of language skills, including an assessment of receptive and expressive language. Finally, the educational evaluation includes an analysis of academic abilities, achievement and acquisition skills.

Basic Characteristics

Hyperactive children are well-known to every elementary school teacher, since one out of every ten elementary school children is hyperactive. The child is likely to be about seven years old when the overactivity first begins to attract notice. The condition was probably not diagnosed during the preschool years and will be present only in its secondary forms by the time he reaches high school. Hyperactivity is truly a condition of elementary school children. Family background, socioeconomic class and other similar variables have little effect on hyperactivity. Boys are five times more likely to be hyperactive than their female classmates (Brummet, 1968; Kenny, 1971).

Hyperactive children belong to that expansive group of youngsters who are commonly identified as experiencing minimal brain dysfunction, yet they differ in many respects from children having typical minimal brain dysfunction. Mentally retarded youngsters are three times as likely to be hyperactive, but hyperactivity in no way causes mental retardation. Children possessing minimal brain dysfunction are ". . . of near average, average, or above average general intelligence with certain behavioral disabilities ranging from mild to severe which are associated with deviations of functions of the central nervous system. These deviations may manifest themselves by various combinations of impairment in perception, conceptualization, language, memory, and control of attention, impulse or motor function" (Clements, 1966, pp. 9-10). What differentiates the hyperactive child from other children suffering from minimal cerebral dysfunction is the readily identifiable cluster of symptoms.

The large number of symptoms and the extensiveness of the diagnostic evaluation recommended are in themselves difficult to integrate into a simple concept of hyperactivity. It appears that what is needed is an understanding of the basic characteristics which could serve as a rule of thumb for identifying the hyperactive child and for responding to his special needs.

Werry (1968) factor analyzed the neurological examinations, the EEG's, the medical histories and the psychological and cognitive test performances of 103 hyperactive children. He found that there was no unitary dimension of hyperactivity. That is, there was no one cluster of causally related symptoms. However, the children exhibited a series of separate, independent developmental deficits that interacted with one another.

In our experience with hyperactivity, we have found the hyperactive child to be characterized by four basic symptoms. Hyperactive children exhibit a *disturbance of activity level*. Under certain conditions these children seem to have difficulty reducing their rate of activity. Many of the children also suffer from *disorders of attention*. They seem to have difficulty remaining at a given task for a specified length of time (attention span). Many of the hyperactive children who have an adequate attention span suffer from deficits in their ability to focus their attention while learning to discriminate between stimuli in their perceptual field. Such children often demonstrate difficulties in selective attention and are highly distractible. Complex perceptual discriminations seem to exceed their abilities. Many hyperactive children experience a variety of *cognitive dysfunctions*. Their pattern of intellectual abilities is characterized by much unevenness and disparity between various abilities. They may experience difficulties with visual and auditory memory as well as deficits in mediation abilities. Such children often exhibit maladaptive response sets and maintain faulty cognitive styles. Their ability to produce an acceptable answer may be impaired by deficits in verbal and motor expression. Finally, we have observed many hyperactive children to be *unduly impulsive*. These children respond quickly during problem-solving tasks and seem to lack the problem-solving strategies used by most children in making a critical evaluation of their response alternatives.

These characteristics (high activity level, deficits in attention-distractibility, cognitive dysfunctions and impulsivity) will serve as our guide in understanding the hyperactive child in the subsequent chapters of this text. In the remaining pages of this chapter, four case histories are presented to exemplify the presence of these characteristics in typical hyperactive children.

Case Histories

The variable which allows us to differentiate those children whom we call hyperactive from the children suffering from other forms of minimal cerebral dysfunction (MCD) is the clustering of symptoms which typify the hyperactive child. More than any other MCD child, the hyperactive child is typified by the presence of several concurrent learning dysfunctions. There is enough scientific evidence to dispel formerly held concepts of hyperactivity as being a syndrome. In other words, it is not safe to assume that the symptoms which characterize the hyperactive child are causally related. Perhaps a better definition of this phenomenon is that the hyperactive child is one who experiences two or more minimal cerebral dysfunctions, one of which is always a heightened activity level. The dysfunctions vary in the degree to which they affect the child's ability to learn. It should always be remembered, however, that even if the other dysfunctions are minimal, the interaction with heightened activity level invariably results in serious learning problems.

A Case of Cognitive Dysfunction in a Hyperactive Seven-Year-Old Boy

Tony was first brought to our office by his mother during the first few months of his enrollment in second grade. His problems with reading during the first grade prompted her request for evaluation. She reported that Tony was unable to improve in reading throughout the first grade. Tony's reading ability had not improved even though he had received extensive help in reading during the first grade. His mother had heard that emotional maladjustment often caused reading problems and had wondered if Tony was emotionally upset and unable to tell her about it.

HOME. Tony's relatively well-controlled behavior in school gave way to irritability, tantrums and heightened activity level at home. At home Tony complained about everything. He was particularly sensitive to loud noises and would hold his ears when the other children at home raised their voices. He complained of headaches while holding the sides of his head. Generally, he was negativistic at home, overreacting to criticism. If his parents raised their voice in response to his behavior, Tony would run from the room and hide for several hours at a time. Occasionally, during an upset, Tony would scream out that he knew that he was stupid. Tony's mother wondered if he was troubled by bad dreams, since he had a history of waking up frequently during the night.

His mother was quite confused by his insistence that everything at home be "perfect." Tony became irritable at the slightest change in the home routine. At the same time, he seemed to lack organization and self-discipline. His negative comments about the untidy state of his brother's room were a source of much conflict at home, yet Tony never seemed to be able to organize his own room. He would fly into a rage whenever this was pointed out to him.

Tony's mother reported that she and her husband had tried a variety of approaches in dealing with Tony. The home situation had gotten to the point where his parents had become sensitized to the situations which caused Tony to overreact. Much of their time at home was spent in avoiding outbursts by directing Tony away from frustrating situations. They had attempted to keep Tony calm by allowing him to do the things at home that he liked. Of course, this brought on many complaints from Tony's brother who could not see why such an irritable child should have so many privileges. Tony's mother and father did find that talking to him calmly during tantrum periods helped. Their experiences with verbal threats, spanking and offering rewards all proved negative.

DEVELOPMENT. In reviewing the early developmental history, Tony's mother reported that she did experience some minor problems during the pregnancy. She recalled that the delivery was three weeks past the predicted due date. She had made several trips to the hospital with false labor pains during the eighth month of the pregnancy. She commented that other than the fact that "the baby's head was turned," the delivery was normal. Her description of delivery suggested that Tony was born in the breech position.

Tony's motor development seemed to lag. He did not sit up until age eight months. He started to show initial signs of walking at sixteen months but was not fully ambulatory until he was two years old. His speech development was also immature. He did not begin to use sentences until age twenty-four months. Toilet training presented many problems for Tony. He was two and one-half before he had mastered toilet training during the daytime hours. Enuresis continued until age five.

The medical history was generally unremarkable. However, Tony did have two convulsions at age eighteen months. These were grand mal convulsions, but they were diagnosed by the family doctor as being associated with high fever.

SOCIAL BEHAVIOR. Tony was described as relating poorly to all male and female peers. Regardless of the situation, Tony insisted on having the leadership role. He seemed to become upset when he could not direct the interactions of his playmates.

His parents felt that he enjoyed play because it placed few restrictions on his activity level. They noticed that whenever it was time to change from a high activity level game to one which required attention and patience, Tony began to develop problems in relating to the other children.

Tony was not enthusiastic in making friendships. He usually withdrew when meeting new children. He seemed to want reassurance that they would accept him. Yet he resisted any interpretation that the reluctance of other children was a reaction to his play habits.

His relationship with his younger brother was the cause of many conflicts at home. Tom complained that Tony, with his negative attitude and behaviors, did not deserve the privileges that he received. He did not wish to play with Tony nor did he wish to have Tony around when he was playing with his friends. He claimed that Tony's bossiness and his explosiveness made Tom's friends want to stay away. Tony, on the other hand, complained bitterly that Tom was lackadaisical and that he did not do things properly. Their arguing was continuous.

Tony seemed to relate best to his mother. He brought problems to her and generally sought her out when he wanted affection. Tony's father was not distant, but his employment did keep him away from home a great deal. He was a tolerant man but generally not demonstrative in his affection. Evidently, this was enough to encourage Tony's withdrawal. Tony did not receive discipline well from either parent. Demands for conformity usually resulted in tantrums. Tony's mother complained that family activities were curtailed by Tony's disruptiveness. His inability to sit still had been the source of much unhappiness on family trips. During the previous summer Tony's mother and father had agreed that they would no longer make the long drive to Tony's grandparents house for their annual vacation.

Many of their other leisure-time activities were curtailed. Tony's mother even complained that his overactivity in church was a source of weekly embarrassment.

SCHOOL. The school history was marked by numerous problems in adjustment. Although there had been no retentions, Tony's reading problems seemed to be the source of much underachievement in all of the academic areas. His teacher described him as very fatigued in school. He seemed fretful and complained that other children spoke too loudly. He exhibited number and letter reversals and had much difficulty in simple motor tasks such as lacing his shoes. Tony's teacher thought that these problems might be related to the fact that Tony seemed to exhibit mixed dominance. By the time he reached second grade he was still unable to tell time or read a clock.

The chief complaint seemed to center around Tony's difficulty in bringing his activity level under control. His teacher wondered if his reading would not improve dramatically if his activity level was better controlled. Tony's attendance in school was good, but during the three weeks preceeding his first appointment at our office his requests to stay home had become an increasing problem on school days.

EVALUATION. The pattern Tony presented was quite typical of a hyperactive child with a cognitive dysfunction. Tony's parents accepted the recommendation that a full evaluation of his cognitive abilities, visual motor abilities and personality development be made.

Tony's test pattern was very typical of the performances exhibited by hyperactive children. His overall performance on the intelligence test indicated that his intellectual potential was in the bright normal range. However, there was a wide variability between several of his cognitive abilities. His word knowledge ability and his ability to collect, store and retrieve information were found to be nearly at the mentally defective level. In contrast, his ability to use previous experiences in dealing with novel situations and his immediate short term auditory memory ability were found to be in a superior range. His low scores on several measures of verbal abilities tended to counterbalance his exceptionally high scores in the remaining verbal ability areas. His overall verbal ability was within the average range. This contrasted greatly with his exceptionally well developed nonverbal abilities. However, even within this group of abilities the degree to which each of the abilities was developed varied greatly. Tony's ability to comprehend social situations, for instance, was in a very superior range while several other of his nonverbal abilities did not exceed the average range. The difference between his ability to perform on a verbal and nonverbal level was significant.

Tony exhibited a borderline performance on measures of perceptual-motor development. As his teacher had pointed out, his demonstrated mixed dominance, rotations, substitutions and difficulty in reproducing angles typified his attempts to reproduce visual images.

Apparently, he also experienced minor deficits in his ability to identify the locus of tactile stimulation. During this phase of the testing, with his eyes closed, Tony was unable to identify various body locations that were touched by the examiner.

In view of Tony's deficits in visual motor development and tactile ability, a special opthalmalogic examination was recommended. Tony was referred to an opthalmalogist who specialized in the diagnosis of vision problems in learning disabled children. The results of his examination indicated that Tony experienced deficits in visual recognition and visual memory. His ability to fixate and converge his vision on reading materials was at an immature level. He was confused over concepts of directionality. In particular, Tony had no concept of the difference between right and left.

Tony's difficulty in identifying the locus of tactile stimulation, along with his complaints that loud noises caused headaches and his history of convulsions, prompted referral to a pediatric neurologist for further evaluation. Tony's parents were very relieved to find out that his neurological status was normal.

Tony's performance on several measures of auditory ability indicated that his level of auditory reception and verbal expression were somewhat underdeveloped for his chronological age. Several of his psycholinguistic abilities were found to be at a lower level of maturity, however. Here again his pattern of abilities was one in which extremely well developed abilities were offset by several poorly developed abilities.

Tony's performance on the various personality tests indicated that even at this young age hyperactivity had begun to affect his self-image. His performance on one of the measures of self-concept indicated that he felt inferior to his younger brother. His negative feelings over his own ability tended to aggravate his competitiveness with Tom. He viewed himself as unable to compete with Tom. Many of his fantasies centered around being an only child. He tended to view himself as a highly anxious youngster and considered himself to be of low intelligence. He saw himself as alienated from both parents, believing that they disliked him. He felt that he was the brunt of other people's anger and believed that others scapegoated him.

On a broader measure of personality assessment, Tony's responses indicated that he felt stress in almost every area of interpersonal involvement. He tended to view himself as in need of help in order to be successful. He seemed to feel frustrated in his competitiveness with other children. He tended to view himself as an "ugly" child and saw himself as the least-liked member of his family. He seemed very conflicted in his perception of his relationship with his mother. He tended to view himself as wishing to please her in order to earn her approval. At the same time, he seemed to wish to be free of dependencies on her. He was confused by the fact that he perceived her as submissive in her relationship with his father and yet she seemed powerful and controlling in her relationship with him. Just prior to being evaluated he had come to fear that his uncontrollable behavior at home would result in his placement. Many fears about separation from his mother had developed. He seemed to maintain a strong wish that she care for him and protect him. This wish was a source of conflict in his relationship with peers where he thought of himself as wanting to be a leader.

Tony was having much difficulty in integrating his needs for independence with his strong wish to be taken care of. These conflicts were complicated by the fact that he had developed a constellation of fearful feelings about family life. He worried that his behavior had begun to cause family disintegration. Evidently he had developed many fears of separation which he pictured in his fantasies as being brought about by both parents conspiring to abandon him. He developed a very unrealistic picture of his parents' feelings towards him. He came to believe that they were continuously angry with him. At the same time, he developed little insight into the many ways in which he had provoked hostility in others. He maintained a counterfantasy in which he saw himself as the most powerful member in the family. He daydreamed of being able to summon his parents at his beck and call.

Needless to say, Tony was a very anxious youngster. He maintained no insight into the cause of this problem. The reactions of others to his hyperactive behaviors led him to believe that he was unwanted and unlikeable. From a learning point of view, his problems in reading abilities stemmed both from the uneven pattern of his cognitive development and from his developmental lag in visual motor development and auditory reception and verbal expression. The combination of his overactivity and his cognitive dysfunctions seemed to be overwhelming to him and acted to confuse others.

A Case of Severe Overactivity

Ronny was six years old and already in special education classes. By the time his mother brought him for evaluation, she described him as uncontrollable both at home and at school. She complained that no form of discipline had been able to curb his overactivity. She described him as being in "perpetual motion." As might be expected, his attention span and degree of concentration were limited. Ronny was easily frustrated. He seemed to act out his hostility on toys. His mother complained that they had stopped purchasing toys for him because of his destructiveness.

His overreaction to his mother's leaving home for several days to care for a sick relative precipitated her request for evaluation. During her absence he complained of a continuous stomach ache. He was irritable and had returned to bedwetting.

HOME. Ronny's mother reported that his limited needs for

sleep had been a major source of problems at home. It was common for him to require less than five hours sleep. Quite often he would awaken during the night and play by himself. On one occasion this almost ended in near tragedy when he caught his hair on fire on the kitchen stove. His parents had resorted to having him sleep in the same room with them.

Ronny's mother had complained that no technique had been successful in curbing his overactivity. She had tried reasoning with him and spanking with no success. At one time she had held out some hope for controlling his behavior by sending him to his room when he became particularly disruptive. At first this seemed to help, but on one occasion he became so irritable and explosive over having to remain in his room that he broke the slats on his bed. Family life was adjusted to his overactivity. Television programs were closely monitored, for instance, as he became more overly active in watching exciting television shows.

DEVELOPMENT. In describing her pregnancy Ronny's mother reported that due to a series of illnesses, the obstetrician had warned her that the pregnancy was in danger. Ronny's mother described the delivery as a very difficult one. He was born with the umbilical cord wrapped around his neck and, according to the doctor, the child experienced minor damage to his spleen in the birth process. It was later discovered that he also sustained injury to his left eye during the delivery.

Generally, the developmental history was within normal limits. Ronny sat up at four months and walked at nine months. He was speaking in sentences by the time he was eighteen months old. Toilet training was delayed until thirty-six months with bedwetting continuing to be a problem. The medical history contained no major illnesses but was marked by a series of minor injuries, most of which seemed to be related to clumsiness.

SOCIAL BEHAVIOR. Ronny's mother described him as highly aggressive in his relationship with peers. Indeed, he seemed to relate only to the most passive children. When in the company of other children he tended to be aggressive and boastful. The stimulation of meeting new peers seemed to bring on an even greater degree of overactivity. Many of the neighborhood children were not permitted to play with him because his aggressive acts and lack of judgement had caused many accidents.

Of Ronny's three brothers, only his thirteen-year-old brother, Leon, was still living at home. Leon was a rather passive teenager who showed remarkable patience with Ronnie. The relationship between the two was a positive one. Ronny seemed to be closest to his mother. He was very guarded about his relationship with her. He seemed to not wish to share her attention with others, including adults. She noted that he would become frantic when she would leave his sight. Many home incidences were recounted in which tantrums were linked to his refusal to accept her going out of the house. Ronny's mother described her husband as distant in his relationship with Ronny. He was an older gentleman who dealt with Ronny's continuous activity and irritability by avoiding contact with him.

SCHOOL. Even though Ronny was only six, the school history was quite an extensive one. In anticipation of his problems in adjusting to kindergarten, Ronny's mother had entered him into a preschool program. His overactivity in the preschool program became especially apparent whenever he was required to decrease his activity level. During free play and active games he tended to be more active than the other children but relatively better controlled than was his usual custom. During organized group activities, such as learning to form a line and rest period, he became overly excitable and, at times, belligerent. He seemed to adjust better to the socialization aspects of the kindergarten program. Any attempts at structured academic learning invariably resulted in much frustration on Ronny's part. He seemed to do much to attain negative attention from his teacher. Even though he was just completing the last month of school in the first grade special class program, he could not count past ten. He had much difficulty conforming to the discipline of even this relatively unstructured classroom situation. He could remain in his seat for only brief periods of time. Even while sitting, he was observed to shift his weight from one side to the other and to tap the top of his desk with his pencil.

EVALUATION. Psychological testing included a measure of intelligence, measures of perceptual motor development, auditory reception and verbal expression. Tactile learning ability was tested in addition to a full personality assessment. Special tests included opthalmalogical and neurological examinations.

Ronny's performance on the intelligence test indicated that his intellectual potential was in the average range. His overall verbal performance and his overall nonverbal performance were relatively well matched. However, the differences between various verbal abilities and the difference between various nonverbal abilities were significant. Immediate short-term auditory memory, abstract thinking ability and arithmetic reasoning ability were found to be in a defective range. Abilities in eye-hand coordination, comprehension and details were also found to be significantly below average.

Ronny's qualitative performance on the intelligence test was probably indicative of his general approach to learning tasks. He had much difficulty in following instructions. Whenever confronted with a change in instructions, he would revert to the previous set of instructions. On the vocabulary subtest he substituted words. For instance, he dealt with the stress of not knowing the definition of the word "gamble" by insisting that the examiner had asked for a definition of the word "camel." He experienced sequencing problems in arranging pictures in their proper order and arranged them from right to left. He also exhibited many reversals in writing as well as in verbal expression. He was overly distractible at times during the evaluation.

His performance on the auditory test indicated that he experienced deficits in the area of auditory learning. He obtained a language age of five years three months, a score which placed his language ability well over a year behind his chronological age. His perceptual-motor functioning also appeared to be impaired. He showed severe deficits in the area of substitutions, rotations and perseveration. He seemed to be little able to distinguish between different sizes and shapes. He had particular difficulty in reproducing objects in relationship to one another. No deficits were found in his tactile abilities. Evidently, he was well able to learn through his sense of touch.

Personality testing indicated that Ronny's hyperactivity was having a devastating effect on his self-concept. He tended to view himself as unlikeable and as the object of ridicule. He seemed to feel that the only way to gain approval of others was to align himself closely with his mother, whom he viewed as successful and as well-accepted by others. He tended to think of himself as different from other children and seemed to feel that the only way he could be assured of a response from others was to provoke anger. He exhibited many concerns over his own aggressiveness. He tended to dislike himself for his hostility but at the same time felt unable to control his own behavior. On a deeper level, Ronnie viewed himself as not having enough of his parents' love. He tended to respond to what he viewed as a lack of affection with anger.

He was very conflicted regarding dependency. He seemed to want to gain his parents' affection through dependency but feared that he would fail at doing so. He considered his mother's attempts to set limits on him as an indication of her anger. He seemed to be confused by the limit setting of adults. He tended to view this as rejection rather than as an encouragement of his independency. Much of his difficulty in adjusting seemed to center around his feelings about school. He tended to view school as a punishment and had come to believe that his mother had sent him there as a means of rejecting him.

In view of his clumsiness and frequent complaint of headaches, a neurological examination was recommended. The results of the neurological exam indicated the presence of only "soft signs" of neurological impairment. A special opthalmological examination was also advised in view of his reported eye injury at birth and his poor performance on the tests of perceptual-motor ability. He was examined by an optometrist specially trained in diagnosing learning disabilities. He was found to have deficits in visual accommodative ability. His ability to fixate on visual stimuli was also found to be deficient. Eye-hand coordination abilities were at a low level of development, and he was found to have difficulty in perceiving the form of visual stimuli. Finally, his visual recognition skills were quite limited.

Ronny's overall performance was quite typical of a highly active child with additional cognitive dysfunction. His conflicts over independence and his needs to identify with his mother, whom he saw as his only link with success, presented serious problems to his adjustment. A multi-approach treatment plan was necessary. Special learning assessment and special academic programming was begun. Visual training was conducted at home by Ronny's mother under the direction of the opthalmologist. The family doctor prescribed medication which helped to control activity level and seemed to improve attention span and concentration ability. Ronny was also seen for several months in weekly psychotherapy to help him work through his struggles with independence. Ronny's mother was seen weekly in a parents group in which she learned more effective child management skills.

A Case of a Hyperactive Impulsive Boy

By the time Kenny was seven years old he had his parents at their wits' end. He was brought to the office by his mother who described him as a "nervous and hypertensive child." She complained that he became hysterical whenever scolded. His tantrums had been the source of much disagreement between relatives who accused the mother of having spoiled him. She described his restlessness and inability to sit still as a major problem in school. She had received many notes from the teacher describing Kenny as unable to sit down and as unwilling to control his behavior. Evidently, Kenny was verbally overproductive also. She described his incessant talking as "nerve wracking." His ability to follow instructions was impaired, and she noted that in the last school report the teacher commented that instructions needed to be repeated several times before Kenny could complete them. He exhibited many fears, especially a fear of the dark. While there was no sleep disturbance, he was reluctant to sleep alone at night. Apparently, his self-confidence had been weakened as he complained continuously that he was unable to do things.

Low frustration tolerance was another problem area. He was

not a particularly aggressive child but did become angry with only slight provocation. Kenny's mother's strongest complaint was related to his "quickness and poor judgment." She complained that Kenny would begin to respond to requests before the instructions had been completed. She described him as being a child who "never thinks things through." Evidently, his quick responses were characterized by little critical evaluation of alternative responses. Kenny's mother and father felt that they had exhausted every means of bringing his behavior under control. In fact, their referral was prompted by the fact that Kenny became hysterical at any mention of discipline.

DEVELOPMENT. There was a history of complications in the birth process. Kenny was premature by six weeks; however, the delivery went normally. Kenny was born with a deformed palate. At three months he was hospitalized for one week for corrective surgery. The developmental history was generally unremarkable. Sitting, walking and talking all occurred within the normal time ranges. Toilet training lagged behind by six months. The medical history was a rather extensive one due to Kenny's needs for corrective surgery. He had been hospitalized three times in relation to treatment for his deformed palate.

SOCIAL BEHAVIOR. The combination of Kenny's impulsivity, hyperactivity and speech problems made peer relationships difficult. He was the object of ridicule by his classmates to such an extent that he refused to ride on the school bus. He did seem to relate better when playing with one other child. In most of his peer relationships, Kenny tended to be passive. He seemed to show little willingness to express himself and generally was reserved when meeting new children. Kenny related well to his younger brothers. While this was one positive area of relating to children, Kenny tended to act immature when playing with them.

Kenny seemed closest to his mother and tended to bring problems to her and sought her out for affection. He did seem to enjoy his father's company and was reported to look forward to weekends so that he could help his father with repairs around the house. Generally, Kenny was affectionate with adults. He seemed to feel more secure with them than with peers.

SCHOOL. Kenny's problems in school were quite extensive. Evidently, they did not become manifest until first grade when he was required to complete academic assignments. He showed deficits in handwriting and reading. The teacher described him as a behavior problem saying that he refused to stay in his seat. His impulsivity was a major area of concern. He tended to respond before instructions were completed. His teacher felt that his "inability to think things through" obscured his intelligence, which she believed to be average. At one point, his impulsivity made the teacher question whether Kenny had a hearing problem. She began to think that he was unable to hear all of her directions. However, a hearing test conducted by the school nurse was negative.

EVALUATION. A full psychological test battery was administered. Kenny's performance on the intelligence test was indicative of learning disability. His pattern of intellectual ability was characterized by wide variability between various abilities. Verbal and nonverbal abilities were not well matched. In the verbal area, for instance, his ability to use and understand the meanings of words was in a superior range while his arithmetic reasoning ability was found to be at a near mentally defective level. The scatter between the nonverbal abilities was not quite as dramatic, but nevertheless it represented a handicap to learning. His performance on the test was suggestive of impulsivity. His initial responses to questions were of poor quality. It was necessary to present test questions several times before Kenny produced the correct answer. He gave the impression of valuing the quick response over the correct response. It appeared as if his poor understanding of instructions was related to the rapidity with which he responded. It was difficult to attain an accurate measure of intelligence due to these factors. He did, however, perform at at least an average level. He exhibited sequencing problems on several of the subtests. He seemed to be unable to follow instructions in their proper order. In addition, he had difficulty changing from one set of instructions to another. It almost appeared as if Kenny was looking for the quickest response and that the shifting from one set of instructions to the other was an intolerable delay.

The measure of perceptual motor development indicated that he experienced significant difficulties. He was observed to rotate perceptual designs. This trait seemed to be linked to his tendency to perseverate in his responses. Kenny would tend to make the same response repeatedly. Other errors were indicative of poor organization in his approach to problem-solving tasks. Here again he seemed to have little appreciation for evaluating response alternatives. When asked to reproduce a circle, Kenny was as likely to draw a square. He seemed to pay little attention to the differences between various forms.

His performance on a measure of his tactile recognition abilities suggested minor problems in this area. He seemed to have difficulty identifying the locus of tactile stimulation. Evidently, he became confused over concepts of right and left. He was able to talk about direction but seemed unable to translate these concepts into motor movements.

His performance on tests measuring his auditory abilities indicated that Kenny was about six months behind his chronological age in verbal expression. Evidently, his understanding of the usages of words was excellent but his ability to express himself was being affected by his birth defects.

Achievement testing indicated that Kenny was learning in the classroom even though his behavior, his difficulty in following instructions and his impulsivity made it appear as if he could be absorbing little. His achievement scores in math, reading and spelling were average.

Neurological and opthalmological results were within normal limits. There was no indication of the presence of any serious neurological problem. While visual problems were indicated on the test in perceptual motor development, the overall opthalmological examination was within normal limits. Apparently, Kenny's performance on the visual motor test reflected the effects of his impulsivity on test performance.

Fortunately, Kenny's performance on the measures of personality development indicated that his emotional conflicts were not more serious than that of an adjustment reaction. Self-concept was negatively affected. He tended to view himself as a child who lacked self-control and he thought poorly of his ability to follow through. He seemed to have come to equate impulsivity with being a bad person. He was generally negativistic toward school, seeing the classroom as a source of frustration. Generally, his attitudes toward adults were positive. He seemed to accept his own needs for dependency, but at the same time saw little need to be more independent. Kenny showed many signs of doubting his own ability to succeed. He had come to view himself as being not as intellectually capable as his classmates. His general attitude was negativistic. He seemed to be angry most of the time. Evidently he was frustrated both by his inability to control his responses and by the reactions of others.

Kenny's overactivity combined with impulsivity had acted to alienate him from others. He tended to react as others viewed him. Even though his problems were held to a moderate level, his improvement would require a series of positive experiences, over an extended period of time, at school and at home.

A Case of Severe Attention Deficits in a Hyperactive Boy

Michael was referred to our office by the school psychologist following an incident shortly after his entrance into second grade. During the second week of school he became irritable and explosive with his classmates. After striking another child, he raced down the hall in an attempt to escape from his teacher. He entered the school gymnasium and threatened to jump from the stage to the floor if anyone tried to touch him. Michael's mother was called to the school and was able to calm him after a short talk with him. His irritability and overreaction to classroom experiences had been apparent in the first grade, but had not been a cause of concern as it was in second grade.

HOME. Michael's parents were interviewed prior to his evaluation. They expressed serious concern over his recent behaviors. They described Michael as suffering from an extremely short attention span and as having difficulty in bringing his excitability under control. They had reported that from an early age, he seemed unable to attend to even the most interesting of tasks for more than a few minutes. They claimed that unless he was extremely well motivated, his difficulties with attention and weakness in concentration prevented his meaningful involvement in any activity. He seemed to be very easily frustrated, especially by motor tasks. When working on projects he tended to become explosive. He usually was overly affectionate after one of these episodes. His mother described him as a child who clung to her. He often required a great deal of parental reassurance and attention. At other times he seemed excitable and tended to show off. This was especially true whenever he was in a group setting. Much of Michael's parents' description of him was suggestive of hyperactivity with attention deficits. They reported a history of tantrums which seemed to predominate his adjustment at home in the past. While they described him as being an overly active child, neither parent considered Michael to be hyperactive. Their main concern was for his irritability which seemed to stem from his inability to attend to any task long enough to see it through successfully. There were no reported problems with sleep, but he did seem to be restless at night. His overactivity was expressed mainly in the form of fidgeting. His parents also reported that he tended to become fixated on specific ideas and that it was very difficult to change his perseverative thinking centered around fears. They reported that he maintained fears of airplanes, birds, being out of his parents' sight and the sight of blood. It had only been within the past few weeks before coming to the office that Michael had been willing to go out of the house alone. Even then he insisted on having the family's pet dog with him. Both parents felt that they had tried every method of behavioral management but with no success. The general approach was to be positive with Michael. However, both parents admitted that when this approach failed they tended to become discouraged and, at times, punitive. Actually, punishment seemed to be the only form of behavioral management to which Michael seemed to respond. His parents were perplexed as they reported that at times he almost seemed to request that they punish him.

DEVELOPMENT. The developmental history left no clues as to possible causes of Michael's problem. Both the pregnancy and the labor went smoothly with no complications and there were no birth defects reported. The developmental milestones were generally within normal limits. Sitting, walking and talking all occurred at the appropriate times. There was a minor lag reported in toilet training with enuresis continuing until age five years. Michael's parents reported that his enuresis was related to the fact that he was a particularly heavy sleeper. The medical history was clear with no contributing medical problems.

SOCIAL BEHAVIOR. In his relationships Michael tended to be more at ease with girls than with boys. He seemed to relate fairly well to boys only in a one-to-one situation. However, in a small group setting or a triad, he became extremely irritable and seemed to be unable to participate meaningfully in organized games or in any task that required him to follow a sequence of instructions. His extremely short attention span for peer group activities made him unpopular with other children who, at the second grade level, began to take an active interest in organized sports and team cooperation. At times, he attempted to assume a leadership role with peers. It seemed that he always failed miserably at this task, as the combination of his overactivity and short attention span caused him to be too distractible to direct others. In play he tended to become aggressive, especially with boys. He seemed to be delighted with throwing toys and knocking blocks down.

His parents described him as having a very positive relationship with his older sister. They claimed that he seemed close to her and seemed to enjoy having her read to him. Michael accepted her supervision when babysitting and generally seemed to look to her for support. At the same time they described him as being very jealous of her; the difference in her ability to complete tasks was obvious to him. Apparently he was particularly competitive with her over his needs for parental attention. Michael's sister, on the other hand, seemed to be somewhat less positive about her relationship with him. She viewed him as a source of family disruptiveness and complained that his competitiveness caused her to lose parental attention.

Michael seemed closest to his mother. Both parents agreed that this was due to the fact that his father was away from home on business much of the time. They also both agreed that Michael was eager to be with his father. He seemed very excited when his father returned home from work daily. Both parents seemed saddened by the fact that Michael brought his problems to no one. Even when hurt he would prefer to be alone than to seek parental assistance. Both parents agreed that Michael accepted discipline equally well from both of them. He seemed very contrite and apologized profusely for his transgressions. However, his parents had come to expect that problems would begin again not long after punishment.

School. The school history was marked by early indications of behavioral and cognitive dysfunction. Out of recognition for Michael's needs for further experience at organized activities, his parents had enrolled him in a prekindergarten program. Needless to say, he did not do well. At the end of the year the teacher advised that his entrance into first grade be delayed by a year. In the prekindergarten program he tended to be immature and excitable. He seemed to lack an ability to organize his activities. Predominate among these characteristics was the fact that he seemed to be unable to remain at any task for more than a brief time. When he was able to bring his attention span under control, he seemed to lack the skills necessary for focus of attention. Selective attention abilities also seemed to be underdeveloped.

Problems in school centered around these attention problems, in conjunction with his inability to remain in his seat and his tendencies to become overly excitable. The classroom teacher also reported that Michael tended to spin himself around in circles frequently. This was especially noticeable whenever a new person entered the room. At times his twirling became a management problem. Michael's performance during the first grade paralleled his prekindergarten experiences. In addition, he was no longer accepting of authority. He would frequently exhibit tantrums in the classroom and also shouted at his teacher. He seemed to like school and was never reluctant to attend. However, he did have much trouble completing homework assignments. Incompleted assignments seemed to contribute to his dawdling in the mornings. Missing the school bus had become an increasing problem at home. Prior to being referred for evaluation, he had become more regressive both in school and at home. During periods of relatively minor stress, such as being home with chicken pox, he reverted to eating with his fingers.

In first grade Michael was described by his teachers as a discipline problem during most of the year. His response to any form of teacher disapproval was to cry hysterically or to withdraw to some "hiding place." During one such incident he cried while telling the teacher that he "tried to be good but it didn't always come out that way." She noted that it took several minutes to bring his overactivity under control in the mornings. Generally he would run into the classroom and immediately start to disrupt other students. During the afternoon he would complain of being tired and would ask if he could lie down. When permitted to do so he would not remain for very long. By the time Michael had entered second grade his teachers and the school psychologist advised his parents that they suspected emotional problems.

EVALUATION. Michael's performance on psychological testing was indicative of a learning disability associated with hyperactivity and attention deficits. Intelligence testing revealed a wide disparity between Michael's various cognitive abilities. Both his verbal and nonverbal abilities were unevenly matched, and the differences were significant. For example, his ability to think abstractly was in a superior range while his ability to collect, store and retrieve information and his immediate short-term memory ability were at a defective level. Nonverbal abilities showed a similar pattern. Based on his performance on this measure of cognitive abilities alone it was not difficult to understand why school proved to be a frustrating experience for Michael. His ability to perform well at some tasks while failing at other tasks proved to be a source of frustration to him.

His qualitative performance on the intelligence test was highly suggestive of attention deficits. Indeed, he had to be reminded frequently to complete instructions. He seemed to have difficulty keeping goals in mind. When he was able to give an adequate amount of time to a specific task, he seemed to have difficulty focusing his attention on the test materials. Complex discrimination seemed to frustrate him. He became irritable and verbally hostile on two of the subtests which called for making complex stimulus discriminations.

Performance on the measures of perceptual and motor development were indicative of learning disabilities associated with hyperactivity. Eye-hand coordination was observed to be poor. In addition he exhibited mixed dominance. His ability to reproduce visual stimuli was deficient. He seemed to have difficulty reproducing the spacial relationship between various stimuli in his perceptual field.

Minor deficits were also observed in his psycholinguistic abilities. Although measures of his basic abilities indicated that his ability to understand words was within average limits, his ability to associate words with visual images was found to be at a level that was developmentally six months behind his chronological age.

Evidently, problems in learning extended to his tactile sensory system. With his eyes closed he was unable to identify the location of areas of tactile stimulation. He seemed to have difficulty developing concepts through the sense of touch.

Special examinations included a neurological evaluation and an analysis of visual functioning. The neurological examination proved negative for any active neurological disturbance. Several "soft signs" indicative of minimal cerebral dysfunction were evidenced in the area of eye-hand coordination and figure-drawing abilities. The initial visual evaluation indicated deficits in usable vision for both eyes. During the second phase of visual testing, Michael also exhibited problems with visual fusion. His overall performance was indicative of visual motor dysfunction usually associated with underachievement in reading.

Personality assessment revealed that Michael experienced difficulties both with self-concept and with his relationship with adults. His self-concept tended to be very negative. He seemed to view himself as unable to control his responses. Apparently the combination of poor attention skills and hyperactivity had left him with the feeling of lack of mastery. He viewed himself as ineffectual and as being disliked by others. Evidently his future self-image was also affected as he pictured himself as unable to find a job. Needless to say, he projected much hostility onto others. He tended to view his teachers and his parents as angry and rejecting. This negativism extended to the test battery itself. Even with much praise and encouragement, he was reluctant to complete the personality testing. His overall test performance was suggestive of much emotional turmoil. He seemed not to be able to remain objective about the events which took place in his life. He tended to personalize events around him to the point that he explained the cancellation of a school field day as due to his acting out. He seemed to have difficulty in censoring his own impulses. He made frequent references to hostility towards others. Much of his confusion seems to center around his perception of his own state of health. Evidently his irritability and his inability to adjust both at home and in the classroom led him to believe that he was ill. Many fears centered around his anxiety that he had contracted a fatal illness. From Michael's point of view, only something as catastrophic as a fatal illness could explain his behavior. The fact that he was seen by several doctors including a psychiatrist, a neurologist and the family pediatrician confirmed for him that he was seriously ill.

The treatment plan in this case was extensive. Special programs within the classroom were established for him by the teachers. The school psychologist assisted in monitoring Michael's progress. The family doctor prescribed medication designed to lower activity level while facilitating attention abilities. Michael's parents were seen for several supportive family counseling sessions in order to help them understand the nature of his disabilities. In view of his fear that he was suffering from a major illness, no direct therapy was offered to him. His parents were advised, however, that should he not adjust to changes in school and in the home after several months he would need to be seen for child psychotherapy.

SUMMARY

The children described in the preceding four brief case histories are typical of the learning and emotional adjustment problems experienced by hyperactive children. The remaining chapters in this text have been designed to acquaint the teacher with both the research and the treatment approaches to each of the four primary characteristics associated with hyperactivity: high activity level, deficits in attention (distractibility), cognitive dysfunctions and impulsivity.

The second chapter of the text presents a more comprehensive concept of hyperactivity and an overview of the major treatment modes. Each remaining chapter gives a detailed account of one of the characteristics associated with hyperactivity and examples of appropriate treatment strategies. Treatment recommendations incorporating the teacher's knowledge of educational programs, academic materials and learning theory are made at the end of each chapter.

REFERENCES

Alabiso, F. P.: Inhibitory functions of attention in reducing hyperactive behavior. *American Journal of Mental Deficiency,* 77:259-282, 1972.

Brummet, H.: The use of long-acting tranquilizers with hyperactive children. *Psychosomatics,* 9:157-159, 1968.

Clements, S. D.: *Minimal brain dysfunction: terminology and identification.* Phase 1 of a 3-phase project. U.S. Dept. of Health, Education and Welfare, 1966, National Institute of Neurological Diseases and Blindness, Monograph No. 3.

Doll, E. A.: "Behavior syndromes of CNS impairment, neurophrenia, cerebral palsey and mental deficiency." *Bulletin of the Devereux School,* 1954.

Gofman, H.: The physician's role in early diagnosis and management of learning disabilities. In Tranopol, L. (Ed.): *Learning Disabilities.* Springfield, Thomas, 1970.

Kahn, F., and Cohen, L. A.: Organic drivenness: a brain-stem syndrome and an experience. *New England Journal of Medicine,* 210:748-756, 1955.

Kenny, T. J.: Hyperactivity. *Journal of Pediatrics,* 79:618, 1971.

Levy, S.: Postencephalitic behavior—a forgotten entity: a report of 100 cases. *American Journal of Psychiatry,* 115:1062-1067, 1959.

Meichenbaum, D.: *The nature and modification of impulsivity.* Paper presented at the First International Congress of Child Neurology, Toronto, Canada, 1975.

Minde, K., Lewen, D., Weiss, G., Lavigueur, H., Douglas, V., and Sykes, E.: The hyperactive child in elementary school: a five-year, controlled follow-up. *Exceptional Children, 38:*215-221, 1971.

Palkers, H., and Stewart, M.: Intellectual ability and performance of hyperactive children. *American Journal of Orthopsychiatry, 42:*35-39, 1972.

Schrager, J., and Lindy, J.: Hyperkinetic children: early indicators of potential school failure. *Community Mental Health Journal, 6:*447-454, 1970.

Schrager, J., Lindy, J., Harrison, S., McDermott, J., and Wilson, P.: The hyperactive child: an overview of the issues. *Journal of the American Academy of Child Psychiatry, 4:*526-533, 1966.

Weiss, G., Minde, K., Werry, J. S., Douglas, V., and Nemeth, E.: Studies on the hyperactive child. VIII. Five-year follow-up study. *Archives of General Psychiatry, 24:*409-414, 1971.

Werner, H., and Strauss, A. A.: Pathology of figure background relation in the child. *Journal of Abnormal Social Psychology, 36:*58-67, 1941.

Werry, G. S.: Studies on the hyperactive child. IV. An empirical analysis of the mental brain dysfunction syndrome. *Archives of General Psychiatry, 19:*9-16, 1968.

CHAPTER 2

THE HYPERACTIVE CHILD

THE HYPERACTIVE CHILD can be identified as experiencing cognitive dysfunction, impulsivity, a heightened level of activity and a disturbance in the attention process. The secondary characteristics associated with the syndrome include aggressiveness, poor concentration, emotional lability and failure in social relationships. Academically, these children appear to suffer from a general impairment which prevents their progress in almost every academic area. Neurologically, they seem to suffer from a variety of disorders. A consensus appears to be that the majority of hyperactive children experience some form of neurological dysfunction originating in the brain stem. However, there is sufficient evidence to show that a small number of hyperactive children suffer from some form of cerebral cortex malfunction. Although it has been difficult to separate the emotional characteristics resulting from this syndrome from those which seem to cause the syndrome, hyperactive youngsters often appear to be withdrawn and overaggressive. They exhibit changes of mood and a low tolerance for frustration. These children often find themselves socially isolated and ostrasized by their peer group and they are characterized by poor self-image and damaged self-concept. To provide a more complete description, this chapter presents a review of research findings regarding the characteristics of the hyperactive child and a discussion of the etiology of the syndrome. The more prevalent treatment modes are then explored.

CHARACTERISTICS OF THE SYNDROME

Since its identification as a syndrome separate from mental retardation (Strauss and Werner, 1941), numerous behavioral, physiological, emotional and intellectual characteristics have been identified with the disorder. As knowledge about hyperactivity has increased over the years, it has become increasingly apparent that the syndrome be viewed as a combination of behavioral, cognitive, emotional and physiological dysfunctions. Anderson (1963) defined the hyperactive child's behavior as being characterized by short attention span and distractibility. He also emphasized that these children were stimulus-oriented. That is, they seemed to become disorganized whenever any new stimulus was introduced into their field of vision. Cognitively, these children were described as having the greatest difficulty in reading and mathematics. Emotionally, they seemed to lack fear and exhibited a low tolerance for frustration. Physiologically, hyperactive children were described as being characterized by premature birth, a high incidence of anoxia and a developmental history interrupted by infectious disease.

In studying the characteristics of hyperactive children with a history of damage to the diencephalon, Burks (1957) observed that on a behavioral level these children were impulsive, exhibited irratic behaviors and were restless. Burks was particularly impressed by their high level of activity, poor concentration and extreme aggressiveness. Explosiveness was the overriding emotional characteristic of the children studied. Academically, these children manifested perceptual difficulties which led to general academic underachievement in all areas.

Cruickshank et al. (1966) reported on hyperactive children suffering from damage to the reticular formation. On a behavioral level, he described them as suffering from motor disinhibition. Emotionally, these children exhibited what he described as a catastrophic reaction. Such children were found to overreact to even the slightest disappointment or frustration. Academically, Cruickshank et al. observed these children to have a disturbance of the relationship between figure and ground resulting in poor reading and mathematics ability.

Still another dimension was added to the characteristics of the syndrome by Horenstein's (1957) observation that children whose hyperactivity was the result of an encephalitic infection exhibited "social inferiority" as well as all the primary characteristics of the syndrome. Near the same time, Ingram (1956) observed that characteristics of children whose hyperactivity was caused by damage to the temporal lobe appeared to be shallow emotionally. They exhibited little fear of danger and were highly resistive to punishment as a means of behavioral control. A predominant behavioral characteristic was their tendency to place objects in their mouth.

Noble (1962) studied the reactions of hyperactive children in whom no physiological cause could be found. Emotionally, these children were depressed, apathetic and generally sullen. They were also found to be moody and exhibited much withdrawal.

Stewart et al. (1966) added several other characteristics in describing those children whose hyperactivity appeared to be the result of emotional conflicts. He observed these children to be eneuretic and antisocial. A high incidence of public masturbation was also reported in this population. Stewart also observed these children to have a general impairment of speech and vision which he theorized led to general academic failure. Werry et al. (1969) supported Stewart's findings. They noted that nonorganic hyperactive children exhibited a general visual and motor disturbance which resulted in academic underachievement. They also observed these children to be destructive, impulsive and excitable, and reported them to require only a minimum amount of sleep. In earlier reports Werry et al. (1964; 1966; 1968) reviewed the developmental histories of over 1,000 hyperactive children of normal intelligence. They found a high incidence of abnormal delivery at birth, genetic disturbances and biochemical deficits. In addition to the academic, emotional and behavioral characteristics reported by other authors, he described these children as extremely hostile and as having poor motor coordination along with an impaired drawing ability.

More recently, Mindle et al. (1971) reported on the academic performance of thirty-seven school children diagnosed as hyperactive. All of the subjects had been identified as having been hyperactive for at least four years. These children were compared to their nonhyperactive classmates and were found to have significantly higher failure rate in all academic subjects. They were also rated by their teachers as displaying far more behavioral problems than their peers. Palkes and Stewart (1972) studied the relationship between intelligence, school achievement and perceptual motor development in hyperactive elementary school children. The children studied showed significantly lower IQ scores than the control group. However, when the group's lower level of intelligence was taken into consideration, they were found to learn at a rate equal to that of a control group. In other words, Palkes and Stewart suggested that although some hyperactive children are of lower intelligence, they learn at a rate that is normal for their level of intelligence.

The variables of sex and age also seemed to play as important role in the development of hyperactivity. Numerous researchers have observed hyperactivity to be more prevalent in boys than in girls. Girls seem to develop the characteristics of the syndrome at a later age than boys, and in general neither sex exhibits the primary symptoms of hyperactivity beyond puberty. Brummet (1968) found hyperactivity to be six times as frequent among elementary school boys as it was among elementary school girls. Patterson (1964) surveyed referrals of children to mental health clinics and found significantly greater numbers of boys to have been diagnosed as hyperactive.

Over the past decade, there has been much controversy over the relationship between intelligence and hyperactivity. In general, there is agreement among researchers and practitioners that while hyperactivity does occur more frequently in mentally retarded children than in the general population, there is no cause-effect relationship between hyperactivity and lowered intelligence.

The hyperactive child presents a complex picture. Whether we view him as a youngster suffering from some physiological deficit, as a child lacking in ego development or as reacting against intense depression, the primary emotional characteristics of the hyperactive child seem devastating. Such children are irritable, have a low tolerance for frustration, are often aggressive and are weak in forming relationships with peers. The reaction from adults to their irritating behaviors teaches them early in their lives to depend less on teachers and parents for guidance and support. Often their aggressiveness and their impulsivity result in rejection or in a sense of alienation. Such children learn early in life not to count on peers or the environment for support. The effect of the emotional component of the syndrome seems to be that of gross alienation. On all levels the hyperactive child finds himself feeling like a misfit. Typically, his earliest school experiences are filled with criticism and punishment. He senses the frustration of adults who come into contact with him. Many such children, although of average or above intelligence, are often held back academically during the first three years of school. Their frustration is intensified by handicaps to their ability to learn. It is no wonder that many hyperactive children come to think of themselves as stupid. Usually within the first few years of his classroom experience the hyperactive child comes to view himself as a failure. Such children do not allow themselves to hope for success. In fact, many of these children come to despise success. They come to see the smallest success as so out of contrast with the rest of their emotional experience that it becomes too threatening to accept. As the alienation increases, resentfulness toward adults and rebelliousness join the already damaged personality structure. Such children often seem to be almost comfortable with rejection. When threatened by acceptance, they seem to work endlessly at provoking a hostile reaction from others.

While there is a consensus that the primary characteristics of hyperactivity diminish with age, recent studies by Weiss et al. (1971a, b) suggest that by the time the hyperactive child enters adolescence, the residual effects of the handicap are devastating. Of the children studied, a significantly high incidence of social and intrapsychic difficulties along with severe learning disorders were found to persist well into adolescence. By the time they reach adolescence, they have come to view themselves as lonely and isolated. Their failures in relationships with peers and adults and their history of academic failure leaves them poorly prepared for the tasks of adolescence. With this seemingly endless backlog, it is little wonder that many hyperactive children withdraw from the task of transferring their dependency from their family to their peer group. Very few of these children deal adequately with the complex task of identifying and preparing for a career choice. By the time the hyperactive youngster reaches adolescence, the primary characteristics of the syndrome generally are no longer manifest. Several authors have documented the remission of the primary characteristics associated with the syndrome during adolescence (Laufer and Denhoff, 1957). The residual effects, however, unfortunately persist into adulthood.

Mendleson et al. (1971) interviewed the parents of adolescents who had been diagnosed as hyperactive while in elementary school. They found the primary characteristics (overactivity, distractability, impulsivity and irritability) to have decreased. However, difficulties in adjusting to family life and school maladjustment were found to be severe. Parents complained that their children refused to obey rules at home. They described their own children as moody and suffering from a lack of self-esteem. These parents' own alienation from their children was reflected in the fact that about 40 percent of the parents studied had seriously considered sending their children to military school. Another 46 percent of these parents were unable to identify a career for which their children were suited. Antisocial activities were also found to present major problems. A significant number of the children studied had histories of lying, stealing, fighting and destructiveness. These children were identified as being high risks for becoming sociopaths as adults. They had much difficulty in conforming to rules. Fifty-nine percent of these children had had some contact with the police by age fourteen. Their school records were marked by failure. Fifty-eight percent of the children studied had failed one or more grades. Fifty-seven percent were reported as having reading difficulties. Over 70 percent were found to have difficulties in concentration, perseverance and attention. Mendleson et al. (1971) summarized their findings by concluding that although hyperactive children generally behave in a more normal manner by the time they enter adolescence, the primary symptoms of high activity level, distractability, impulsivity and excitability remain to a lesser degree. By the time the hyperactive child is an adolescent, the primary maladaptive behaviors become those of disobedience, rebelliousness at home and at school, antisocial behavior and apathy. Academic failure and low self-esteem characterize their school attitudes.

In a sense hyperactive children become victims of their own cure. That is, as they approach physiological maturation and as higher cortical centers take over the complex tasks of processing incoming and outgoing impulses across the nerves, the primary characteristics of the syndrome are no longer present. Usually, by the mid-teens, perceptual and motor deficits are no longer present, the high rates of activity have subsided, attention span and concentration have improved, distractability is no longer a problem. In effect, they are not even left with an excuse for their sense of alienation and failure.

ETIOLOGY OF HYPERACTIVITY

Understanding the causes of hyperactivity is a formidable task. Although the syndrome was identified over 100 years ago, it has only been within the past two decades that research has been able to uncover some of its causes. To date, knowledge about the syndrome indicates that hyperactivity may have one of three causes. There is a large body of research which indicates that hyperactivity is primarily a physiological condition which is caused by a disturbance of the functioning of the brain stem. Other research has demonstrated a relationship between damage to the frontal area of the brain and hyperactivity. Finally, there is some indication that in a smaller percentage of hyperactive children the cause is primarily psychogenic.

Reticular Activity System

By far the greatest incidence of hyperactivity has been linked to a disturbance in the functioning of the reticular activating system (the brain stem). This subcortical center has the primary functions of relaying incoming impulses to the brain and transmitting impulses from the brain back to the sense organs. Within the reticular formation lie the thalamus and the hypothalamus. These centers of the nervous system serve as terminals for incoming and outgoing nervous impulses. It is this part of the human nervous system that is responsible for human arousal. Researchers interested in this area of the nervous system functioning discovered that hyperactivity in animals could be directly attributed to a dysfunction of the reticular activating system (Adametz, 1959; Amassian and DiVito, 1954; French, Amerongen and MaGoun, 1952; French, Hernandez-Peon and Livingston, 1955; Moruzzi and MaGoun, 1949; Scheibel, Scheibel, Mollica and Moruzzi, 1955). The work of these investigators stimulated interest in the role of the reticular activating system in controlling activity level in human beings. Early research in this area by Strazel, Taylor and McGoun (1951) revealed that stimulation of certain brain centers activated the reticular formation. Ensuing drug studies demonstrated that activity level in normal subjects could be lowered by using a general anesthetic. This finding had strong implications for the cause of hyperactivity. Such anesthetics worked directly on the synapse (the link between nerve endings). Further investigation along these lines by Alexandris and Lundell (1968) revealed that activity level could be reduced by inhibiting synaptic transmission within the reticular activating system. Theoretically, activity rate could be reduced by altering the chemical composition of the synaptic fluid, as illustrated in Figure 1. Impulses travel along the afferent nerve pathways and are transmitted from one nerve to the other by traveling through the fluid at the synapse. Tranquilizing drugs act to change the chemical composition of this fluid in such a way as to retard the rate at which the impulses are transmitted. The result is that activity level becomes markedly decreased.

It is well known that for most hyperactive children, tranquilizing drugs result in only minor improvement. In their study of the functions of the thalamus and the hypothalamus, Laufer and Denhoff (1957) hypothesized that the hyperactive child already experienced a blockage at the synapse. As a result, incoming or outgoing nervous impulses tended to gather at the

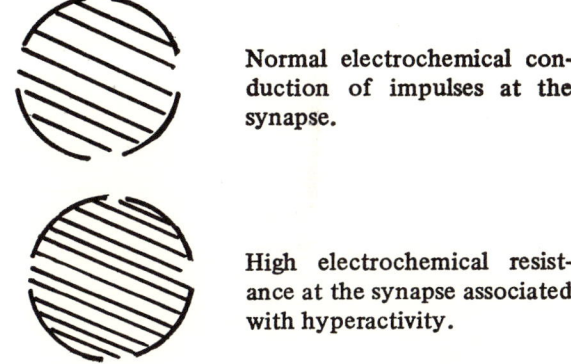

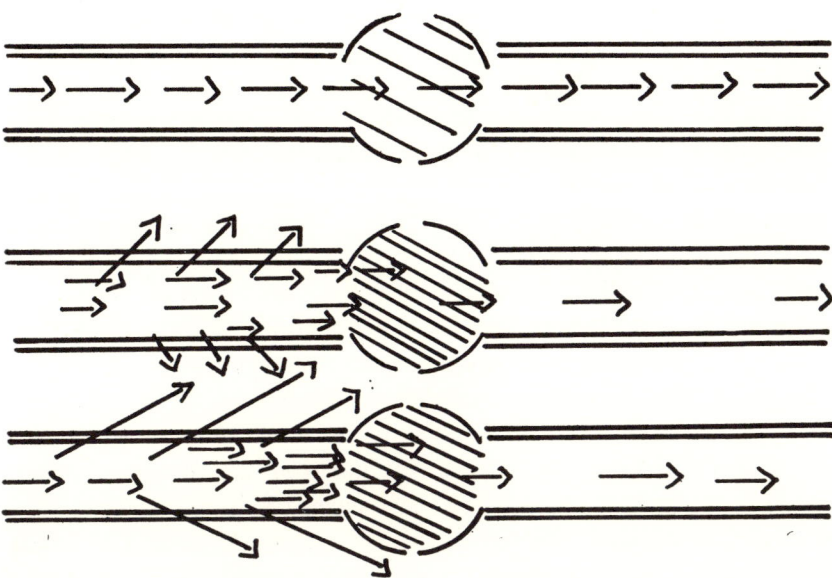

Figure 1. Electrochemical resistance to synaptic transmission of nervous impulses.

synapse and to irradiate to other nerves in such a way as to increase activity level. A good analogy is that of a turnstile. The more slowly the stile turns in a busy subway station, the greater the backup of passenger traffic. Eventually, as the line gets too large, travelers begin to spill over into other passageways.

Figure 1 demonstrates this on a neuronal level. Laufer and Denhoff used this theory to explain the role of amphetamines. This class of psychostimulants acts directly on the synapse in the reticular formation. It reduces electrical resistance at the synapse so that incoming and outgoing nervous impulses can travel from one nerve pathway to another at a more rapid rate than usual. In normal subjects, this promotes activity level. In hyperactive subjects, however, it acts to neutralize the process, which causes the impulses to "back up" and "spill over." In normal subjects amphetamines act to speed activity level, but in hyperactive subjects they permit the level of activity to fall within normal limits.

While it is possible that hyperactivity which has been caused by a malfunction of synaptic transmission within the reticular formation could be caused by injury or by infection, research in this area suggests that developmental lag is responsible for the majority of cases of hyperactivity. The Developmental Lag Theory places emphasis on the process of maturation. This theory attributes dysfunction of the reticular formation to uneven physiological development. It suggests that as the hyperactive child grows and matures, higher brain centers take over the relay functions which the thalamus and hypothalamus perform inadequately. This theory would then account for the fact that as the child grows older, i.e. matures, the symptoms of hyperactivity become less prevalent until adolescence, at which time only the secondary symptoms usually remain. According to the Developmental Lag Theory, various parts of the nervous system develop at uneven rates. In the case of hyperactivity, the Developmental Lag Theory would hypothesize that the brain (cerebral cortex) is developing at a normal rate while the brain stem (reticular formation) is maturing at a slower rate.

Brain Damage

The role played by the cerebral cortex in causing hyperactivity is not as clear-cut as the role played by the dysfunction of the reticular formation. Early research on the relationship between the brain and activity level in animals revealed that temporal lobe lesions significantly increased activity level while reducing fear (Kulver and Bucy, 1939). Further research in this area by Gastaut, Vigouroux and Naquet (1952) revealed that temporal lobe lesions not only increased activity level but also resulted in unusual states of both fear and rage. Little is known about the neuronal causes of hyperactivity in children with temporal lobe disturbances. However, Ingram (1956) did observe that hyperactive children who suffered from temporal lobe lesions exhibited high rates of activity along with little fear of danger, and aggressiveness. An important characteristic of temporal lobe disturbances was the observation that in such disturbances there was excessive tendency to place objects in their mouths. In recent years, there has been little published research on the relationship between hyperactivity and temporal lobe malfunction.

In one of the most recent studies on the subject, Buckley (1972) hypothesized that hyperactivity was directly related to a disturbance in the ability to inhibit and control temporal lobe activity. This two-stage theory suggested that one form of hyperactivity may result from a combination of temporal lobe malfunction in conjunction with a disturbance of the activity of the brain stem.

Another smaller subgroup of hyperactive children may suffer from malfunctioning of the prefrontal lobes of the brain. Early research on the relationship between damage to the prefrontal regions and activity level in animals confirmed that high rates of activity may be associated with damage to these cerebral areas (Bianchi, 1922; Brickner, 1936; Ferrier, 1876; Jacobsen, 1931; Kennard, Fullton, Jacobsen, 1932). In an impressive study on the relationship between prefrontal lobe damage and hyperactivity, Levin (1938) was able to link hyperactivity to prefrontal lobe damage resulting from epilepsy in 279 hyperactive children.

Genetic Causes

Several more recent theories have associated hyperactivity in children with a genetic disturbance. In one such study, Morrison et al. (1973) hypothesized a polygenetic theory of causation. In a study of fifty-nine families of hyperactive children,

Morrison found a significant incidence of hyperactivity in the parents of the children included in the study. These parents reported that as children they themselves suffered from hyperactivity. In addition, a significant incidence of alcoholism was found in the families of these children. Morrison suggested that hyperactivity may be caused by more than one genetic variable operating at the same time. However, to date, no study has shown a clear-cut relationship between genetic disturbance and hyperactivity. The work of Warren et al. (1971) reports that chromosome studies of ninety-six hyperactive children resulted in the finding of no abnormalities. In addition, a higher incidence of hyperactivity in boys could not be attributed to sex-linked chromosomal differences. Much research needs to be carried out in order to substantiate a genetic theory of hyperactivity.

Psychogenic Causes

Much of the current research on drug therapy makes reference to the fact that psychogenic hyperactivity in children is not responsive to treatment with psychostimulants. Such children have been found to respond more favorably to tranquilizers. Current theories as to the emotional causes of hyperactivity have tended to view hyperactivity as either a response to a maladjusted home environment or as a reaction formation against underlying feelings of depression. In one such study Conrad et al. (1967) found a significant relationship between hyperactivity in children and a disturbance in the parent-child relationship. Generally, those parents who were either psychologically disturbed themselves or found to be socially incompetent tended to have hyperactive children. Cantwell (1972) studied the parents of fifty hyperactive children. He found hyperactivity to be prevalent in children whose parents suffered from alcoholism, personality disorder or hysteria. Ten percent of the parents studied also reported having suffered from hyperactivity themselves as children. Several texts on depression have cited hyperactivity as linked to depression in children (Jacobsen, 1971; Rie, 1966; Beck, 1972). In one such study Zrull (1970) hypothesized that hyperactivity acts as a reaction formation against depression in children. In other words, for some children whose hyperactivity is not organically based, hyperactivity may be a reaction to underlying feelings of depression. This theory suggests that the hyperactive child defends himself against lethargy and other feelings of depression by becoming overactive. In one recent study Kissel and Freeling (1974) rated fifty-seven hyperactive children on the Kissel-Freeling Depression Scale. They found a significant relationship between hyperactivity and degression. In general, those children who received high hyperactivity scores were also described by their teachers as being unusually sad and lonely, crying easily, being easily provoked to tears, lethargic, feeling sorry for themselves, being pessimistic and making frequent self-discouraging remarks. Much further research needs to be done in order to explore the relationship between hyperactivity and depression. In addition, other psychogenic causes need further exploration.

Other Possible Causes

A variety of other less researched causes have been hypothesized. In one study Minde et al. (1968) discovered a relationship between hyperactivity and conditions at the time of birth. They discovered that the probability of hyperactivity increased significantly with the use of forceps in the delivery along with an abnormally long or an abnormally short labor period.

In another study Rapoport et al. (1970) linked hyperactivity to a mulfunction of the endocrine glands. His research was able to demonstrate an inverse relationship between the amount of adrenaline in the urine and hyperactivity. In other words, as the amount of adrenalin in the urine increased, hyperactivity was found to decrease. He also discovered that symptom improvement decreased as the amount of adrenalin in the urine decreased. The results of his study strongly suggest that higher amounts of adrenalin found in the urine act to reduce hyperactivity.

Perhaps the most ignored theories of hyperactivity are those which view hyperactivity as a purely psychological reaction to emotional stress. Shortly after its identification as a syndrome distinct from mental retardation, hyperactivity came to be viewed as an emotional maladjustment stemming from weakness in ego development (Sheer, 1954). These early theories suggested that the child's ability to inhibit and censor his primitive impulses represented a faulty development of the ego. Hyperactivity was considered to be an ego defense which could be treated in a setting which allowed the child to release his inhibitions and express his emotional conflicts in the presence of an adult who served as the child's censor (Shainman, 1951).

There appear to be several possible causes for hyperactivity. Although a specific cause may not be identified, knowledge of some possibilities may help in understanding the child. Whatever the cause, the hyperactive child is described as experiencing cognitive dysfunction, impulsivity, a heightened level of activity and a disturbance in the attention process. Focus is now directed to several treatment aproaches that have been used with hyperactive children.

MODES OF TREATMENT

Treatment approaches for the hyperactive child have developed along three main lines. By far, the greatest volume of research has been done in the area of chemotherapy. Specialization in educational programming, i.e. academic therapy, has undergone several stages of development. More recently, theorists have applied the principles of learning theory to provide for a social environment which maximizes the hyperactive child's motivation. While these three forms of therapy have developed along separate lines, the most effective treatment approach for the hyperactive child occurs when the three of them are brought together. For many hyperactive/learning-disabled children, the combination of intervention at the physiological, social, emotional and academic levels is effective in negating many of the behavioral, cognitive and emotional characteristics associated with the syndrome. A brief overview of several modes of treatment is presented here, and then applied to each aspect of the syndrome in a separate chapter.

Chemotherapy

During the past two decades, psychotropic drugs have predominated the treatment of hyperactivity. It is only within the past ten years that the full impact of drug treatment has come to light. By far, the greatest single source of present day knowledge about this disturbance emanates from drug research.

At present, there are three main classes of drugs used to treat the condition. Psychostimulants (amphetamines) have their effects mainly on the brain stem and are most useful in the treatment of hyperactive conditions arising from unevenness in physiological development. Tranquilizing agents may act either on the brain stem or on the cerebral cortex itself. This category of drugs is most often prescribed for hyperactive children whose condition is primarily psychological. Finally, anticonvulsant drugs are sometimes prescribed for hyperactive children whose conditions are associated with a seizure disorder. No single drug or single mode of treatment acts on a panacea. Each category of drug works or has a specific action on certain brain centers. No single form of drug treatment is capable of controlling all of the symptoms of hyperactivity simultaneously. Perhaps the best testament to the effectiveness of chemotherapy is the frequency with which drugs are used in the treatment of hyperactive children. In one study (Hundert et al., 1974), 69 percent of the hyperactive children in a public school system were being treated with some form of psychostimulants. An additional 11 percent of the hyperactive children studied were taking a major tranquilizer. The 20 percent remaining were being treated with a variety of other medications.

PSYCHOSTIMULANT DRUGS. Within the area of drug treatment, the use of psychostimulants predominates the medical picture As described in an earlier section, these drugs reduce hyperactivity by permitting impulses to travel more freely between the nerves in the brain stem. While a variety of psychostimulants have been tested in order to determine which particular type is most effective, researchers generally agree that methylphenidate (Ritalin®) is the most effective chemical agent in this category of drugs.

In one such study, Burks (1964) tested the effectiveness of amphetamines on two groups of hyperactive children. The first group was identified as being hyperactive primarily due to a disturbance in the functioning of the brain stem. The second group's hyperactivity was directly attributed to damage to the brain itself. Most of the children who made up this second group suffered from some form of seizure disorder. Both groups showed a significant improvement in motor control. Activity level seemed to decrease in both groups of children. The greatest gains were made by those children whose hyperactivity was associated with a subcortical disturbance. Other than improvement in activity level, no improvement in academic thinking abilities was found. In addition to decreases in activity level and improvement in motor coordination, Conners (1966) found that dexedrine improved the hyperactive child's ability to discriminate while learning. He also found that the children who received dexedrine therapy demonstrated an increased ability to perceive and organize their own behaviors. A very important conclusion of this study was that drug therapy seemed to facilitate learning ability. In a comparison study, Sprague et al. (1970) measured the effects of placebo, tranquilizers and psychostimulants on a group of emotionally disturbed hyperactive boys. The psychostimulant group (ritalin group) showed the greatest gains in reduction of activity level and improvement of learning. An additional variable in this study found that the drug acted to improve reaction time. Weiss et al. (1971a) compared the effectiveness of ritalin with tranquilizing drugs. These researchers found that ritalin was superior to all other forms of medication in controlling hyperactivity. A surprising finding was that tranquilizing drugs were effective for a majority of the children but that they acted only to reduce activity level. Evidently, when hyperactivity had a subcortical base, tranquilizing drugs were not effective in reducing distractibility, aggressiveness or excitability. Ritalin was by far the most effective in producing goal-oriented behavior and reducing distractibility.

The widespread use of these drugs has brought forth a recognition of the need for close evaluation of their long-term effects. In 1971 the Department of Health, Education and

Welfare published the results of a longitudinal study on the effects and usages of stimulant drugs in the treatment of behaviorally disturbed school children. This report advised that the prolonged use of psychostimulants be closely monitored medically. This recommendation was made in view of the finding that the long-term use of amphetamines tends to suppress growth in children. Certain amphetamines were strongly advised against by the Federal Drug Administration (Maynard, 1970). These drugs produced serious side effects including damage to internal body organs. The use of this particular subgroup of psychostimulants in the treatment of hyperactive children is rare. However, the more generally used psychostimulants such as Ritalin and dexedrine have been shown to affect the child's growth pattern in a number of ways. Safer et al. (1972) reported on the use of amphetamines in hyperactive school-age children. The results of his research indicated that amphetamines caused a suppression of weight gain and a depression of growth and height in the children studied. The differences in height and weight between students who were being treated with medication and a control group of normal students was noticeable in as little as nine months. However, Safer did report that both weight gain, growth and height reappeared spontaneously when the medication was discontinued. These researchers suggested that the medications be discontinued during school vacations and on weekends. The beneficial effects of drug therapy in the treatment of hyperactive children is considered to outweigh the harmful side effects reported. However, the importance of close medical supervision in the medication regime cannot be underestimated in view of the side effects.

TRANQUILIZING DRUGS. For those children whose hyperactivity is not caused by a malfunction of the brain stem, tranquilizing drugs have been shown to produce beneficial effects. This general category of drugs, known as phenothiazines, is frequently used in the treatment of emotional disturbance in adults. Unlike the psychostimulants, these drugs act to inhibit processing of nervous impulses. In a child whose hyperactivity is related to brain stem malfunction, these drugs tend to have no effect on activity level and in some instances they may even increase activity level.

Several studies have shown improvement in hyperactive children whose hyperactivity is psychogenic. Weiss et al. (1971a) found chlorpromazine (a major tranquilizer) to be effective in reducing activity level in a number of hyperactive children. However, the medication was found to have no demonstrable effect on distractibility, aggressivity or excitability. Two forms of amphetamine were administered to two matched groups of control subjects. They were found not to be as effective in reducing activity level as chlorpromazine. However, they did result in significant improvement in goal-oriented behavior and a reduction in distractibility. Brummet (1968) administered chlorpromazine to 134 hyperactive children whose hyperactivity was determined to be related to a malfunction of parts of the brain other than the brain stem. All the subjects were found to have an abnormal EEG pattern. This study demonstrated that this medication was effective in controlling the high activity levels of the children studied for a six- to twelve-month period. Other researchers have reported similar findings.

The main limitations of this category of drugs in the treatment of hyperactive children are in their narrow range of effectiveness and in their potential side effects. Reported side effects include an increase in irritability, loss of sleep, loss of appetite and psychomotor retardation. The major area of effectiveness seems to be that of reduction of activity level. The other characteristics associated with hyperactivity seem not to be significantly altered by the administration of these drugs.

THE RELATIONSHIP BETWEEN CHEMOTHERAPY AND LEARNING. The relationship between drug treatment and academic learning is complex. Several theories have emerged regarding the relationship between learning and the effects of drugs. Studies evaluating the interaction between these two variables must take into account several factors. Firstly, the effects of the drug itself must be evaluated. That is, it may be found that the medication affects certain complex motor behaviors but does not directly affect learning. In general, studies which have observed an improvement in learning due to improvement of psychomotor control infer that the learning process has been improved as a result of the medication treatment. However, such inferences may be misleading. The most reasonable conclusion from such studies is that improved psychomotor control as a result of medication treatment may permit the learning process to occur more readily. The type of medication used is a second important variable. Several studies have shown that psychostimulants affect learning in a very different way than do the tranquilizing drugs. Finally, one must take into consideration the cause of the hyperactivity under investigation. In other words, to evaluate the effectiveness of the treatment one must take into consideration whether the medication directly affects the learning process itself or whether it improves one of the primary characteristics of hyperactivity, thereby permitting learning to occur more readily. One must also take into consideration the type of medication applied and the cause of the hyperactivity being studied. Evaluations of the complex interaction between these variables have produced several theories regarding the effectiveness of drug treatment on learning.

Some research proposes that chemotherapy directly influences learning. These studies generally report a correlation between drug treatment and academic improvement. In general these studies have compared matched groups of hyperactive subjects being treated with either psychostimulants, tranquilizers or a placebo. In one such study, Sprague, Barnes and Werry (1970) compared the effects of tranquilizing drugs, psychostimulants and a placebo on three groups of nonorganic hyperactive boys. In this particular group, tranquilizing drugs were found to facilitate learning. Similar studies have shown that learning improves in emotionally disturbed hyperactive children treated with tranquilizing drugs. Conners (1966) found that both fine motor coordination and discrimination learning ability were significantly improved in organically impaired hyperactive youngsters who were treated with psychostimulants. Conners concluded that the medication affected hyperactive children in such a way as to increase their ability to perceive and organize their behaviors. In a prior study, Conners and Eisenberg (1963) compared two groups of subjects on three pre- and posttest measures of learning ability. The psychostimulant group of hyperactive children showed significant improvement in learning over the placebo group. In still another study Conners (1972) compared improvement in academic achievement and cognition in two groups of subjects. Each group received a different type of psychostimulant. Both groups showed significant improvements on several measures of cognitive development and academic achievement. Sykes, Douglas, Weiss and Mindle (1971) Confirmed Conner's (1966) finding that psychostimulants improved discrimination learning in hyperactive children. In a more recent study, Braddard and Rapoport (1974) compared the effectiveness of various forms of treatment. In this particular study they treated one group of hyperactive children with behavior therapy while the other group received psychostimulants. While both groups showed an improvement, the drug treatment group showed the greatest gains in IQ performance and academic achievement in math and spelling. This study was particularly important in view of the questions it raised about what was actually being improved in the children treated with psychostimulants. Of the studies cited, it was not possible to determine whether the drugs affected intelligence, learning or academic performance. These studies raise questions regarding the specific cause of the improvement in the children. Do such drugs improve intelligence, thereby resulting in greater academic achievement? Do they control attention and activity level in order to permit the child to learn at a rate that he was not capable of maintaining prior to the administration of the drug? Do the drugs affect some general cognitive learning process which then permits academic achievement to occur? Research findings in this area warrant close scrutiny.

From this line of research, a second school of thinking regarding the relationship of drugs and learning in hyperactive children has emerged. Research in this area has shed some light on the relationship between drug treatment and learning and between drug treatment and intelligence. In one such study, Finnerty, Soltys and Cole (1971) administered psychostimulants to a group of twenty hyperactive children enrolled in regular elementary school classes. The Wechsler Intelligence Scale for Children and the Wide Range Achievement Test were administered before and after the administration of the drug. These researchers found a significant improvement in the children's IQ scores. However, there was no change in academic achievement.

While it is not possible to conclude on the basis of a few studies that drug treatment affects intelligence, this and other findings do suggest that drugs may positively affect some general cognitive process. This general improvement may not affect any specific area of academic learning, but may permit improvement in specific learning areas where improvement was not possible before. The work of Campbell, Douglas and Morgenstern (1971) seems to support such a theory. These researchers compared hyperactive and normal children on four dimensions of cognitive style: reflection-impulsivity, field dependence-independence, constriction-flexible control and automatization. The pretest of the two groups showed the hyperactive children to be more impulsive, more field-dependent, more constricted in their ability to control attention and slower on measures of automatization than the control subjects. Subsequently, psychostimulants were administered to the hyperactive children. A significant improvement was found in two of the cognitive areas studied. In a more recent study, Connley (1973) investigated the effects of psychostimulants on six basic cognitive processes: visual motor functioning, short-term auditory and visual memory, auditory and visual attention span, work recognition and retention skills. Those hyperactive children treated with psychostimulants showed significant improvements in all of these cognitive abilities. While no measure of intelligence or academic achievement was made in this study, the results did indicate that the basic learning skills under study did improve as a result of chemotherapy.

The results of these studies must be interpreted with caution. There are probably as many studies which show no improvement in either IQ or learning as a result of drug treatment (Burks, 1964). Probably, the most practical theory about the interaction of drugs and learning is one which measures the effectiveness of the learning environment as well as the effectiveness of the medication administered. That is, improvement in learning is thought to be a result of the interaction between the drug administered and the effectiveness of the academic techniques employed. The research of Forward (1972) lends support to an interaction theory. This study measured the interaction of five variables on reading, spelling and math achievement in hyperactive school children. Between three and five factors seem to make the critical difference in improvement in reading and math. Medication was only one of these critical factors. The other critical factors included such variables as the average time per day spent on homework assignments, parent interest and intelligence.

At this point none of the schools of thought regarding the relationship between learning and drug treatment have provided conclusive evidence to support their tenants. It remains unclear whether drugs actually improve intelligence, whether they facilitate some cognitive process or whether they simply control the symptoms of the syndrome in such a way as to permit learning or achievement to occur. It is unlikely that any process as central to learning as intelligence itself is significantly affected by drugs alone. Whether chemotherapy affects learning and academic achievement directly or whether it affects academic achievement indirectly by improving cognitive skills, it seems unlikely that significant improvements in learning could occur without a well-executed academic program. The lack of full understanding of the interaction between drugs and learning is well summarized in Sprague's et al. (1970) statement that, "The nature of covariance of learning and activity level is quite obscure . . . it might improve some aspects of learning and thus reduce drug overflow or it might reduce activity level and thus decrease distractibility . . . or it might change some central process such as mood state with motor activity and learning both changing as a result" (p. 626).

Psychological Theories

Prior to the popularization of psychoanalytic theory, hyperactivity was viewed as a disorder of the central nervous system.

During this prepsychoanalytic period, hyperactive children were classified as mentally retarded. They were thought to be mentally deficient and incapable of benefiting from public education. Quite often hyperactive youngsters who were able to demonstrate adequate intellectual ability were considered to be deranged. Prior to the advent of the mental hospital, treatment for such children consisted of confinement to home. They were excluded from the everyday social and academic activities available to other children their age. Later, as mental hospitals were built and children's units were added, these children were institutionalized. Unfortunately, such institutions offered little more than incarceration. Strict behavioral controls were the only forms of "treatment." The condition was thought to be a disease associated with childhood which went into remission at adolescence. For many years it was thought to be part of a psychotic condition. Unfortunately, practitioners failed to recognize that much of the psychotic-like behavior exhibited in such children was probably a reaction to years of institutionalization.

PSYCHOANALYTIC THEORY. Conditions improved somewhat with the advent of psychoanalytic theory. According to this theory, hyperactivity was viewed neither as a physiologic condition nor as a psychotic process, but rather it was viewed as resulting from faulty personality development. Freud has postulated that personality functioning was governed by three main processes. The id was the source from which all primitive and primary impulses erupted. The super ego represented the internalization of social ideals and parental sanctions. The ego's function was to serve as the censor of the primary and primitive urges stemming from the id and at the same time it acted to prevent the super ego from dominating the personality. It was the ego that was hypothesized to keep the personality system in balance. According to Freud the hyperactive child represented faulty ego development. He inferred that their impulsivity and their aggressiveness were the result of a weak ego, that is, one which failed to control id impulses. Such children were thought to be in constant emotional conflict. Since the ego was unable to adequately do the job of striking a balance between id impulses and super ego ideals, the personality was thought to be in continuous internal conflict between primitive impulses and parental expectations for conformity of behavior. Hyperaction was viewed as a symptom of the continuous conflict between these two personality forces (Allen, 1942).

Treatment consisted of permitting the hyperactive youngster to release his inhibitions while acting out his impulses in the presence of an accepting adult (Shainman, 1951). Theoretically, in such therapy sessions the therapist acted as the child's ego. It was the task of the therapist to construct the child's ego by externally censoring his primitive impulses while not encouraging him to become overly conforming to parental standards. Naturally, very little has been reported regarding the effectiveness of this approach. Most of what has been reported has been theoretical in nature with little emphasis on evaluation of the effectiveness of the technique (Sheer, 1954). Actually, the value of this approach remains questionable.

SELF THEORY. The self-theorists add still another dimension to the psychological understanding of the hyperactive child. These theorists viewed the hyperactive child as an individual whose true (acceptable) self would emerge given the proper therapist/client relationship. Theirs was a very Rousseauian conceptualization of the personality of the hyperactive child. It was believed that given the proper adult/child relationship and the proper environment, a well-adjusted personality would emerge. Treatment involved the establishment of a nonthreatening therapist/child relationship. Within this therapeutic relationship the therapist was nondirective. He made no value judgments about the rightness or wrongness of the child's behavior. The therapist helped the child to evaluate alternate forms of behavior by reflecting back to him his feelings and helping him to clarify his thoughts. Perhaps the most important contribution made by this group was the recognition that the hyperactive child responded better to treatment within a controlled environment. Working with the child in an environment which was devoid of excessive stimulation was considered an essential part of the treatment (Jacob, 1951).

LEARNING THEORY. The most current psychological theory

regarding the cause and treatment of hyperactivity has its roots in learning theory. Learning theorists accept the developmental lag theory of hyperactivity. However, such theorists also accept that hyperactivity may be linked to a variety of other conditions (damage to the cerebral cortex, reaction formation against depression and endocrine disturbance). Regardless of the "internal" cause, this approach emphasizes the environmental stimuli which elicit and reinforce hyperactive behaviors. Consequently, the hyperactive child is viewed as a youngster who differs from other children only in the frequency with which he exhibits certain behaviors. That is, the five primary characteristics of the syndrome are found in all children, but to a much lesser extent than are exhibited by the hyperactive child. This concept is a very important one in the history of psychological approaches to hyperactivity. It views the hyperactive child as differing from normal children only in the frequency with which he exhibits the primary characteristics of the syndrome. This whole concept elevates the hyperactive child from previous theories which viewed him as either mentally incompetent or as emotionally maladjusted.

This form of therapy involves the application of respondent and operant learning principles. Behavior modification with hyperactive children relies heavily on the use of environmental control and reinforcement techniques in order to shape and extinguish the hyperactive child's excess behaviors. The efficacy of this technique has been attested to by the voluminous literature reporting improvement in hyperactive children. Using operant techniques, Anderson (1964) was able to significantly reduce the frequency of out-of-seat behaviors by making teacher attention contingent on sitting behaviors. The effectiveness of withholding reinforcement following negative behaviors was pointed up by the work of Madsen, Becker, Thomas, Koser and Pager (1968). Their research demonstrated that sitting behavior in hyperactive children could be increased significantly when the teacher intermittently praised those children who were sitting while ignoring those who stood up. A number of other high-frequency behaviors associated with the syndrome were shown to be brought under control through the systematic use of positive reinforcement (Alabiso, 1975).

The relatively easily understandable concepts as well as the efficiency with which behavior modification techniques can be mastered by both therapist and teacher have provided a natural bridge between education and psychotherapy. In many respects the history of educational approaches to the hyperactive child parallel the history of psychological approaches to him.

Educational Approaches

Educational programming for the hyperactive child has long been recognized as a formidable task. Helping the hyperactive youngster to learn challenges the classroom teacher on many levels. Academically, the teacher is faced with understanding the child's specific learning deficits and the various techniques used to overcome his handicaps. On a social level, she is confronted with managing the child's peer group. Quite often hyperactive children are ostracized by their peers. Reversal of this process within the classroom is a complex and personally demanding task. Keogh (1971) pointed out the complexity of trying to teach the hyperactive child. Her review of the literature in this area revealed that the classroom teacher is faced with at least three general explanations of the hyperactive child's learning problems. One explanation presented to the teachers is a medical/neurological situation in which the teacher is reassured that the child's problem is a physical one and mainly out of her control. A second theory suggests the child's heightened activity level disrupts his ability to attend to the relevant information to be learned, and therefore he fails to achieve. Finally, the classroom teacher may be told that the hyperactive child fails to learn at a rate comparable to his peers because his impulsivity prevents him from making decisions necessary for the critical evaluation of what is presented to him in the classroom.

A historical review of the educational approaches to the hyperactive child helps to bring academic approaches into focus. Prior to the classic work of Strauss and Werner (1941), hyperactivity was viewed as either mental retardation or dementia.

Like the prepsychoanalytic therapists, educators viewed the hyperactive child as mentally incompetent. Educational programming ranged from a school program which was primarily custodial in nature to exclusion from the classroom. Many such children simply never attended school, an action based on the theory that they were unable to learn.

The work of Strauss and Lehtinen (1947) constituted a turning point in educational programming for hyperactive children. Their research demonstrated that hyperactivity was a syndrome distinct from mental retardation. It also demonstrated that this syndrome could exist in children of normal or higher intelligence. Their initial research demonstrated that at least part of their difficulty in learning could be attributed to a malfunctioning of the visual-perceptual system. These children were found to have a disturbance in their ability to separate figure from ground in their visual perceptions. Their research set the trend for other investigators to examine the relationship between hyperactivity and the disturbance of the child's ability to receive and to respond to visual, auditory and tactile stimulation. Early educational approaches centered on the use of destimulation techniques (Jolles, 1956; Kirk, 1953). This approach focused on helping the hyperactive child to learn by freeing the classroom from as many distractors as possible. This approach was based on Strauss' and Lehtinen's observation that a portion of the child's difficulty in learning resulted directly from his inability to inhibit impulses to distracting stimuli.

During the 1950's and 1960's, educational planning for the hyperactive child took on a greater degree of sophistication. Such children came to be classified technically as being learning disabled, and hyperactivity came to be viewed primarily as being caused by a lag in the child's development of the physiological systems necessary for adequate learning. The child's learning dysfunction was attributed to a disturbance of one or more of the primary sensory systems. Special tests were developed to measure the child's ability to accurately perceive what he sees and to translate those perceptions across the optic nerve to the brain in order to produce a visual image of the object. His ability to execute fine and gross motor movements was also evaluated. In addition, his ability to accurately perceive the sounds that he hears and to translate those sounds into mental images was closely evaluated. The child's inability to understand and use words representative of these mental images constituted another area of specific learning disability which is affected by hyperactivity. Finally, his ability to learn through his sense of touch was established as an area in need of thorough evaluation. A child's ability to learn might be negatively affected by failure to recognize objects according to shape, size and texture through his sense of touch.

Another important development stemming from the concept of the hyperactive child as a youngster who is learning disabled was the recognition that the hyperactive youngster may suffer from an uneven development of intellectual abilities. In other words, such children may be of average intelligence or above. However, they may demonstrate very high scores on measures of certain intellectual abilities while very low scores on measures of other intellectual abilities. Such children, for example, may have very well developed abilities to use and understand words and to recall the sounds that they hear, while at the same time they function at a nearly mentally defective level in their ability to think abstractly and to use previous experiences in dealing with novel situations. The concept of the hyperactive child as a child who suffers from an unevenness in the development of intellectual abilities is a relatively new one. Nevertheless, there is much merit to this conceptualization.

Academic programming for these children calls for individualization in instruction. Initially, special classes for learning-disabled children were established. Over the years, controversy developed over the negative effects of separating these children from their normal classroom peers. In recent years there has been an educational trend toward maintaining the hyperactive child in the regular classroom and having him attend special learning modules in order for him to receive remedial instruction in the specific areas of his learning disabilities. This approach relies heavily on helping the hyperactive child learn through his sensory systems, which are fully intact. In other words, a child who has difficulty with visual perception may receive reading instruction which complements the instructional program by providing tapes which accompany the reading material. Thus, the child is encouraged to compensate for his deficits in visual perception by relying on his intact auditory system. As early as 1955, Kaliski reported the need for training in perceptual skills, auditory acuity and kinesthetic responsiveness. Later Cruickshank et al. (1966) developed a special educational program for reducing distractibility, motor disinhibition, dissociation, figure-ground disturbance and perseveration.

Current trends in educational programming have emphasized the value of combining the principles of learning theory with the concept of learning disability. Schrager et al. (1966) for instance recommended that educational programming and academic training for the hyperactive child include limitations on classroom stimuli, the presentation of a structured program in which changes were slowly and carefully introduced, patient repetition of information, concrete rather than abstract presentation, breaking down of processes to small manageable segments, a sensitivity to the child's most efficient sensory channels and heightened tolerance for otherwise troublesome behavior on the part of the teacher. Shortly afterwards, Werry (1969) recommended the use of behavior therapy in the treatment of specific behavioral and learning disturbances in the hyperactive child. He proposed that the use of behavior modification techniques would be helpful in increasing attention span and reducing distractability in improving perceptual motor skills.

An early forerunner of the combination of educational programming and behavior therapy was the work of SantoStefano and Stayton (1967). These researchers taught parents and teachers behavior modification techniques in order to help hyperactive children improve their visual-motor coordination and concept formation abilities. Both teachers and parents rated the program as being exceptionally successful. Pihl (1967) was able to obtain significant gains in classroom sitting behavior in nonbrain-injured hyperactive children through the use of reinforcement techniques. Patterson, Jones, Whittier and Wright (1965) made the important transition from behavioral control to improvement in the academic areas by reinforcing hyperactive children for remaining in their seats and for working in their workbooks. In another related article, Patterson (1965) defined hyperactivity in terms of the high frequency of certain classroom behaviors. He was able to use primary reinforcement and peer group approval in order to increase classroom sitting behavior. An important observation of this study was that reinforcement for in-seat behavior alone was not sufficient to improve the child's performance on academic tasks. Patterson recommended that reinforcement for correct academic responses accompany classroom behavior modification programs. DuBrose (1966) recognized the importance of Patterson's statement that reinforcement for sitting behavior alone would not increase the hyperactive child's performance on academic tasks. He reinforced hyperactive children in the classroom on three academic tasks over a twelve-day period. He found that the high rates of behavior associated with hyperactivity decreased significantly, while learning in specific academic areas which were reinforced increased.

Martinson (1967) recommended that special education programs concentrate on training hyperactive children in the component behaviors from which academic and social skills are formed. Several authors doing early research in this area had reported increases in social and academic skills when chemotherapy, behavior modification and special education programming were combined (Bradley, 1950; Horenstein, 1957; Millichap et al., 1967; Schulman and Clarinda, 1964; and Ziziemsky, 1964).

The combination of chemotherapy, behavior modification and specialization in academic programming provide the most effective classroom environment for the hyperactive child's education. The positive effects of chemotherapy in the areas of behavioral control and learning, along with the application of learning principles assist specialized techniques used in educational programming for the learning disabled child.

SUMMARY

It is only within the past three decades that hyperactivity has come to be viewed as a condition separate from mental retardation or insanity. While there are numerous behavioral, cognitive and emotional characteristics associated with the syndrome, most researchers agree that the condition is primarily characterized by cognitive dysfunction, impulsivity, excessively high activity level, and deficits in the distractibility and attention process. The other characteristics reported to accompany the syndrome seem to vary greatly according to the cause of the hyperactivity and the locus of the neurological impairment.

Several areas of research have proven fruitful in drawing attention to possible causitive factors. However the relationship between genetic disturbance and hyperactivity remains vague. Research in this area points toward a theory which suggests that hyperactivity may be the result of multiple genetic variables. At this time a polygenetic theory seems most feasible. Other areas of research, however, have proven more fruitful in shedding light on the causes of the syndrome. Investigation of the relationship between the cerebral cortex and hyperactivity has demonstrated that a malfunctioning of either the temporal or frontal lobe areas may result in hyperactivity. Damage to these areas may be the result of infection, tumor, lesion or trauma. Whatever the cause, the research tends to suggest that damage to either of these areas alone is usually not sufficient to cause hyperactivity.

The most convincing body of literature regarding the cause of hyperactivity stems from the research on the activity of the reticular formation. Research in the area of the brain stem suggests that hyperactivity may result as a disturbance of synaptic transmission. This body of data indicates that the hyperactive child suffers from a physiological disturbance in which impulses are blocked from traveling from one nerve to the other. This blockage appears to be the result of a chemical imbalance at the terminal between the end of one nerve and the beginning of the next. As a result, incoming and outgoing nervous impulses spill over, stimulating other nerves which in turn result in heightened activity level. This understanding of hyperactivity as being caused by a disturbance in the child's physiological development has led to a general developmental lag theory. This theory proposes that in some children certain neurological centers develop at uneven rates. The hyperactive child suffers from an uneven development of the centers contained in the brain stem. According to the developmental lag theory, as the child grows older, the development in the impaired areas quickens. In addition, higher brain centers take over the functioning of the centers which are lagging in development. In other words, the higher brain centers compensate for the lag in development.

Psychogenic theories of hyperactivity suggest that the characteristics of hyperactivity represent an ego defense against underlying feelings of depression. The hyperactive child's heightened activity level, his constant motion, his racing mood and racing behavior are all viewed as defensive reactions against underlying feelings of depression. Research in this area has been limited; however, there is a substantial body of literature that suggests that these theories hold merit for some hyperactive children.

Chemotherapy has provided the most effective unilateral treatment approach to the condition. While medication alone is not as effective as the combined educational/psychological/medical approach, it has proven highly effective in controlling many of the primary characteristics of the syndrome. Tranquilizing drugs appear to be most effective for those children whose hyperactivity is psychogenic. These emotionally disturbed children tend to respond best to a general sedative-type medication. In these children the primary positive effect reported is a reduction in activity level. By far the majority of hyperactive children respond best to psychostimulants. This category of drugs acts directly on the brain stem to correct deficits in synaptic transmission. Both categories of drugs, however, can be the cause of harmful side effects.

The relationship between chemotherapy and learning is obscure. Three general theories have been proposed. One such theory suggests that the drugs directly affect intelligence. A more likely theory is the one which suggests that drugs control the symptoms of hyperactivity in order to permit the child's native intellectual abilities to function properly. A third theory suggests that medication not only controls the symptoms, but that it affects some central cognitive process which allows the child to function more adequately in the academic areas. While all of these theories have some substance in the research literature, many questions remain unanswered. In all likelihood, a combination of medication therapy along with environmental stimulation and environmental structuring is the most effective means of promoting learning.

The history of psychological approaches in the treatment of hyperactivity reveals several distinct trends. The psychoanalytic formulation of hyperactivity as a deficit in ego development gave rise to other forms of treatment. Hyperactive youngsters were viewed as being in need of therapy. Treatment called for the establishment of a relationship by an accepting adult who served as the child's ego until the child reached the stage in therapy where he was able to internalize this relationship. In effect, the therapist censored the child's primitive impulses while at the same time discouraging him from the excessive internalization of parental standards and ideals.

The self-theorists viewed the hyperactive child from a different viewpoint. Theirs was a very Rousseauian concept of the hyperactive child. They hypothesized that, given the proper adult/child relationships and the proper environment, the child's natural personality would emerge. This emergent personality would be more like that of the average child who did not suffer from hyperactivity. Two significant contributions of this theoretical approach involved its emphasis on understanding the hyperactive child's emotional adjustment in terms of his negative self-concept and the realization that such children function best when the environment is structured. The most current and most effective psychological approach to hyperactivity is that of learning theory. The hyperactive youngster is viewed as responsive to the principles of operant and respondent conditioning regardless of the origin of the hyperactive behavior. This behavior modification approach applies the principles of learning theory to the child's behavior. An important aspect of this theory was that it viewed the hyperactive child as neither pathological nor sick. The hyperactive youngster's characteristics are viewed in terms of their freqeuncy of occurrence. This theory emphasizes that all the behaviors exhibited by the hyperactive child are also found in normal children. It is only the frequency of occurrence which makes their behavior out of the ordinary.

Educational approaches have gone through a period of evolution over the years. Research in the 1940's by Strauss and his colleagues served as a turning point in educational programming for the hyperactive child. From an academic point of view, these youngsters were no longer considered to be mentally incompetent. Shortly thereafter, they came to be viewed as learning-disabled youngsters. Educators came to recognize that such children may be of average or above intelligence and yet maintain cognitive disabilities. Much emphasis was placed on the child's ability to learn through his senses. Special academic programs were developed to take into consideration that the child may have a deficit in one or more sensory areas. Special programming centered around training in the deficient area of sensory reception or expression as well as training the child to use his fully functioning sensory areas to compensate for the deficit in the impaired area. These programs utilized the techniques of individualization of instruction and destimulatization of the classroom environment. Special academic programs have been developed to help the child compensate for deficits in his visual perception and motor expression, auditory reception and vocal expression and in his tactile reception and proprioceptive expression.

Current educational programming emphasizes the combination of special education techniques applied to learning-disabled children along with the utilization of learning theory and medication management. This multi-disciplinary approach is the most effective form of medical/psychological/academic therapy. The majority of hyperactive children are then viewed as suffering from an unevenness in their physiological development. These children are considered to be abnormal only in the frequency with which their behaviors occur. Academically, these children are considered to need special educational programming which takes into account their deficits in sensory reception and motor expression.

REFERENCES

Adametz, J. L.: Rate of recovery functioning in cats with rostel reticular lesion. *Journal of Neurosurgery, 16*:85-98, 1959.

Alabiso, F. P.: Operant Control of Attention Behaviors: A Treatment for Hyperactivity. *Behavior Therapy, 6*:39-42, 1975.

Alexandris, A. R., and Lundell, F. G.: Effects of thioridazine amphetamine and placebo on hyperkinetic syndrome and cognitive area in mentally deficient children. *Canadian Medical Association Journal, 98*:92-96, 1968.

Allen, F.: *Psychotherapy with Children*. New York, W. W. Norton, 1942.

Amassian, B. B., and DiVito, R. T.: Unit activity in reticular formation in nearby structures. *Journal of Neurophysiology, 17*:575-603, 1954.

Anderson, D. B.: *Application of behavior modification techniques to the control of the hyperactive child*. Unpublished Master's thesis, University of Oregon, 1964.

Anderson, W. M.: The hyperkinetic child: a neurological appraisal. *Neurology, 13*:968-973, 1963.

Beck, A. T.: Depression: Causes and Treatment. *University of Pennsylvania Press*, 1972.

Bianchi, L. T.: *The mechanisms of the brain in the functions of the prefrontal lobes*. New York, William Wood and Company, 1922.

Braddard, G. S., and Rapoport, J. L.: Minimum brain dysfunction with hyperactivity: comparison of behavioral and cognitive effects of pharmacological and behavioral treatments. Personal Communication, 1974.

Bradley, C. E.: Benzadrine and dexadrine in treatment of children's behavior disorders. *Pediatrics, 5*:24, 1950.

Brickner, R. E.: *The Intellectual Functions of the Frontal Lobes*. New York, Macmillan, 1936.

Brummet, H.: The use of long-acting tranquilizers with hyperactive children. *Psychosomatics, 9*:157-159, 1968.

Buckley, R. E.: A neurophysiological proposal for the amphetamine response in hyperkinetic children. *Psychosomatics, 13*:93-99, 1972.

Burks, H. P.: The effect of learning on brain pathology. *Exceptional Children, 24*:169-172, 1957.

Burks, H. P.: Effects of amphetamine therapy on hyperkinetic children. *Archives of General Psychiatry, 11*:601-604, 1964.

Campbell, S. B., Douglas, B. I., and Morgenstern, G.: Cognitive styles and hyperactive children and the effect of methylphenidate. *Journal of Child Psychology and Psychiatry and Allied Disciplines* (London), *1*:55-67, 1971.

Cantwell, D.: Psychiatric illness in families of hyperactive children. *Archives of General Psychiatry, 27*:414-417, 1972.

Conners, C. K., and Eisenberg, L.: The effects of Methylphenidate on symptomtology and learning in disturbed children. *American Journal of Psychiatry, 120*:458-464, 1963.

Conners, C. K.: The effects of Dexedrine on rapid discrimination and motor control of hyperactive children under mild stress. *Journal of Nervous and Mental Disease, 142*:429-433, 1966.

Conners, C. K.: Symposium: Behaviour modification by drugs. II. Psychological effects of stimulant drugs in children with minimal brain dysfunction. *Pediatrics, 5*:702-708, 1972.

Connley, D. P.: *Effects of Ritalin on hyperkinetic children attending the Glendale Elementary School.* (Doctoral dissertation, Arizona State University) Ann Arbor, Michigan. University Microfilms, 1973, No. 73-20427.

Conrad, W. G.: Anticipating the response to amphetamine therapy in the treatment of hyperactive children. *Pediatrics, 40*:96-99, 1967.

Cruickshank, W. T., Bentzen, F. P., Retzenberg, F. L., and Tannenhauser, M. M.: *A Teaching Method for Hyperactive and Brain-Injured Children.* Syracuse, Syracuse UP, 1966.

DuBrose, S. G., and Daniels, G. T.: An experimental approach to the reduction of overactive behavior. *Behavior Research and Therapy, 4*:251-258, 1966.

Ferrier, D. L.: *The Functions of the Brain.* New York, Putnam, 1876.

Finnerty, R. J., Soltys, J. J., and Cole, J. O.: The use of D-Amphetamine with hyperactive children. *Psychopharmacologia* (Berlin), *3*:302-308, 1971.

Forward, T. C.: *Factors relating to an increase in achievement in hyperkinetic children who are on a combined program of motor perceptual training and drug therapy.* (Doctoral dissertation, Case Western Reserve University) Ann Arbor, Michigan, University Microfilms, 1970, No. 70-25957.

French, J. T., Amerongen, F. S., and MaGoun, H. H.: An activating system in the brain stem of the monkey. *Archives of Neurological Psychiatry, 68*:577-590, 1952.

French, J. T., Hernandez-Peon, R. O., and Livingston, R. F.: Projections from cortex to cephalic brain stem (reticular formation) in monkey. *Journal of Neurophysiology, 18*:75-95, 1955.

Gastaut, H. O., Vigouroux, R. N., and Naquet, R. P.: Lesions amygdalocampiques. Provoquees chez le chat par injection de creme d'alumine. *Revue Neurologique, 87*:607-613, 1952.

Horenstein, S. R.: Resparine and Chlorapromazine in hyperactive mental defectives. *American Journal of Mental Deficiency, 61*:525-529, 1957.

Hundert, J., Gibbons, C., Weir, C., Denton, L., and Hillcoat, B.: *The prevalance of drug treatment for hyperactive children.* Unpublished research, 1974.

Ingram, T. P.: A characteristic form of overactive behavior in brain damaged children. *Journal of Mental Science, 102*:550-558, 1956.
Jacob, W. O.: Mental retardation: The educator's quandary. *Training School Bulletin, 48*:59-67, 1951.
Jacobsen, E.: *Depression: Comparative Studies in Normal, Neurotic and Psychotic Conditions.* International University Press, 1971.
Jacobsen, C. T.: A study of cerebral function in learning: the frontal lobes. *Journal of Comparative Neurology, 52*:272-281, 1931.
Jolles, I. L.: A public school demonstration class for children with brain damage. *American Journal of Mental Deficiency, 60*:582-588, 1956.
Kantwell, D. P.: Psychiatric illness in families of hyperactive children. *Archives of General Psychiatry, 27*:414-417, 1972.
Kaliski, L. E.: Educational therapy for brain-injured retarded children. *American Journal of Mental Deficiency, 60*:71-76, 1955.
Kennard, M. T., Fullton, J. L., and Jacobsen, C. C.: A note concerning the relation of frontal lobes to posture enforced grasping in monkeys. *Brain, 3*:524-530, 1932.
Keogh, B. K.: Hyperactivity and learning disorders: a review and speculation. *Exceptional Children, 38*:101-109, 1971.
Kirk, S. P.: What is special about special education?: The child who is mentally retarded. *Exceptional Children, 19*:138-142, 1953.
Kissel, S., and Freeling, N. W.: *A brief note on the relationship between hyperkinesis and depression.* Rochester Mental Health Center, Winter, 1974.
Kulver, H. U.. and Bucy, P. A.: Preliminary analysis of the functions of the temporal lobes in monkeys. *Archives of Neurology and Psychiatry, 6*:979-978, 1939.
Laufer, M. W., and Denhoff, E.: Hyperkinetic behavior syndrome in children. *Journal of Pediatrics, 50*:463-474, 1957.
Levin, T. M.: Restlessness in children. *Archives of Neurology and Psychiatry, 39*:764-770, 1938.
Madsen, C. A., Becker, W. B., Thomas, D. H., Koser, L. E., and Pager, E. K.: An analysis of the reinforcing function of "sit down" commands. In Parker, R. R. (Ed.): *Readings in Educational Psychology.* Boston, Allyn, 1968.
Martinson, M. E.: Education of a trainable child: An opportunity. *Exceptional Children, 34*:293-297, 1967.
Maynard, R. C.: FDA warns against use of "behavior" amphetamines. *Washington Post*, October 17, 1970.
Mendelson, W., Johnson, N., and Stewart, M. A.: Hyperactive children as teenagers: a follow-up study. *Journal of Nervous and Mental Disease, 4*:273-279, 1971.

Millichap, J. E., and Boldruy, B. D.: Studies in Hyperkinetic Behavior. II. Laboratory and Clinical Evaluations of Drug Treatments. *Neurology,* *17*:467-471, 1967.

Minde, K., Webb, G., and Sykes, D.: Studies on the hyperactive child. IV. Prenatal and paranatal factors associated with hyperactivity. *Developmental medicine and child neurology* (London), *10*:355-363, 1968.

Morrison, J. R., and Stewart, M. A.: Evidence for polygenetic inheritance in the hyperactive child syndrome. *American Journal of Psychiatry, 130*:142-147, 1973.

Moruzzi, G. O., and MaGoun, H. M.: Brain stem, reticular formation and activation of EEG. *Journal of Neurophysiology,* 6:471-489, 1949.

Noble, M. I.: Psychopharmacology for the hyperkinetic child: dynamic consideration. *Archives of General Psychiatry,* 6:198-202, 1962.

Palkes, H., and Stewart, M.: Intellectual ability and performance of hyperactive children. *American Journal of Orthopsychiatry, 42*:35-39, 1972.

Patterson, G. R.: An empirical approach to the classification of disturbed children. *Journal of Clinical Psychology, 20*:236-237, 1964.

Patterson, G. R.: An application of conditioning techniques to the control of the hyperactive child. In Ullman, L. M., and Krasner, L. H. (Eds.): *Case Studies in Behavior Modification.* New York, HR&W, 1965.

Patterson, G. R., Jones, R. W., Whitter, J. E., and Wright, M. A.: A behavior modification technique for the hyperactive child. *Behavior Research and Therapy, 2*:217-226, 1965.

Pihl, R. F.: Conditioning procedures with hyperactive children. *Neurology, 17*:421-423, 1967.

Rapoport, J. L., Lott, I. T., Alexander, D. F., and Abramson, A. U.: Urinary nor-adrenalin and playroom behavior in hyperactive boys. *Lancet, 2*:1141, 1970.

Rie, H.: Depression in children: A survey of some pertinent conditions. *Journal of Academy of Child Psychiatry,* 5:653-686, 1966.

Safer, D., Allen, R., and Barr, E.: Depression of growth of hyperactive children on stimulant drugs. *New England Journal of Medicine, 5*:217-220, 1972.

SantoStefano, S. P., and Stayton, S. N.: Training the preschool retarded child in focusing attention: a program for parents. *American Journal of Orthopsychiatry, 37*:732-743, 1967.

Scheibel, M. P., Scheibel, A. D., Mollica, A. H., and Moruzzi, G. M.: Convergence and interaction of impulses on single units of reticular formation. *Journal of Neurophysiology, 18*:309-330, 1955.

Schrager, J. M.: The hyperkinetic child: an overview of the issues. *Journal of American Academy of Child Psychiatry,* 5:526-533, 1966.

Schulman, J. L., and Clarinda, M. K.: The effect of promazine on activity level of retarded children. *Pediatrics, 33*:272, 1964.

Shainman, L. D.: Vocational training for the mentally retarded in the schools. *American Journal of Mental Deficiency, 56*:113-119, 1951.

Sheer, D. P.: Is there a common factor in learning for brain injured children? *Exceptional Children, 21*:10-12, 1954.

Sheer, D. R.: *The effect of frontal lobe operations on tension process.* (Doctoral dissertation, University of Michigan) Ann Arbor, Michigan. University Microfilms, 1959, No. 59-2648.

Sprague, R. L., Barnes, K. R., and Werry, J. S.: Methylphenidate and Thioridazine: Learning reaction time, activity and classroom behavior in disturbed children. *American Journal of Orthopsychiatry, 40*:615-628, 1970.

Stewart, M. T., Pitts, F., Craig, A. D., and Dieruf, W. T.: The hyperactive child syndrome. *American Journal of Orthopsychiatry, 36*:861-867, 1966.

Strazel, T. K., Taylor, C. E., and MaGoun, H. H.: Collateral afferent excitation of reticular formation of brain stem. *Journal of Neurophysiology, 14*:476-496, 1951.

Strauss, A., and Werner, H.: The mental organization of the brain injured, mentally defective child. *American Journal of Psychiatry, 97*:1194, 1941.

Strauss, A., and Lehtinen, L. B.: *Psychopathology and Education in the Brain Injured Child.* New York, Grune, 1947.

Sykes, D. H., Douglas, V. I., Weiss, G., and Minde, K. K.: Attention in hyperactive children and the effects of methylphenidate (ritalin). *Journal of Child Psychology and Psychiatry and Allied Disciplines* (London), *2*:129-139, 1971.

Tizard, B. E.: Observations of overactive imbecile children in controlled and uncontrolled environments. II. Experimental studies. *American Journal of Mental Deficiency, 72*:548-553, 1968.

Warren, R. J., Carduc, W. A., Bussaratid, S., Stewart, M. A., and Sly, W. S.: The hyperactive child syndrome: Normal chromosome finding. *Archives of General Psychiatry, 24*:161-162, 1971.

Weiss, G., Minde, K., Douglas, V., Werry, J., and Sykes, D.: Comparison of the effectiveness of chloropromazine, dextroamphetamine, and methylphenidate on the behavior and intellectual functioning of hyperactive children. *Canadian Medical Association Journal, 104*:21-25, 1971a.

Weiss, G., Minde, K., Werry, J. S., Douglas, V., and Nemeth, E.: Studies on the hyperactive child: VIII. Five-year follow up. *Archives of General Psychiatry, 24*:409-414, 1971b.

Werry, J. S., Weiss, G. O., and Douglas, V. R.: Studies on the hyperactive child. I. Some preliminary findings. *Canadian Psychiatric Association Journal, 9*:120, 1964.

Werry, J. S., Weiss, G. O., Douglas, V. R., and Martin, J. T.: Studies on the hyperactive child. II. The effect of chlorapromazine on behavior and learning. *Journal of the American Academy of Child Psychiatry*, 5:292-312, 1966.

Werry, J. S.: Studies on the hyperactive child. IV. An empirical analysis of minimal brain dysfunction syndrome. *Archives of General Psychiatry*, 19:9-16, 1968.

Werry, J. S.: Developmental hyperactivity. In Chess, S. E., and Thomas, A. B. (Eds.): *Annual Progress on Child Psychiatry and Child Development*. New York, Brunner-Mazel, 1969.

Werry, J. S., and Sprague, R. L.: Hyperactivity. In Costello, C. G. (Ed.): *Symptoms of Psychopathology*. New York, Wiley, 1970.

Ziziemsky, D. D.: Some considerations of the hyperactive syndrome in children. *Acta Psiquiatrica Y Psichological America Latina*, 10:132-138, 1964.

Zrull, J. P., McDermott, J. F., and Pozmanski, E.: Hyperkinetic syndrome: the role of depression. *Child Psychiatry and Human Development*, 1:33-41, 1970.

CHAPTER 3

ACTIVITY LEVEL IN HYPERACTIVE CHILDREN

Hyperactivity is a primary characteristic of the disorder. Indeed, if the child does not display a heightened activity level but evidences the other characteristics ordinarily associated with the disorder, he is diagnosed as suffering from minimal cerebral dysfunction rather than from hyperactivity. Activity level is the one factor which seems to differentiate between the hyperactive child and other brain-dysfunctional children. Lewis' (1963) thumbnail sketch of the hyperactive child brings attention to the importance of this characteristic. "He tends to be hyperactive, disinhibited and impulsive. He jumps around often and unexpectedly. He is highly distractable so that his attention jumps around too. He is often anxious . . . he seems to have few restraints," (p. 6). Lourie's (1962) description further rounds out the picture. "These children are born without brakes, and once the impulse starts they keep on reacting . . . a pat becomes a slap, a hug becomes a hurtful squeeze," (p. 3). Lourie points out that on a behavioral level overactivity seems the most difficult characteristic to cope with. "We make this diagnosis ('hyperkinetic child') in the waiting room usually. While the youngster is poking over the shoulders of the secretary pulling the paper out of the typewriter, the mother is saying helplessly 'Now Johnny you know you shouldn't do that,' " (p. 13).

Schrager et al. (1966) reviewed over forty major articles which reported on the characteristics associated with hyperactivity, and concluded that there was a high consensus among all articles reviewed that activity level was a predominant characteristic of the disorder. Actually, considering how often this characteristic is cited as the primary characteristic associated with hyperactivity, little is known about activity level. Researching the nature of activity levels and the variables which affect them is very complex. For example, the neurological centers responsible for activity level must be identified. This is a highly complex task requiring a sophisticated knowledge of neurophysiology. Even when the brain centers which control activity level have been identified, several other variables must be evaluated. The nature of activity level must be studied in a variety of bodily states. Is activity level only affected during wakefulness, or does disturbance of activity level carry over into sleep? If it does not, might there be some mechanism in the physiology of sleep that could provide us with insight into how to bring activity level under control during the daytime hours? Another variable involves the measurement of activity level. Does the evaluation of activity level depend on the judgment of an observer? If so, would all observers equally agree as to what activity is hyper and what is not? If a pediatrician, a parent and a classroom teacher were to observe the same child under the same circumstances, would they all agree on the extent to which a child is hyperactive? It is unlikely that they would. In fact, research in this area indicates that there is a poor consensus among observers of hyperactive children (Kaspar and Schulman, 1972). The question of which factors to measure adds complexity to the problem of studying activity level. Does one measure activity level by observing it, or can activity level be measured by monitoring heart rate? Is movement the predominant unit of measurement? If so, does the area of the body which is under observation make a difference? Would measures of hand movement differ significantly from measures of trunk movement in the hyperactive child? If we are able to identify the neurological center responsible for activity level, control for instrumentation and observer differences, what is the relationship between level of activity and the demand characteristics of the environment in which the child finds himself? Are hyperactive children more active in high-stimulus environments? Does stimulation increase or decrease activity level? Is activity level affected by the introduction of other children into the environment? All of these factors are important variables in understanding the relationship between activity level and the other characteristics identified with the disorder.

Chapter 3 will review the research on the neurology of arousal and activity level. The variables which affect activity level and a description of the instruments used in assessing it will be discussed. Psychological studies on the nature of activity level will be reviewed along with a summarization of the research related to control of activity level.

Much emphasis will be placed on the utilization of behavior modification within the classroom setting. Several approaches to the control of activity level within the classroom will be described and practical issues in applying these techniques to the classroom setting will be discussed.

ETIOLOGY OF ACTIVITY LEVEL

Over the past three decades several different types of theories have emerged as a result of research attempts to identify the causes of activity level disturbance.

The motor neuron theories associate overactivity with a malfunctioning of the motor neurons. This theory is based on a construct which proposed that activity level is a function of motor neuron firing. Consequently, atypical neuronal discharges are thought to result in excessive motor activity. The neuronal malfunction may be the result of lesion, genetic mutation or infectous disease. In their review of these theories, Cromwell, Baumeister and Hawkins (1963) pointed out that such theoretical formulations leave many unanswered questions. For example, there has been no clear theoretical explanation which would allow one to predict the differential effect between diffuse lesions and focal lesions on activity level. The precision of this theory in predicting activity level is also obscured by the fact that there has been little information regarding the differential effect of neuronal malfunctioning in the afferent tracks as opposed to neuronal malfunctioning in the efferent tracks. In other words, it is not clear from this theory whether any of the neuronal malfunctioning for incoming nervous impulses would have the same effect on activity level as a disturbance of neuronal activity in the tracks that control outgoing impulses.

A second set of theoretical formulations dates back to the early research of Strauss and Lehtinen (1947). Their early research acted as a prototype for the psychophysiological theories of activity level which maintain popularity today. This group of theories infers brain injury. The basic premise of this set of theories is that a series of intervening events occurs between the reception of external stimuli and the motor response which follows. The brain is viewed as being required to complete a cycle between incoming stimulus impulses and the output of a motor response. Strauss and Lehtinen proposed this as a five-stage process. The first stage involves reception of external stimuli by the sense organs. Stage two involves the neurological organization of the stimuli in order to present a meaningful pattern in the brain (that is, perception). Stage three is a cognitive step which requires the individual to interpret his perception in light of his needs. Step four calls for a selection of an adaptive motor response. It is the fifth step which requires the actual production of the overt behavior by the skeletal muscles. According to Strauss and Lehtinen, the overactive youngster experiences some physiological interruption in one or more of the five steps in the cycle. Failures in perception, deficits in motor execution and production of perseverative responses, all represent one or more neurological defects in the execution of the five-stage process. A key concept central to this theory is that, at whatever locus in the process that the deficit occurs, the full amount of energy required to process the entire response through its five stages is not utilized. Hence, the child builds up a store of excess energy. Consequently a reservoir of excess energy is accumulated, resulting in overactivity. It must be remembered, in considering such theories, that much of what has been hypothesized has been inferred from observing overt behavior. Whether the disturbance occurs on an internal physiological level is unknown. While such theories have their weaknesses, they have proven very fruitful in helping us to develop educational programs for the hyperactive youngster.

Other theories have linked overactivity to deficits in the receptor-effector systems. Such theories focus on the relationship between the visual motor, auditory motor, visual autonomic and auditory autonomic receptor and effector systems (Gellner, 1959). Developmental theorists such as Zaporozhet (1957, 1960) have viewed overactivity as a compensatory response to a block in physiological development. According to such theories, each child goes through a natural progression in which he makes a transition from exploring his environment through his tactile sense, to use of language to explore and adapt to environmental conditions. According to such theorists, hyperactive children represent that population of youngsters who have been unable to make a successful transition from the tactile exploration of environment to the verbal exploration of environment. Such children compensate for this deficit by "overusing" their motor-touch association system.

More recently some theorists have begun to view the overactive child as an individual who may experience varying degrees of difficulty in sorting out relevant from irrelevant responses (Bindra, 1961). Such children, regardless of the internal cause of their hyperactivity, are hypothesized to be unable to differentiate between relevant and irrelevant behavior responses. Their hyperactivity is viewed as a deficit in the ability to discriminate between these two types of behaviors. In recent years psychological theories have been developed to take into account the simultaneous interaction of social variables as well as internal physiological processes (Kaspar, 1971, 1972, 1973, 1974).

The translation of psychological theories into research findings has been anything but conclusive. For instance, Payne (1962) reported that about 75 percent of the children who had exhibited minimal brain damage in his study were found to show definite abnormal neurological signs. Just three years prior to Payne's report, Knobel, Wolman and Mason (1959) found no positive, significant correlation between minimal cerebral dysfunction developmental history, neurological examination, psychological tests or EEGs. Schulman et al. (1965) added to this apparent inconsistency by reporting that there was no significant correlation between ratings of minimal brain damage on a neurological evaluation and any of the seven measures hypothesized to be measures of brain injury.

Research on the relationship between hyperactivity and abnormal EEG status has also produced contradictory results. A number of studies of children who have been prediagnosed as not suffering from organic brain damage have shown varying degrees of abnormal EEG status. In a population of subjects with no known neuropsychopathology, the percentage of abnormal EEGs ranges from 10 percent to 55 percent (Secuda and Finley, 1942; Solomon, Brown and Deutsch, 1944; Miller and Lennox, 1948; Gibbs, Rich, Foice and Gibbs, 1960).

Another set of explanations have been incorporated into Drive Theory as an explanation for activity level. Using the Hull-Spence theory of learning as a function of reduction in drive, Cantor (1963) and Hilgard (1956) have proposed that overactivity represents a high drive for activity level. According to this theory, the higher the drive, the more rapidly learning will occur. Cantor hypothesized that subjects with a high drive for activity level tend to have difficulty in learning complex motor responses. The effects of this difficulty are thought to be intensified by the fact that the high drive for activity level results in a multiplication of learned incorrect habits. The unique aspect of this group of theories is that they place almost no emphasis on internal neurophysiological processes, but rather seek to explain and predict the course of activity level solely on the basis of one type of learning theory. To date, this line of research has failed to contribute significantly to our understanding of the relationship between hyperactivity and learning.

Current Research

Kaspar (1971, 1972, 1973, 1974) has provided a great service by summarizing the research on activity level over the past several decades. Due to the lack of consistent, high correlations between hyperactivity and measures of minimal brain dysfunction, Kaspar concluded that hyperactivity represents a biosocial response rather than a physiological condition. Based on this review of the literature and three of his own studies, he refuted the previously held theories that hyperactivity is a "convergent syndrome." That is, he reported that all of the primary characteristics associated with minimal brain dysfunction are not automatically associated with hyperactivity. He has advocated for an approach to understanding hyperactivity which views the primary characteristics associated with the "syndrome" as being separate but parallel processes that are not necessarily significantly correlated with one another. Viewing control of activity level as one of a number of possible areas of disturbance, he hypothesized that hyperactivity represents an inability on the part of the subject to adjust his activity level to the demand characteristics of the situation. Kaspar hypothesized that each individual possesses a homeostatic control mechanism for activity level. He theorized that there is a mean optimal activity level for each person. According to this hypothesis, an individual's activity level may vary with the social situation and his bodily state. While an individual's activity level may range from excessive activity to minimal activity under varying circumstances, the intact homeostatic control mechanism controls overall activity level in such a way that the individual's activity level over time averages out to an optimal activity level. The brain-injured youngster suffers from a deficit in his body's ability to adjust activity level. According to Kaspar, in such children the homeostatic control mechanism has been damaged. Kaspar thus defines hyperactivity as a deficit in the ability to shift activity level upward or downward rather than as an unalterable body state which produces the syndrome. Kaspar further refined his theory to point out that the major problem for such individuals seems to be in shifting their activity level downward. It is well known that hyperactive youngsters have no problem increasing their activity level. However, when required by situational demands to shift activity level downward, the result is usually heightened activity level. According to Kaspar, any attempt to shift activity level downward tends to increase activity level rather than decrease it. Kaspar cited the work of Stevens, Stover and Backus (1970) as supporting his theories. Stevens and his colleagues compared groups of hyperactive and nonhyperactive children on a speed tapping test under incentive and nonincentive conditions. They observed that the hyperactive youngster maintained basically one response tempo (moderately fast). Normal control subjects were observed to be able to shift their response tempo upward and backward with relative ease. On a physiological level the research of Villa Blanca (1972, 1974a, b) and Villa Blanca and Marcus (1972, 1973, 1974a, b) lends support to this theory. Villa Blanca's research pointed out that the ascending tracks of the reticular formation regulate activity level while the descending tracks of the reticular formation serve to inhibit activity level. It is quite possible that in the hyperactive child the ascending tracks of the reticular formation function adequately, while the descending tracks are impaired in such a way as to make a downward shift of activity level not possible without producing overactivity.

Perhaps of equal importance to this theory was Kaspar's (1973) conclusion that the importance of activity level in understanding the overall condition of hyperactivity has been greatly overrated. Indeed, his own studies led him to conclude that the characteristic of distractibility seems to be more central to the condition of hyperactivity. This conclusion finds support elsewhere in the literature. For instance, Cromwell, Baumeister and Hawkins (1963) concluded that "Any attempt to build a theoretical framework to handle activity level as a unitary or homogeneous phenomenon would probably be futile" (p. 652). More recently, Walker (1974) prefaced his review of the literature on hyperactivity by stating, "Hyperactivity is a collection of symptoms, not a disease. It has a number of causes. Without exhaustive diagnostic tests, a physician may grab the expedient pill, mask the real problem, and let the child down hard" (p. 43).

The electrophysiological theories such as those of McGoun (1952), Gastaut (1950), and Villa Blanca (1972, 1974a, b) and Villa Blanca and Marcus (1972; 1973; 1974a, b) proposed that overactivity is a result of a malfunctioning of synaptic transmission in the reticular formation control human arousal and thus activity level. The emphasis of these theories is on disturbance of electrophysiological functioning in the process of synaptic transmission. Overactivity is thought to be the result of high electrochemical resistance at the synapse. This resistance slows the transmission of incoming nervous impulses to the extent that impulses are thought to "spill over" from one tract to another, resulting in heightened activity level. This has been the most vigorous area of research in recent years and has proved to be the most fruitful explanation of overactivity in terms of its ability to generate testable hypotheses.

The early work of Moruzzi and McGoun (1949) linked human arousal with the functioning of the brain stem. In a later article, McGoun (1952) suggested that overactivity was associated with a malfunctioning of the ascending tracts of the reticular activity system (the brain stem). These early studies led other investigators to examine the relationship between the reticular activating system and activity level. Several researchers were able to create hyperactivity in laboratory animals by altering the functioning of the brain stem (Adametz, 1959; Amassian and DeVito, 1954; French, Amerongen and McGoun, 1952; French, Hernandez-Peon, and Livingston, 1955; Scheibel, Scheibel, Mollica and Moruzzi, 1955). The success of these researchers in linking disturbance of activity level to an alteration of the functioning of the reticular formation led Berkson and Mason (1963) and others (Hernandez-Peon, 1966a, b; Lindsley, 1966; Windle, 1966a, b) to investigate the functions of the reticular activating system in human arousal.

Woodburn (1967) summarized the early research by pointing out that the reticular activating system serves as a coordinating mechanism for all incoming and outgoing nervous impulses. It is the nervous pathways of the ascending tracts of reticular activating system that are responsible for arousal. A disturbance of these nervous pathways may lead to heightened activity level. The descending tracts of the reticular activating system are responsible for inhibiting impulses. In other words, the reticular formation acts as a terminal for nervous impulses traveling from the receptors of the sense organs to the cerebral cortex. It further acts as a terminal for those impulses traveling from the cerebral cortex back to the sense organs. It is the job of the ascending tract to increase activity level while the function of the descending tracts is to inhibit activity level.

There has been little research with human subjects. Most of our knowledge about the role of the reticular activating system in human arousal comes from research with animal subjects. Several authors have demonstrated a direct relationship between removal of the thalamus and hyperactivity in dogs and cats (Emmers, Chung, and Wang, 1965; Goltz, 1892; Kleitman and Camille, 1932). The reticular formation is composed of bundles of nerve fibers located in the area known as the brain stem. These bundles are located adjacent to one another and pass through a subcortical center known as the thalamus. It is this subcortical center which serves as the terminal through which incoming and outgoing impulses travel. Animal research on hyperactivity has been accomplished by altering the structure of the thalamus either by complete removal or by partial impairment of the nerve fibers which comprise it. Over the past decade, the research of Villa Blanca has been exemplary in exploring the relationship between activity level and the reticular formation.

Villa Blanca (1972; 1974a, b) and Villa Blanca and Marcus (1972; 1973; 1974a b) completed a series of studies in which they investigated the relationship between the reticular formation and walking activities in animals. Their findings indicated that a disturbance of a reticular formation creates a state of persistent activity called *obstinant progression.* Any attempt to stop obstinant progression increased activity level. This finding in itself draws a striking parallel to the behavioral reactions observed in hyperactive children when attempts are made to decrease their activity level. Their research findings also included the observation that sleep time decreased while irritability and rage reactions became more frequent. Other effects of experimental alteration of the reticular formation produced clumsiness and overreaction to external stimuli. Interestingly enough, all the subjects in the Villa Blanca study showed a normal EEG pattern indicating that hyperactivity may be experimentally produced in animals without disturbing the activity of the cerebral cortex. This in itself may be one plausible explanation why EEG reports have been unreliable in identifying hyperactivity in human subjects.

Similar effects on behavior and activity level were produced by surgical alteration of the frontal lobes. Here again, the parallel to hyperactivity in human subjects with frontal lobe damage was striking. In one of the studies, Villa Blanca et al. administered psychostimulants to the animals in which the reticular formation was surgically interrupted. Behavioral improvements were observed. Perhaps most important for purposes of this text were the studies in which Villa Blanca studies the relationship between disturbance of the brain stem and learning. He reported that surgical alteration of the brain stem resulted in a tendency to fixate on the last response before a reward was given. In other words, once a subject has received a reward for learning the correct response, he became fixated on that response even though no further reward was available. In addition, the alteration of the brain stem resulted in an inability to shift to a new response pattern. Once the animal had learned a given response he seemed unable to learn a new response. Responses during learning tasks also became perseverative and an inability to make reversals was noted. All of these deficits in responding have been observed in hyperactive children.

While there has been no comparable research with human subjects, the findings of Villa Blanca and his colleagues have strong implications for our understanding of hyperactivity. His observations regarding activity level, obstinate progression, exaggerated overresponsiveness, irritability, stereotyped behaviors, perseveration and inability to shift responses seem to find their counterpart in the hyperactive child. Hopefully, this line of research will provide us with the sophisticated technology necessary to identify the specific locii in the human reticular formation responsible for these deficits.

MEASUREMENT OF ACTIVITY LEVEL

In spite of its status as the characteristic which differentiates a hyperactive child from his brain-damaged peer, very little is known about the nature of activity level. In their review of the literature, Cromwell, Baumeister and Hawkins (1963) concluded that the body of knowledge about activity level had been limited and disorganized. A lack of standards in the measurement of activity remains as an obstacle to increasing our knowledge in this area. No valid and reliable measure of activity has been devised. There has been no consistent definition of activity. Defining activity in terms of observable, measurable human behaviors has been a painstaking and largely dissatisfactory endeavor.

Even if there were consistent agreement among researchers and practitioners as to the definition of activity, the development of an instrument to measure it would be a very complex and demanding task. A review of the literature brings the conclusion that such an instrument would need to meet seven criteria to be effective. Firstly, the instrument would have to be standardized on both hyperactive and nonhyperactive children at various age levels and at various levels of development. This means that the instrument should be able to discriminate between brain-damaged and nondamaged children at various age levels and at various levels of development. Secondly, an instrument would have to be appropriate for use with all types of children. This would mean that it should be able to discriminate overactivity from normal activity in various subgroups. Such a measure should be able to discriminate between hyperactive and non-hyperactive physically handicapped youngsters. Thirdly, the measure would have to take into account various qualitative differences in activity level. Some hyperactive children exhibit a pattern associated with what seems to be continuous prolonged activity, while other children diagnosed as hyperactive may exhibit intervals in which activity level seems normal. These intervals may be interspersed with "bursts" of activity in which activity level increases rapidly and intensively and then drops off quickly. This aspect of measurement relates closely to the fifth characteristic. The instrument must be able to measure activity level as a series of discreet acts rather than as a continuous process. This presents a very important concept to the measurement of activity level. The better able the instrument in defining activity level in terms of separate, discreet behaviors, the more powerful it is in discriminating hyperactive from nonhyperactive subjects. A sixth variable has to do with environmental factors. Our ideal measure of activity level would take into account that activity level varies under different social and environmental conditions. Finally, as is true with all measurements, the instrument would have to be reliable as well as valid. In other words, such variables as differences in observer ratings would have to be controlled. Unfortunately, no such measure of activity level exists.

Rating Scales

Numerous attempts have been made to construct rating scales in which the child's level of activity is determined based on the judgments of an observer. These scales vary in complexity and in detail; however, they share certain characteristics. The primary characteristic of all such scales is that they focus mainly on rating the frequency of certain behavior. A second requirement of measurement includes a frequency count during a specified time interval. In effect, the "hyperactivity score" reflects the frequency of occurrence of certain behaviors over the amount of observation time. Further refinement has been added to these scales by using a time-sampling technique. That is, the frequency of occurrence of certain behaviors is observed for a number of specified random intervals. Still other refinements have been added by having the child observed by more than one observer in a variety of settings.

In recent years, a number of rating scales have been developed which evaluate hyperactive behavior by observing the child at random intervals within the classroom (Conners, 1969) and in a variety of settings outside of the classroom (Mendelson, Johnson and Stewart, 1971). More recently, scales developed by Patterson et al. (1970) and Davids (1971) have added to our skill in rating hyperactivity by treating each of the hyperactive child's behaviors as separate, discreet events. In a review of the literature on such scales dating back to 1954 (Horowitz), Kaspar (1974) concluded that observer rating scales are usually unreliable. They have been characterized by low interscorer reliability as well as discrepancies in the scores when the test was repeated at various time intervals.

In an attempt to develop more objective measures of activity level several investigators have developed automated devices in the hope that such instruments would meet the criteria necessary for an effective rating scale (Cromwell et al., 1963). Utilization of such instruments as the free space transversal apparatus (Tizard, 1968a, b), the kinetometer (Schulman and Reisman, 1959), the actometer (Schulman, Lipkin, Clarinda and Mitchell, 1961; Bell, 1967) and fidgetometer (Castanera et al., 1955) and balistograph (Foshee, 1958); Morgan and Stellar, 1950; McConnell, Cromwell, Bailer, and Son, 1964) have failed to provide valid and reliable measures of activity level.

To date, all attempts at developing an objective, accurate measure of activity level seem to be encumbered by disadvantages. While the direct observation measures permit the observer to record the quality as well as the quantity of the subject's behaviors, they have been shown to be highly subjective and, in many instances, of poor reliability. The use of instrumentation in order to gain objectivity has presented its own set of disadvantages. Difficulties in measuring the qualities of behavior as well as loss of reliability and lack of correlation with other measures of hyperactivity represent some of the disadvantages of this approach. Current attempts at more objective, more reliable measures of activity level have called for the use of more sophisticated multi-modal measures of activity level. The value to these approaches has yet to be demonstrated. Regardless of the existence of such a measure of activity level, it is not possible to accurately record activity without documenting the circumstances in which it occurs. Several sets of experimental variables and subject variables affect activity level in different ways. No measure of activity can present an accurate picture of the child's performance unless we know the circumstances under which it occurs. It is likely that the classroom teacher's own subjective impression of the degree to which a child's activity level exceeds the norm is as valid and as reliable as any other measure. In reality the teacher's subjective impression of the degree to which a child is overactive is probably what will determine if he is labeled an overactive child.

VARIABLES AFFECTING ACTIVITY LEVEL

In addition to the neurological variables associated with heightened activity level, a myriad of other intrasubject variables have been found to co-vary with activity level. Such physical conditions as vein engorgement, low level of glucose in the blood, low level of calcium, cyanosis, mixed dominance and allergic reaction to artificial coloring in foods have been found to be closely associated with overactivity (Walker, 1974). The characteristics of the child himself are also determining factors in activity level. Such variables as age, developmental level, sex, intelligence and socioeconomic class have been studied in order to determine their relationship to activity level. Even so, it is clear that activity level cannot be defined independently of the circumstances and the environmental conditions under which it occurs. Such variables as the social situation, visual stimulation and auditory stimulation have been shown to directly affect the level of a child's activity.

Environmental Stimulation

The work of Kalverboer (1970; 1971a, b, c; 1973a, b; 1975) has been particularly helpful in understanding the relationship between activity level and various environmental conditions. In order to control for individual personality differences resulting from negative school experiences, Kalverboer studied the relationship between various environmental conditions and activity level in preschool children. All of the youngsters studied were diagnosed as suffering from minimal brain dysfunction. In these studies, Kalverboer observed activity levels in a free field setting. The children were permitted to move freely within the observation room. Activity level was recorded with the use of a video tape recorder and then rated by a panel of judges who reviewed the video tapes. The behaviors of the children studied were assigned to one of six categories: sensory motor, posture, coordination, choreiform movements, maturation of functions, and maturation of responses. All children were observed in the same playroom setting at different times. The video tape recordings were analyzed by two independent observers and the interscorer reliability was determined to be significantly high. The childrens' activity levels were rated under six different environmental conditions: 1) they were observed together with their mothers in an unfamiliar, empty room; 2) they were observed in an empty room by themselves for the first time; 3) this was followed by an observation period in which the children were free to play with blocks in the presence of a passive observer; 4) the children were observed in an empty room for the second time; 5) following this they were observed alone in a room with a variety of toys; and 6) the final condition was one in which they were observed alone in the room with one "nonmotivating" toy. Of course, the length of time in each of these observation periods was standardized. The significant environmental variables differentiating between each of the six conditions were: novelty of the environment, the presence of a social figure, and the amount and variety of stimulation. As might be expected, each of the environmental conditions produced a variety of different behaviors occurring at various frequencies. For instance, in the empty room situation alone (Condition two) the children's activity levels were categorized into the following patterns: room exploration, passive waiting, body-oriented activity, one-way screen reaction, close contact and visual contact. Condition five (alone with a variety of toys) produced the following pattern: low- and high-level play, exploratory play, no play, activity, gross body activity, body-oriented behavior and room-oriented behavior. These behavior patterns seem to vary with the environmental conditions at the time of the observation. No one pattern seemed to maintain itself throughout the six observation conditions. This observation in itself strongly supports the hypothesis that environment has a profound effect on activity level.

The relationship between the subjects' sex and their activity levels, and the relationship between degree of neurological impairment and activity levels were studied for the six observation conditions. In general, boys were found to exhibit more exploratory activity and a higher frequency of verbal behavior when the variables of social figure and novelty were introduced. Girls exhibited significantly more body-oriented behaviors than did boys under all six observation conditions. The boys on the other hand were observed to have a significantly higher frequency of gross bodily activity under all six of the conditions. While the differences in activity level between sexes were found to be negligible, there did appear to be qualitative differences between boys' and girls' reactions to these environmental conditions. Some minor sex differences were also observed regardless of exhibited higher activity level associated with the sensory motor and postural categories. Girls exhibited higher frequencies of behavior associated with the categories of maturation of function and maturation of responses.

The interaction between neurological status and type of environment was found to be an important one. For example, children with low neurological scores showed a pattern of high exploratory activity level in the novel room situation, with low exploratory activity level in a familiar setting. However, when a variety of toys were introduced (Condition five), the children with low neurological scores displayed a higher activity level than the children who were identified as having a more serious neurological impairment.

In his most recent research summarizing the results of all previous studies, Kalverboer (1975) concluded that the study of activity level required close specification of the situational context in which the behavior occurred. He also reported that the analysis of interaction between the degree of neurological impairment and the environmental conditions was paramount. One interesting conclusion from this study was the inverse relationship between degree of neurological impairment and activity level under Condition five. That is, activity level seemed to decrease when the more severely impaired children were observed in the setting with a variety of toys. This observation challenges the long-held rule of thumb among educators that minimization of classroom stimulation decreases activity level in hyperactive, brain-dysfunctional children. The concept that hyperactive children are overly active at all times and in all situations does not seem to hold up under the stress of research.

Based on ten years of research, Kaspar (1971, 1972, 1973, 1974) concluded, "It would appear that the term hyperactivity has a large social connotation in that there is an acceptable activity level for each situation which is defined by adults, and when a child is designated as hyperactive it is on the basis of his ability to regulate his level of activity to that which is expected or permitted in the circumstances in which he finds himself" (1972, p. 25). In one recent study, Kaspar (1974) challenged the concept that activity level represents a fixed physiological condition which is unresponsive to the environment. Two groups of children matched for age and sex were studied under two social conditions. The experimental group contained thirty-six hyperactive youngsters while the control group children were free of neurological impairment. Activity level was rated by judges who observed each of the two groups during structured and unstructured activities in the same playroom. No significant differences between the activity levels of the control subjects and the experimental subjects were observed during the unstructured activity period. During the structured activity, however, significant group differences in activity level emerged. The neurologically impaired group produced approximately twice as much activity as the control group. A major conclusion of this study was that structured activity situations produce a higher activity level in neurologically impaired youngsters. This finding suggests that activity level decreases with a decrease in the structuring of classroom activity. Indeed, certain types of increased stimulation may even act to decrease activity level. Gardner, Cromwell and Foshee (1959) reported on the effects of varying amounts of visual stimulation on the activity level of groups of mentally retarded subjects. Institutionalized, brain-injured and non-brain-injured mentally retarded youngsters matched for mental age and chronological age were rated on activity level under varying conditions of distal stimulation. No significant difference in activity level in the brain-injured and non-brain-injured groups was observed. The most noteworthy finding of this study was the observation that both the brain-injured and the non-brain-injured youngsters were more active under conditions of reduced visual stimulation than when exposed to high amounts of visual stimulation. In a sequel to this study, Gardner et al., compared hyperactive and hypoactive groups under the same conditions reported in the first part of the experiment. Gardner et al., concluded that both hyperactive and hypoactive subjects were significantly more active under conditions of reduced stimulation. They concluded that one possible explanation for this might be that hyperactive subjects compensated for their lack of exteroceptive stimulation by initiating proprioceptive stimulation. This again challenges a long-held educational concept that the hyperactive child functions best in a highly structured educational program.

In another study, Kaspar (1974) failed to find a relationship between activity level and IQ or academic performance. In a similar study Kaspar (1973) studied the relationship between activity level, distractibility and performance on the Wechsler Intelligence Scale for Children in a group of five- to eight-year-old minimally brain dysfunctional children. Performance of the experimental subjects was compared with a matched group of control subjects. There was no significant relationship between activity level, distractibility or performance on the IQ test. Here again, Kaspar concluded that the concept of activity level as an unchangeable physiological state has little value in understanding the condition of hyperactivity.

Auditory Stimulation

Auditory stimulation has also been found to affect activity level. Early research on the relationship between auditory stimulation and activity level has resulted in contradictory theories. One widely held view proposed that heightened activity level represented a drive for increased stimulation. This theory hypothesized that external auditory stimulation would reduce the drive for self-stimulation and thereby decrease activity level (Berkson and Mason, 1963; Berkson and Davenport, 1962). Other theorists proposed that auditory stimulation would increase activity level. This hypothesis was based on the belief that hyperactive children have a heightened drive for activity. The research of several authors showed activity level to increase under conditions of auditory stimulation (Rieber, 1965; Levitt and Kaufmann, 1965). Still other research has suggested that the relationship between auditory stimulation and activity level is determined primarily by the type of auditory stimulation to which the subject has been exposed. Kuhnke (1952) for instance reported that activity level decreased rapidly and momentarily when loud, unexpected noise was introduced. Three other studies demonstrated that sedative music decreased activity while activity level was found to escalate rapidly under conditions of stimulative music (Slaughter, 1954; Sears, 1954; Shatin, 1958). The work of Reardon and Bell (1970) helped clarify the relationship between activity level and auditory stimulation. An observer rating scale was used to count the frequency of fourteen separate, distinguishable behaviors, under four different conditions of auditory stimulation, in a population of mentally retarded hyperactive youngsters. The activity level of the experimental subjects was observed under the four conditions over a thirty-two-hour period. During the experiment, each of the subjects was exposed to four different conditions (Condition 1: no noise; Condition 2: the sound of a man's voice reading from a book; Condition 3: stimulative music; Condition 4: sedative music). An analysis of the data revealed that activity level was related to both the degree of the novelty of the stimuli and to the type of auditory stimulation presented. The most clear-cut finding of the study was that activity level was found to decrease significantly when the subjects were exposed to stimulative music. Just as is the case with visual stimulation, these findings regarding auditory stimulation challenge the long-held concept that activity level decreases under conditions of destimulation. It would appear that the greater the reduction in auditory, visual and social classroom stimulation, the higher the rate of activity level.

The one clear fact that emerges from all of these research findings is that activity level cannot be defined independently of the circumstances and the environmental conditions under which it occurs. For example, recent research on the environmental variables which affect activity level has demonstrated a relationship between the amount of Xrays emitted by the cathode ends of fluorescent lights and the degree of hyperactivity in the classroom. Ott (1974) proposed that in certain children the ultraviolent wave lengths emitted by fluorescent lighting tended to aggravate a pre-existing condition of hyperactivity. His theory was substantiated in two separate studies involving 370 school children. The children in the control group were exposed to standard fluorescent lighting while the activity level of subjects in the experimental group was monitored in open field classroom situations in which the classroom fluorescent lighting had been altered to include lead foil shields over the cathodes to prevent Xrays from escaping. Videotaped time samples of the children's activity level over a ninety-day period were analyzed. The activity level of the subjects in the experimental group was found to be significantly below the activity level recorded for the control group.

BEHAVIORAL CONTROL OF ACTIVITY LEVEL

The application of learning theory to the control of activity level is a relatively new concept. Prior to the introduction of behavior modification techniques into the classroom, educational programming for the hyperactive child involved a combination of a special remedial program complemented by "destimulation" of the classroom and the use of medication. While this approach seemed to help somewhat, the value of controlling activity level by destimulating the classroom, in view of the research presented in this chapter, is questionable. Medication continues to play an important role in the treatment of hyperactivity. However medication alone does not provide the youngster with an opportunity to learn specific appropriate classroom behaviors. These approaches have not provided a mechanism for generalizing behavioral control to other, less highly structured environments.

Clarizio and Yelon (1967) outlined behavioral modification

techniques for classroom use with hyperactive children. Positive reinforcement was described as the method of choice for increasing appropriate positive classroom behaviors. This technique calls for reinforcing the child immediately after appropriate behaviors have been demonstrated. In the case of activity level, positive reinforcement is often used to increase responses that are incompatible with high rates of activity. Extinction is the technique to be used to reduce high rates of undesirable behaviors. According to this technique, the environmental contingencies are arranged in such a way that the undesirable behavior cannot be followed by any reinforcing event. In the case of activity level, extinction is used in combination with positive reinforcement of incompatible behaviors to bring activity level under control. Clarizio and Yelon also described appropriate conditions for the use of negative reinforcement, i.e. punishment. They advised that punishment only brings temporary control of the undesirable behavior. That is, punishment acts to suppress undesirable behaviors but not to extinguish them. In addition, the fear and tenseness a child associates with punishment may serve to inhibit his adaptive responses. They warn that teachers often become frustrated by the failure of punishment to produce the desired results. However, negative reinforcement does have a proper place. This technique is used primarily to bring an immediate suppression of adverse, inappropriate classroom behaviors. Finally, Clarizio and Yelon reported on the importance of using social modeling as a technique for bringing classroom behaviors under control. This technique, like positive reinforcement, is used primarily to increase the frequency of desirable behaviors. According to social modeling theory, the imitation of the behaviors of others occurs spontaneously and is often self-reinforcing. Modeling is viewed as the primary component of the socialization of appropriate behaviors.

Patterson, Shaw and Ebner (1970) pioneered the use of behavior modification techniques in reducing activity level. In their review of the literature, they introduced three important concepts which underlie the use of behavior modification in the reduction of activity level. First, these authors pointed out that, from a behavioral point of view, hyperactivity is to be defined as the high frequency of certain behaviors. Second, they stressed the concept that the behaviors of hyperactive children differ from normal children only in their frequency. Qualitatively the behaviors of both groups of children are similar. Finally, they introduced the important concept that activity is to be viewed as a series of discreet responses. This concept differed significantly from previously held concepts of hyperactivity, in which activity was viewed as an ongoing process. In making this point, these authors pointed out that the reduction of one or more discreet high-frequency responses does not guarantee that the gains will generalize to other behaviors. In other words, the reduction of out-of-seat behaviors does not guarantee that fidgeting or squirming will also automatically be reduced. Patterson succinctly summarized these observations in his statement that ". . . (hyperactivity is) a gross summary term referring to a complex set of observable responses . . . the specific responses which make up the pattern eliciting the label 'hyperactive' are not qualitatively different from the behaviors which are observable in nonhyperactive children" (p. 22).

Patterson (1965) presented a prototype for future studies using behavior modification to reduce high-frequency behaviors. In this study Patterson used a baseline-reinforcement-return to baseline model for bringing high rates of inappropriate high-frequency behaviors under control in a minimally brain-damaged hyperactive nine-year-old male student. He used a point system for tabulating the frequency of talking, pushing, pinching, hitting, looking about the room, moving out of location and moving in location, i.e., tapping, squirming, etc., during a twenty-minute baseline observation period. During the baseline observation the frequency of occurrence of each of these responses was tabulated for each thirty-second interval. The subject was given one point for each of the target behaviors which persisted for a duration of one or more seconds. Hyperactivity was then defined in terms of the number of points accumulated over a twenty-minute period. The training took place in an examining room. The examiner sat across from the student, who was to complete an assignment in his workbook. A light was flashed and a candy reinforcement was given for each ten-second interval that the youngster attended to the workbook without exhibiting any of the target behaviors. After the training sessions were completed the youngster was again observed in the classroom under conditions of nonreinforcement. Patterson reported a significant decrease in the high-frequency target behaviors when the frequency of these behaviors during baseline was compared with the frequency of these behaviors during reinforcement. The decrease in target behaviors also generalized to the classroom. Patterson observed that the decrease in high-frequency behaviors remained intact for a fifteen-day classroom observation period after the reinforcement phase of the experiment had been completed. Indeed, the approach was so successful that when compared to three control subjects during the last phase of the study, the "hyperactive" youngster exhibited fewer of the target behaviors. Finally, Patterson concluded that, although the high-frequency behaviors decreased, in-classroom learning did not seem to be affected by this change. Here again, Patterson's research points out that improvement in one or more of the characteristics associated with hyperactivity does not assure improvement in other areas of classroom functioning.

Other authors have reproduced Patterson's findings using a variety of other techniques and different target behaviors. Nixon (1966) and Grindee (1970a) used primary reinforcement to control out-of-seat behaviors in hyperactive youngsters. Allen, Henke, Harris, Reynolds and Baer (1967) and Grindee (1970b) replicated Patterson's research using social reinforcement to bring high-frequency behaviors under control. Still other authors (Ebner, 1968; Anderson, 1964; Phil, 1967) have used combinations of primary and secondary reinforcement to effectively reduce out-of-seat behaviors as well as other high-frequency behaviors associated with hyperactivity.

The literature has emphasized not only the techniques for bringing high-frequency behaviors under control but also the importance of the role of the classroom teaching in controlling hyperactivity. In the next section, four classroom strategies representing different behavioral techniques will be described. Each of the strategies emphasizes the dramatic improvement that can occur in the reduction of high-frequency behaviors with a minimum of teacher effort. The strategies presented are by no means exhaustive; however, they do represent the major categories of approaches to bringing high-frequency behaviors under control. The number of strategies that could be generated are limited only by the teacher's creativity and imagination.

Classroom Reinforcement Strategies

STRATEGY I: EXTINCTION OF A HIGH-FREQUENCY CLASSROOM BEHAVIOR THROUGH THE SYSTEMATIC APPLICATION OF POSITIVE REINFORCEMENT AND THE WITHHOLDING OF REINFORCEMENT. One of the high-frequency classroom behaviors associated with overactivity by both researchers and classroom teachers alike is that of out-of-seat behaviors. While there are several variations of definition as to what constitutes out-of-seat behavior, few researchers would disagree that this behavior consists of not being in the sitting position. This behavior in particular has been one which has been particularly troublesome to the classroom teacher. It not only interferes with the student's learning, but frequently results in the distraction of other students in the classroom.

A frequently used strategy for bringing these behaviors under control is that of getting the child to return to his seat by using a sit-down command. If the behavior is particularly persistent, the teacher may move the child's desk to the front of the room where she can be in closer physical contact with him, or in severe cases she may order him out of the classroom "until he is ready to sit down." An important variable in any technique is the element of teacher attention. Whether the attention be positive or negative, that is, whether it be praise or criticism, it represents a powerful reinforcer. The importance of teacher attention in bringing out-of-seat behaviors under control has been underscored by the research of Madsen, Becker, Thomas, Koser and Pager (1968). These investigators sought to reduce high activity associated with wandering around the classroom by attempting to extinguish out-of-seat behaviors. Forty-eight first grade students, ranging in age from six years two months to seven years two months, were observed in an elementary school classroom. During the prestudy observation period, the authors hypothesized that out-of-seat behaviors were often increased by the teacher's sit-down commands. The subjects were randomly assigned to one of two groups. The teacher was instructed to continue in her usual manner in dealing with out-of-seat behaviors. For those subjects who had been assigned to the control group, the techniques involved reminding the students to return to their seats, moving their desks closer to that of the teacher, or in extreme cases, asking the students to leave the classroom. The out-of-seat behaviors of the experimental subject were responded to in a different manner. From the onset of the experiment, the out-of-seat behaviors of these subjects were totally ignored by the teacher. The teacher was instructed to be very careful to withhold any response to these behaviors. Sit-down commands, watching the child and giving nonverbal signals were withheld. Children in the experimental groups were praised, however, at the moment they returned to their desk and resumed a sitting position. Analysis of the frequency of the out-of-seat behaviors for the two groups of subjects under both conditions revealed a significant improvement in the experimental group. Significant differences did emerge when the classroom teacher withheld attention from out-of-seat behavior. In other words, sit-down commands actually serve to increase the number of times the children left their seats. In this study the classroom teacher was able to reduce the frequency of out-of-seat behavior to a point where these responses approached extinction. While these behaviors were still being exhibited by children in the experimental groups at the end of study, their frequency had decreased significantly. This study demonstrated that teacher attention, whether it be positive or negative, is a powerful reinforcer.

The withholding of teacher attention in the form of ignoring the child's behavior can be a powerful tool in making the classroom environment conducive to academic learning. One of the problems associated with this approach is that the out-of-seat behaviors of many children, even when teacher attention is withheld, are often maintained by the reinforcing attention of other students in the classroom. In addition, such children serve as distractors for other children who otherwise would be attentive. The fact that that attention from peers is highly reinforcing has been well established. It was for this reason that the authors added an additional component to the reinforcement strategy by reinforcing the desired behaviors. That is, returning to one's seat and sitting down was reinforced while out-of-seat behaviors were ignored. As with many classroom behaviors, the withholding of teacher attention alone may not be adequate to bring the behavior under control since the peer group is a significant factor in virtually every child's classroom behavior. In such cases, it is always wise to plan a strategy which involves extinguishing the undersirable behavior by withholding reinforcement, accompanied by a strategy which increases the desired behavior by positively reinforcing its occurrence.

STRATEGY II: CONCURRENT POSITIVE REINFORCEMENT OF APPROPRIATE CLASSROOM BEHAVIORS AND EXTINCTION OF MULTIPLE INAPPROPRIATE CLASSROOM BEHAVIORS. A pattern of high frequency of any classroom behavior may be made more difficult to bring under control by the fact that other symptoms such as distractibility accompany the overactivity. Such children display a pattern of classroom behavior which is characterized by frequent out-of-seat behaviors along with a high frequency of short duration responses. Such children are not only constantly out of their seats, but they also have difficulty remaining at any given task for more than a few minutes at a time. These are the children that the classroom teacher describes as being in "perpetual motion." They flit from activity to activity in a classroom, never remaining at one activity long enough to master it. Such children are highly distractible to others and often are a source for generating much classroom inattentiveness.

Allen, Henke, Harris, Reynolds and Baer (1967) outlined a classroom behavior modification program for such youngsters. In this study social reinforcement, i.e. adult attention, was used to modify the high-frequency behaviors of an overly distractible hyperactive four-year-old girl in the classroom. During the baseline period, this youngster's high-frequency out-of-seat behaviors as well as her high-distractibility behaviors were recorded. During this observation period this child's average time spent at any given activity was only one minute. She was observed in the classroom for a total of twenty-one hours. The basic reinforcement strategy was to reinforce the child with individual adult attention for each one-minute interval that she spent in a single location attending to a single stimulus. The reinforcement strategy also included a contingency for extinguishing responses which occurred outside of the desired location and which were directed to a different stimulus. This extinction procedure involved withdrawal of all adult attention for any response that was not on task and was not on location. The reinforcement program was carried out by the classroom teacher and the researchers within the classroom for a seven-hour period. In order to assess the degree of improvement, positive reinforcement and withholding of a reinforcement were discontinued during a four-hour "reversal" period. Finally, the reinforcement contingencies were reinstated.

In shaping the "on task" behaviors, the researcher who sat in the back of the classroom used a flashlight to signal the teacher whenever the youngster spent ten or more seconds on location at a specified task. The flash of light served as a cue to the teacher to reward the youngster with praise. This method was used until the youngster reached a criteria of five successive ten-second intervals in which her behaviors were on task and on location. Once this criteria was well established by the reinforcement, the child was reinforced only once every sixty seconds for "on task, on location" behaviors. After only seven hours of training, the researchers reported a significant observable increase in the specified behaviors. In addition, other behaviors associated with being off location and off task were significantly reduced. While the replication of this study in the average classroom would be impractical, it presents some important concepts which may be translated into a similar, less demanding program for the teacher to use in reducing high-frequency behaviors.

STRATEGY III: EXTINCTION OF HIGH-FREQUENCY, UNDESIRABLE BEHAVIORS BY USE OF SCHEDULED SECONDARY REINFORCEMENT AND PEER REINFORCEMENT. More often than not, the classroom teacher is faced with bringing the behaviors of several students under control simultaneously. It is the exception rather than the rule that any one child acts in isolation in the classroom. Even the withdrawn youngster's behaviors have an affect on the students around him. Whenever a reinforcement strategy is introduced in the management of one child's behavior, it has an affect on the other students in the classroom. Indeed, a very common complaint is that the child who misbehaved is the one who is rewarded with a reinforcement program. It seems very unfair to the child with desirable behaviors that he is not being rewarded, while the "misbehaving" student is offered a chance to earn rewards.

It is helpful to use a reinforcement strategy which can be applied to the entire classroom. Such strategies allow for the reinforcement of desirable behavior in all of the students, and act to diffuse student complaints that only the children who misbehave are rewarded. Wolf, Hanley, King, and Giles (1970) reported on one such classroom reinforcement strategy. These authors used a combination of token reinforcement, scheduling of reinforcement and peer pressure to decrease the frequency of certain classroom behaviors for an entire group of elementary school children. The target population was a group of sixteen, underachieving, low-income third and fourth graders who were seen for three hours each afternoon in a remedial education program. All of the youngsters were seen daily for remedial assistance for their homework assignment. A behavior modification program was already in effect at the time of the study. Each child was already earning points (secondary reinforcers) for correct answers. Points were also received for completed homework assignments. In spite of this reinforcement program, certain behaviors continued to present a problem to effective classroom management. Several high-frequency behaviors had been identified as being incompatible with progress in the remedial program. Many of the children were observed to exhibit frequent aimless wandering about the classroom with extended stays in the lavatory, prolonged pencil-sharpening and visiting with other students. These behaviors grouped together under the title "out-of-seat behaviors" were targeted for additional behavior modification strategies.

During the baseline period, the entire class' out-of-seat behaviors were recorded over seven one-hour observation sessions. During each of these sessions the observer recorded the number of children exhibiting the target behaviors during 120 thirty-second observation intervals.

The second phase of the experiment involved the introduction of reinforcement for sitting behaviors. In this phase of the experiment a kitchen timer was used. The students were instructed that the timer would be set for an unspecified interval. Each student who was in his seat at the time that the bell rang earned five extra points. The students never knew when the timer was set to go off. In other words, the teacher varied the interval of reinforcement. During this phase of the study, the timer went off on the average of once every twenty minutes. On any given trial the timer might be set for any time interval between zero to forty-minutes.

Finally, the students' out-of-seat behaviors were recorded in the same manner that they were during the baseline period when the "timer game" was no longer in effect. The frequency of out-of-seat behaviors for the entire class decreased significantly. During the baseline period each child averaged seventeen out-of-seat behavior intervals per hour. During the reinforcement period the mean number of out-of-seat behavior intervals was reduced to a mere two per hour. In other words, the frequency of aimless wandering, extended stays in the lavatory, prolonged pencil sharpening and visiting decreased by 80 percent for the class as a whole after only seven hours of the behavior modification program! During the return to baseline period the frequency of out-of-seat behaviors once again averaged seventeen per hour. This was not surprising, however, in view of the fact that there had only been seven hours of training. Had the program continued and had the reinforcement intervals been spaced even further apart, the classroom teacher might have expected to have had out-of-seat behaviors under control for the entire class for a much longer period of time. Eventually the timer game would have been played only occasionally, perhaps as little as once or twice a week.

In another phase of this study, the authors adapted the reinforcement strategy to the special needs of one of the classroom children whose high frequency of out-of-seat behavior persisted in spite of the timer game. This strategy involved the use of positive token reinforcement for completing homework assignments, as well as maintaining the timer game and the introducing a peer reinforcement program. This phase of the study was carried out over a sixty-day period. The child's out-of-seat behaviors were recorded over twenty one-and-a-half hour observation periods using the recording method described in the baseline of the first phase of the experiment. During this observation period no reinforcement was offered.

During this reinforcement period the frequency of out-of-seat behaviors for this individual child decreased markedly from the frequency of the behaviors observed during the baseline period. During the next phase of the experiment the classroom teacher introduced a new reinforcement contingency. For the next ten sessions the student earned no individual points. Instead, she was told that she would start off each session with fifty points. Each time she left her seat she was to lose ten of her fifty points. Whatever points were remaining at the end of the hour were to be divided equally by her and the four students who sat immediately around her. This peer reinforcement phase was followed by a return to the timer game in which she could acquire individual points but no points for her fellow students. Finally the peer reinforcement strategy was reintroduced for seventeen one-hour sessions.

While the frequency of out-of-seat behaviors decreased during the two sessions in which she could earn individual points, the greatest decrease in these behaviors occurred during the sessions in which she divided her points with several of the other children in the classroom. Even though she could not earn individual points during these reinforcement periods, her out-of-seat behaviors were reduced from an average of thirty out-of-seat behavior intervals to an average of five out-of-seat behavior intervals per hour during the last peer reinforcement phase. The effectiveness of this strategy was further pointed out by the fact that during the peer reinforcement phase she received 80 percent more reinforcements than she did during the intervals in which she could earn individual points.

The reinforcement strategy outlined by Wolf et al. could be used with any one of a number of classroom behaviors. The greatest advantage of these strategies is that they permit the classroom teacher to improve the learning environment by decreasing the frequency of undesirable behaviors for all of the students in the class at the same time. The use of the timer made it possible for the classroom teacher not to have to continuously monitor the out-of-seat behaviors of individual children within the classroom. Actually, throughout the entire experiment, the classroom teacher only had to observe out-of-seat behaviors on an average of once every fifteen minutes. This was made possible by the fact that the time interval between reinforcements was varied from trial to trial so that the students could not discriminate when reinforcement would be available to them. It was just as likely that the timer would ring immediately after it went off as it was that it would not ring for forty minutes. The study also brought to light the importance of a principle that most classroom teachers are well aware of. That is, even the most disruptive child can be strongly influenced by the attitudes and acceptance of his classmates. Another advantage of this approach is that it helps to counteract the criticism of nondisruptive students that only "troublemakers" are given a chance to earn rewards.

STRATEGY IV: DIFFERENTIAL REINFORCEMENT OF OTHER BEHAVIORS. Still another method available to the classroom teacher for reducing the frequency of undesirable behaviors is that of differential reinforcement of other behavior. This strategy is used to increase the frequency of behaviors that are incompatible with high-frequency, undesirable behaviors. In other words, instead of reducing high-frequency, undesirable behaviors by attempting to directly extinguish them through either non-reinforcement of negative reinforcement, this strategy attempts to "replace them" with a desirable behavior. The reinforced behaviors are those behaviors which are incompatible with high-frequency, undesirable behaviors. In one study using this technique, Dubrose and Daniels (1966) attempted to reduce the high frequency of undesirable behaviors associated with hyperactivity by reinforcing appropriate play activities in the classroom. Dubrose theorized that the behaviors identified as "hyperactive" could be significantly reduced by simply reinforcing other behaviors which were incompatible with hyperactivity. In this situation no attempt was made to negatively reinforce or punish those behaviors identified as hyperactive. Instead, reinforcement was offered for other nonhyperactive behaviors. Dubrose predicted that the frequency of hyperactive behaviors would be decreased while play activity would become more constructive. Six mentally retarded, hyperactive, elementary school age children were observed in the school's playroom. This room contained a variety of toys along with a token dispenser and a one-way observation mirror. During the baseline period each subject was observed for a fifteen minute period daily, over a two-week interval. Children were scored by an observer for four separate categories of behaviors. These categories included Body Movements, i.e. scratching, biting objects, shuffling feet, etc., Locomotive Behaviors, i.e. walking, climbing, crawling, etc., Destructive Behaviors, i.e. kicking, throwing, pounding, etc., and Communication, i.e. talking, shouting, whistling, etc. The entire experiment consisted of 56 ten-minute sessions over a fifty-day period. The first eight days consisted of preconditioning sessions. During these sessions the children's behaviors were observed and recorded in the experimental playroom but no reinforcement strategies were in effect. During the next thirty-day period, the children received token reinforcement for desirable play behaviors. Tokens were exchangeable at the end of each session for various rewards such as candy and trinkets. The children were instructed that each session was divided into 20 thirty-second intervals. The child could earn a token for each interval during which he displayed appropriate play behaviors. These behaviors were described to the youngsters with appropriate examples given. The children were also instructed that the opportunity to earn rewards would not begin until they had demonstrated that they could control the target behaviors for a period of sixty-five seconds. This particular schedule of reinforcement, called *a limited hold on reinforcement,* helps the child to immediately bring the undesirable behaviors under control by not permitting him access to rewards until he has demonstrated the appropriate behaviors for a specified length of time. During the reinforcement session, all constructive, "nonhyperactive" play behaviors were reinforced. These behaviors were specified as those behaviors which were incompatible with the hyperactive behaviors of "Body Movement, Locomotion, Destructiveness, Communication." This period was followed by a four-day "phase-out" period in which reinforcement for appropriate play behaviors was given less frequently. During the final eight days of the study no reinforcement was available.

The results of this study demonstrated that the hyperactive behaviors, i.e. high frequencies of scratching, biting, shuffling feet, walking, climbing, crawling, kicking, throwing, pounding, talking, shouting and whistling, decreased significantly within the first twelve days of the conditioning phase of the experiment. The frequency of these behaviors continued to decline up to the twenty-first day when they leveled off and remained relatively stable until the end of this experiment. The results indicated that there was also a slight increase in the use of quiet toys as well as a slight decrease in the use of toys that produced loud noises during the conditioning period. This study clearly demonstrated that it was possible to bring a high frequency of undesirable behaviors usually associated with hyperactivity under control by reinforcing incompatible behaviors. Dubrose further commented that the total number of hyperactive responses during the extinction period was less than one third of those recorded during the baseline period. In addition, the conditioning resulted in more appropriate use of the play media. Another interesting finding was that the children who had been observed to be the most hyperactive during the observation period showed the greatest reduction in overactive behaviors. Dubrose reported that the children in this study exhibited a significant increase in such constructive play behavior as puzzle-solving, drawing and writing as a result of the reinforcement strategy.

The advantage of this type of reinforcement strategy is in the fact that it permits the classroom teacher to control the high frequency of undesirable behaviors by focusing attention on the child's positive behaviors. This is not only appealing from the point of view of enhancing the child's self-confidence, but it also maximizes the value of the reinforcement program by using the reinforcement to help the child acquire appropriate, desirable behaviors through specific learning. While the study took place over a fifty-day period, the entire project required less than ten hours to complete. This reinforcement strategy would be easily adaptable to the classroom. It would simply involve setting up a reward program for all desirable behaviors which occur after the overactive behaviors have ceased for a specified time interval.

Practical Issues in Classroom Application

When given the choice, generally the most effective reinforcement strategy is the one that focuses on the reinforcing power of social and peer reinforcement. The use of social and peer reinforcement seems to be one of the most effective and easily implemented strategies for bringing about behavioral change. Such reinforcement strategies, when combined with extinction procedures, maximize the probability of behavioral change. These reinforcement programs are readily accepted by the other children in the classroom when given an opportunity to receive rewards for their good behaviors. The importance of this factor cannot be underestimated. Quite frequently a well-designed strategy for an individual child can be sabotaged by disgruntled classmates who complain that they are not being rewarded by their good behaviors. Another particularly important factor is that such strategies often help to improve the disruptive child's self-image. When classmates share in the rewards of his learning, his self-image quickly changes from that of saboteur to hero.

When the reinforcement strategy must be designed for an individual child, the strategy of choice is the Differential Reinforcement of Other Behaviors strategy, as described by Dubrose and Daniels (1966). Aside from the effectiveness of this reinforcing strategy in its own right, it retains a qualitative value in emphasizing the child's learning abilities rather than his disabilities. Such reinforcement strategies focus on increasing the frequency of desirable behaviors which are incompatible with the behaviors which need to be extinguished. The whole approach is a much more positive one. It begins by contracting with the child to help him improve what he is good at. The emphasis is on mastery and success, experiences which are sorely needed by hyperactive children.

Even a well-planned reinforcement strategy can fail if it does not take into consideration the individual child's personality and emotional needs. For instance, Farson (1966) reported a case of a youngster who rejected praise and any other positive comments directed to him. Clinically this youngster presented a picture commonly found in hyperactive children. His level of self-esteem was so low that he was unable to emotionally accept any positive statements about himself. Children may accept or may reject reinforcement for other emotional reasons as well. Korn (1966) reported on the case of a youngster who could not accept positive reinforcement because he had been taught from an early age that anything less than the highest of achievements was not acceptable. The whole concept of receiving rewards for showing small amounts of change in a positive direction was alien to him.

There is no substitute for knowing the needs of the individual child. An effective reinforcer is one that is valued by the individual. Varenhorst (1969) pointed out that at the high school level many hyperactive and learning-disabled youngsters reject positive attention. Over the years they have learned to place a high value on negative attention, i.e. criticism and scrutiny. Such children have learned from an early age that they cannot count on adults to reward them with praise. Such children come to rely on the consistency with which they receive negative attention. Positive attention seems to threaten them, and often they will reject a reinforcement program in which positive attention is offered as the reward.

The problem of finding effective reinforcers has received attention in recent years (Daley, 1969). In identifying effective classroom reinforcers, Daley pointed out that activities often served as the most effective reinforcer. This observation was based on the Premack Principle (Premack, 1965). According to this principle, for any pair of responses, the more probable one will reinforce the less probable one. In other words, activities that the child frequently and spontaneously engages in often can be used as rewards to increase the frequency of activities in which he rarely engages. For example, children who like to work on math assignments can often be rewarded by contracting with them to be able to do math work as soon as their reading assignment has been completed. Daley observed the classroom activities of five- to eight-year-olds and identified twenty-two reinforcing activities which he termed the *reinforcement menu.* These activities included: talking, writing, coloring, drawing, reading, swinging feet, listening to records, hugging, dancing, walking, drawing on the chalkboard, telephoning, using puzzles, playing with blocks, jumping, drinking, using colored pencils, singing, swinging on the door, moving chairs, erasing the blackboard, looking out the window and selecting their own reinforcers. Daley listed these activities in an illustrated book which he called the *Reinforcement Menu.* At various points during the day, each child was allowed to look over the reinforcement menu and select the activities which he wished to have as rewards for his learning. Selecting the most effective reinforcers and offering them within a social and emotional context that the child can accept are important variables which depend greatly on a teacher's insight and judgement about each student.

SUMMARY

From the time that hyperactivity was identified as a separate diagnostic entity, it has been primarily thought of as a state of physical overactivity. Considering how much importance has been attached to activity level as the primary characteristic of hyperactivity, little is actually known about this variable. Neurological research seems to point to the general theory that disturbance of activity level is a result of a dysfunction of the reticular activating system. Research in this area suggests that the ascending tracts of a reticular activating system are responsible for increasing activity level, while the descending tracts have the responsibility for reducing activity level. The hyperactive child's problem is mainly that of decreasing activity level. For this reason it seems likely that the main area of neurological dysfunction is in the descending tracts of the reticular formation. However, each case of hyperactivity should be considered individually. Variables such as disturbance of the frontal lobes and endocrine disturbance among others, should be considered.

Several theoretical formulations have been developed in order to explain the disturbance in activity level. To date, the psychophysiological and the electrophysiological theories of activity level have generated the bulk of research in this area. Based on this research, it would appear that level of activity may be viewed as a biosocial response which is not necessarily a part of a convergent syndrome. From a physiological point of view, it would appear that the hyperactive child experiences difficulty in decelerating activity level, though his ability to regulate activity level in an upward direction seems unimpaired. In general, it does not appear that activity level is an adequate construct for a total understanding of the hyperactive child.

Psychological research in activity level has indicated that high rates of behavior might be brought under control through the application of reinforcement techniques. Within recent years behavior modification has been found to provide the link between in-classroom learning and adjustment to social situations in the outside world. The application of such reinforcement strategies as positive reinforcement, extinction, social modeling and negative reinforcement have been found effective in bringing activity level under control in the classroom. From a behavioral point of view, hyperactivity may be viewed as the exhibition of a high frequency of behaviors which are within the repetoire of the normal child.

Where a child exhibits a high frequency of various behaviors, it is not safe to assume that these behaviors are causally linked to one another. Instead, behavioral treatment of a hyperactive child considers each high-frequency response as a separate target for reconditioning. Several studies given have been able to show that a variety of behavioral techniques may be used to bring hyperactive behaviors under control in the classroom.

A number of researchers have used a variety of conditioning techniques in the classroom to bring activity level under control. All of these strategies share the common proposition that hyperactivity should be viewed as a series of high-frequency behaviors which are subject to the principles of reinforcement. The most effective reinforcement strategies are those which combine positive reinforcement of appropriate behaviors with the use of extinction techniques to reduce the frequency of undesirable behaviors. These reinforcement techniques have been highly effective and actually require less teacher effort than traditional methods of bringing high-frequency behaviors under control. While a number of reinforcement strategies were presented, a teacher may generate as many of these strategies as his imagination and creativity permit.

The practicalities of applying reinforcement techniques in the classroom must take into consideration the individuality of the child as well as peer reaction. There is no substitute for knowing the needs and reactions of the individual child and the attitudes of his classmates towards reinforcement. No classroom reinforcement strategy can be effective independent of peer support. In applying such strategies the teacher must build in a means of assuring peer support. Other practical issues, such as discovering reinforcers and determining which events are reinforcing for a given child, should also be taken into consideration.

In view of what is known about activity level it is difficult to specify in behavioral terms the differences between heightened activity, lack of attention and distractibility. Yet these terms are commonly interchanged in describing the hyperactive child. Indeed, the hyperactive child is often referred to as a youngster who is highly active, overly distractible and suffering from short attention span. In the next chapter the characteristics of attention and distractibility will be reviewed.

REFERENCES

Adametz, J. L.: Rate of recovery functioning in calves with rostil reticular lesions. *Journal of Neuro-Surgery, 16*:85-98, 1959.

Allen, K. H., Henke, L. R., Harris, S. A., Reynolds, N., and Baer, R.: Control of hyperactivity through social reinforcement of attending behavior. *Journal of Educational Psychology, 58*:231-237, 1967.

Amassian, V. B., and DeVito, R. T.: Unit activity in reticular formation and nearby structures. *Journal of Neurophysiology, 17*:576-603, 1954.

Anderson, D. B.: Application of behavior modification techniques to the control of a hyperactive child. Unpublished master's thesis, University of Oregon, 1964.

Bell, R. T.: *Adaptation of Small Wristwatches for Mechanical Recording of Activity in Infants and Children.* Bethesda, Maryland, Child Research Branch, National Institute of Mental Health, 1967.

Berkson, G., and Davenport, R. K.: Stereotyped movements of mental defectives. I. Initial survey. *American Journal of Mental Deficiency, 66*:849-852, 1962.

Berkson, G., and Mason, W. A.: Stereotyped movements of mental defectives. III. Situation effect. *American Journal of Mental Deficiency, 68*:409-416, 1963.

Bindra, D.: Components of general activity and the analysis of behavior. *Psychological Review, 68*:205-215, 1961.

Blough, D. D.: New test for tranquilizers. *Science, 127*:586, 1958.

Booksen, B. N.: Physiological studies in mental deficiency. In Ellis, N. R. (Ed.): *Handbook of Mental Deficiency.* New York, McGraw, 1963.

Cantor, G. N.: Hull-Spence behavior theory in mental deficiency. In Ellis, N. R. (Ed.): *Handbook of Mental Deficiency.* New York, McGraw, 1963.

Castanera, T. J., Kimeldorf, D. J., and Jones, C. C.: Apparatus for measurement of activity in small animals. *Journal of Laboratory and Clinical Medicine, 45*:825-832, 1955.

Clarizio, H. F., and Yelon, S. M.: Learning theory approaches to classroom management: Rational and intervention techniques. *Journal of Special Education, 1*:267-274, 1967.

Conners, C. K.: A teacher rating scale for use in drug studies with children. *American Journal of Psychiatry, 6*:884-888, 1969.

Cromwell, R. L., Baumeister, A., and Hawkins, W. F.: Research in activity level. In Ellis, N. R. (Ed.): *Handbook of Mental Deficiency.* New York, McGraw, 1963.

Daley, N. F.: The "reinforcement menu": finding effective reinforcers. In Krumbholtz, J. B., and Thorsen, C. E. (Eds.): *Behavioral Counselling.* New York, HR&W, 1969.

Davids, A.: An objective instrument for assessing hyperkinesis in children. *Journal of Learning Disabilities, 4*:499-501, 1971.

Dubrose, S. G., and Daniels, G. T.: An experimental approach to reduction of overactive behavior. *Behavior Research and Therapy, 4*:251-258, 1966.

Emmers, R., Chung, R. M., and Wang, G. H.: Behavior and reflexes of chronic thalamic cats. *Arch Ital Biol, 103*:178-193, 1965.

Ebner, M. J.: *An investigation of the role of social environment in the generalization and persistence of the effect of a behavior modification program.* Doctoral dissertation, University of Oregon. Ann Arbor, Michigan, University Microfilms, No. 68-3979, 1968.

Farson, R.: Praise reappraised. *Exploration, 5*:13-21, 1966.

Foshee, J. G.: Studies in activity level. I. Simple and complex task performance in defectives. *American Journal of Mental Deficiency, 62*:882-886, 1958.

French, J. T., Amerongen, F. S., and MaGoun, H. M.: An activating system in the brain stem of monkey. *Archives of Neurological Psychiatry, 68*:577-590, 1952.

French, J. T., Hernandez-Peon, R. O., and Livingston, R. F.: Projections from cortex to cephalic brain stem (reticular formation) in monkey. *Journal of Neurophysiology, 18*:74-95, 1955.

Gardner, W. I., Cromwell, R. L., and Foshee, J. G.: Studies in activity level. II. Effects of distal, visual stimulation in organic, familials, hyperactives, and hypoactives. *American Journal of Mental Deficiency, 63*:1028-1033, 1959.

Gastaut, H. O.: Combined photic and metrazol activation of the brain. *Electrocephalogy and Clinical Neurophysiology, 2*:249, 1950.

Gellner, L.: *A Neurophysiological Concept of Mental Retardation and Its Educational Implications.* Chicago, G. Levinson Research Foundation, 1959.

Gibbs, E. L., Rich, C. L., Foice, A., and Gibbs, F. A.: Electroencephalogram study of mentally retarded persons. *American Journal of Mental Deficiency, 65*:236-247, 1960.

Goltz, F.: Der Hund ohne Grosshirn. *Pfluegers Archiv: European Journal of Physiology, 51*:570-614, 1892.

Grindee, T. D.: Operant conditioning of attending behavior in the classroom: A case study. In Benson, F. A. (Ed.): *Modifying Deviant*

Behaviors in Various Clasroom Settings. Eugene, Oregon, Department of Special Education, College of Education, Monograph No. 1, 1970a.

Grindee, T. D.: Operant conditioning of attending behaviors in the classroom for two hyperactive Negro children. In Benson, F. A. (Ed.): *Modifying Deviant Behaviors in Various Classroom Settings.* Eugene, Oregon, Department of Special Education, Monograph No. 1, 1970b.

Hernandez-Peon, R. T.: Attention, sleep, motivation and behavior. In Bakan, P. E. (Ed.): *Attention.* Princeton, New Jersey, Van Nostrand, 1966a.

Hernandez-Peon, R. T.: Physiological mechanisms in attention. In Russell, R. T. (Ed.): *Frontiers in Physiological Psychology.* New York, Acad Pr, 1966b.

Hilgard, E. R.: *Theories of Learning.* New York, Appleton, 1956.

Horowitz, I.: *A developmental study of the relationship between motor activity and perceptual processes as measured by the Rorschach Test.* Dissertation Abstract, *14*:1805-1806, 1954.

Kalverboer, A. F., LeCoultre, R., and Casaer, P.: Implications of congenital ophthalmoplegia for development of visual-motor function. *Developmental Medicine in Child Neurology, 12*:642-654, 1970.

Kalverboer, A. F.: Observation of field free behaviour in pre-school boys and girls in relation to neurological findings. In Stoelinga, V. D., and Werff, B. (Eds.): *Normal and Abnormal Development of Brain and Behaviour.* Leiden, University Press, 1971a.

Kalverboer, A. F.: Observation of exploratory behavior of preschool children alone and the presence of mother. *Psychiatria neurologia, neurochirurgia, 74*:43-57, 1971b.

Kalverboer, A. F.: Over de relatie tussen neurologische dysfuncties en gederag bij kinderen. *Wolters-Noordhoff en groningen, 1*:155-176, 1971c.

Kalverboer, A. F.: Vroege Ontwikkelingsdiagnoftiek: Enige Feiten en Vraagtekens. En De Wit, J., Volle, H., and Jessurun Cardozo-Vanhoorn, R. (Eds.): *Amsterdam,* Willing Vroningen, 1973a.

Kalverboer, A. F., Touwen, B. P., and Prechtl, H. F.: Follow-up of infants at rest of minor dysfunction. *Annals of the New York Academy of Sciences, 205*:173-187, 1973b.

Kalverboer, A. F.: *A Neuro-Behavioural Study in Pre-School Children.* London, Heinman, 1975.

Kaspar, J. C., Millachab, J. G., Backus, R., Child, B., and Schulman, J. L.: A study of the relationship between neurological evidence of brain damage in children and activity level and distractibility. *Journal of Consulting and Clinical Psychology, 3*:329-337, 1971.

Kaspar, J. C., and Schulman, J. L.: Organic mental disorder: Brain damage. In Wolman, B. B. (Ed.): *Psychopathology of Childhood.* New York, McGraw, 1972, pp. 207-229.

Kaspar, J. C.: *The relationship between activity level and distractibility and performance on the WISC in a sample of children with neurological dysfunction.* Paper presented at the proceeding of the 83rd Annual Convention of the American Psychological Association, Washington, D.C., September, 1973.

Kaspar, J. C.: *Research in distractibility and activity level: A review.* Paper presented at the 86th Annual Convention of the American Psychological Association, New Orleans, September, 1974.

Kleitman, N., and Camille, N.: *American Journal of Physiology,* 100:474-480, 1932.

Knobel, M., Wolman, M. B., and Mason, E.: Hyperkinesis and organicity in children. *Archives of General Psychiatry,* 1:310-321, 1959.

Korn, C. V.: Refusing reinforcement. In Krumbholtz, J. D., and Thorsen, C. E. (Eds.): *Behavioral Counseling.* New York, HR&W, 1969.

Kuhnke, E.: An objective proof of reflex immobilization in humans. *Psychother Med Psychol,* 6:208-213, 1952.

Levitt, H., and Kaufman, M.: Sound induced drive in stereotyped behavior in mental defectives. *American Journal of Mental Deficiency,* 69:729-734, 1965.

Lewis, R.: *The Brain-Injured Child.* New York, National Society for Crippled Children and Adults, Inc., 1963.

Lindsley, T. C.: Psychopathology in motivation. In Jones, M. (Ed.): *Nebraska Symposium on Motivation.* Vol. 5. Lincoln, Nebraska, University of Nebraska Press, 1966.

Lourie, R.: *The contribution of child psychiatry to the ptho-genesis of hyperactivity in children.* Read at the George Washington University School of Medicine, 1962.

Madsen, C. A., Becker, W. B., Thomas, D. H., Koser, L. E., and Pager, E. K.: An analysis of the reinforcing function of "sitdown" commands. In Parker, R. R. (Ed.): *Readings in Educational Psychology.* Boston, Allyn, 1968.

MaGoun, H. M.: An ascending reticular activating system in the brain stem. *Archives of Neurology and Psychiatry,* 67:145-154, 1952.

Mendelson, W., Johnson, N., and Stewart, M. A.: Hyperactive children as teenagers: A follow-up study. *Journal of Nervous and Mental Disease,* 4:273-279, 1971.

McConnell, T., Cromwell, R. L., Bailer, R., and Sun, C.: Studies in activity level. *American Journal of Mental Deficiency,* 68:647-651, 1964.

Miller, C. A., and Lennox, M. A.: Electroencephalography in behavior problem children. *Journal of Pediatrics,* 33:753-760, 1948.

Morgan, C. T., and Stellar, P.: *Physiological Psychology.* New York, McGraw, 1950.

Moruzzi, G. O., and MaGoun, H. M.: Brain stem, reticular formation and activation of the EEG. *Journal of Neurophysiology,* 6:471-489, 1949.

Nixon, S. J.: *Ways by which overly active students can be taught to concentrate on study activity.* Cooperative Research Project No. 5-379, Office of Health, Education and Welfare, 1966.

Ott, J.: School lights and problem pupils. *Science News,* 105:258-259, 1974.

Payne, R. S.: Minimal chronic brain syndrome in children. *Developmental Medicine and Child Neurology,* 4:21-27, 1962.

Patterson, G. R.: An application of conditioning techniques to the control of a hyperactive child. In Ullman, L. N., and Krasner, L. H. (Eds.): *Case Studies in Behavior Modification.* New York, HR&W, 1965.

Patterson, G. R., Shaw, D. T., and Ebner, M. J.: Teachers, peers, and parents as agents of change in the classroom. In Benson, F. A. (Ed.): *Modifying Deviant Behaviors in Various Classroom Settings.* Eugene, Oregon, Department of Special Education, College of Education, Monograph No. 1, 1970.

Pihl, R. F.: Conditioning procedures with hyperactive children. *Neurology,* 17:421-423, 1967.

Premack, D.: Reinforcement theory. In Lewis, D. (Ed.): *Nebraska Symposium on Motivation.* Lincoln, Nebraska, University of Nebraska Press, 1965, pp. 123-188.

Quast, W.: *Visual-motor performance in the reproduction of geometric figures as a developmental phenomenon in children.* Dissertation abstract, 18:1111, 1958.

Reardon, D., and Bell, G.: Effects of sedative and stimulative music on activity levels of severely retarded boys. *American Journal of Mental Deficiency,* 75:156-159, 1970.

Rieber, M.: The effects of music on the activity level of children. *Psychosomatic Science,* 3:325-326, 1965.

Scheibel, M. B., Scheibel, B. D., Mollica, A. H., and Moruzzi, G. O.: Convergence and interaction of impulses on single units of reticular formation. *Journal of Neurophysiology,* 18:309-330, 1955.

Schrager, J., Lindy, J., Harrison, S., McDermott, J., and Wilson, P.: The hyperkinetic child: An overview of the issues. *Journal American Academy of Child Psychiatry,* 2:526-533, 1966.

Schulman, J. L., and Reisman, K. M.: An objective measure of hyperactivity. *American Journal of Mental Deficiency,* 64:455-456, 1959.

Schulman, J. L., Lipkin, M. P., Clarinda, N., and Mitchell, J.: *Studies on activity level in children.* Paper read at meeting of the American Psychiatric Association, Chicago, May, 1961.

Schulman, J. L., Kaspar, J. C., and Thorne, F.: *Brain Damage and Behavior. A Clinical Experimental Study.* Springfield, Thomas, 1965.

Sears, W. W.: *Music Therapy.* Lawrence, Kansas, Allen Press, 1954.

Secuda, L., and Finley, K. H.: Electrographic studies on children presenting behavior disorders. *Archives of Neurology and Psychiatry*, 47:1076-1079, 1942.

Shatin, L.: The application of rhythmic music stimulation to long-term schizophrenic patients. *Music Therapy*, 6:111-115, 1958.

Slaughter, F. E.: The effect of musical stimuli on normal and abnormal subjects as indicated by pupil area reflexes. *Music Therapy*, 3:27-32, 1954.

Solomon, C. I., Brown, W. T., and Deutsch, M.: Electroencephalography in behavior problem children. *American Journal of Psychiatry*, 101:51-61, 1944.

Stevens, G. A., Stover, C. E., and Backus, J. T.: The hyperkinetic child. *Journal of Consulting and Clinical Psychology*, 34:56-59, 1970.

Strauss, A., and Lehtinen, L. B.: *Psychopathology and Education of the Brain Injured Child*. New York, Grune, 1947.

Thompson, R. L., and Mettler, F. A.: Permanent learning deficit associated with lesion caudate nuclei. *American Journal of Mental Deficiency*, 67:126-134, 1967.

Tizard, B. T.: Observation of over-active imbecile children in controlled and uncontrolled environments. I. Classroom studies. *American Journal of Mental Deficiency*, 72:540-547, 1968a.

Tizard, B. T.: Observations of over-active imbecile child in controlled and uncontrolled environments. II. Experimental studies. *American Journal Mental Deficiency*, 72:548-553, 1968b.

Varenhorst B. B.: Reinforcement that backfired. In Krumbholtz, J. D., and Thorsen, C. B. (Eds.): *Behavioral Counselling*. New York, HR&W, 1969.

Villa Blanca, J. R.: Permanent reduction of sleep after removal of cerebral cortex and striatium. *Brain Research*, 463-468, 1972.

Villa Blanca, J. R.: *Perseverative instrumental behavior in caudatectomized cats*. Paper presented at the proceedings of the Fourth Annual Meeting of the Society for Neuro Science, Bethesda, 1974a.

Villa Blanca, J. R.: Long-term sleep reduction in frontal cats. *The Physiologist*, 17:280, 1974b.

Villa Blanca, J. R., and Marcus, R. J.: Sleep-wakefulness, EEG, and behavioral studies of chronic cats without Neocortex and Striatium: 'The Diencephalic Cat.' *Arch Ital Biol*, 110:348-382, 1972.

Villa Blanca, J. R., and Marcus, R. J.: Effects of bilateral simultaneous abalation of the caudate nuclei in cats. *Fed Proc*, 32:339, 1973.

Villa Blanca, J. R., and Marcus, R. J.: Effects of caudate nuclei removal in cats. Comparison with frontal cortex ablation. In Buchwald, B. A. (Ed.): *Brain Mechanisms and Mental Retardation*. New York, Acad Pr, 1974a.

Villa Blanca, J. R., and Marcus, R. J.: *Is the striatium needed for amphetamine induced stereotype behaviors?* Paper presented at the proceedings of the Western Pharmacological Society, Los Angeles, 1974b.

Walker, S.: "We're too cavalier about hyperactivity. *Psychology Today, 12*:43-48, 1974.

Windle, W. D.: An experimental approach to the prevention and reduction of brain asphyxia. *Developmental Medicine and Child Neurology, 8*:129-140, 1966a.

Windle, W. D.: Role of respiratoid distress in asphyxial brain damage of the newborn. *Cerebral Palsy Journal, 27*:3-6, 1966b.

Wolf, N. V., Henley, E. N., King, L. G., Giles, D. I.: The timer game: A variable internal contingency for the management of out-of-seat behavior. *Exceptional Children, 10*:113-117, 1970.

Woodburn, L. F.: *The Neural Basis of Behavior.* Columbus, Merril, 1967.

Zaporozhet, A. V.: The development of voluntary movement. In Simon, B. (Ed.): *Psychology in the Soviet Union.* Stanford, Stanford, U Pr, 1957, pp. 108-114.

Zaporozhet, A. V.: *Development of Voluntary Movement.* Moscow, Publishing House, Academy of Pedagogical Sciences, 1960.

CHAPTER 4

ATTENTION-DISTRACTIBILITY IN HYPERACTIVE CHILDREN

ATTENTION AND DISTRACTIBILITY represent primary problems associated with hyperactivity. While these characteristics are usually thought of as two separate processes, in this chapter they are treated as characteristics of the same process. The aspect of attention has been presented a great deal more in literature than has distractibility. It is only within recent years that distractibility has come to be a separate subject for research. Historically, the study of attention predominates psychological research. Since the early days at Leipzig (Bekhterev, 1913), psychologists have concerned themselves with the study of attention. Indeed, William James (1890) exhorted his students to make attention the object of their research. However, attention has proved to be a very elusive area of study.

Perspective

In one of the earliest studies on the subject, Obstersteiner (1879) described attention as an inhibitory function of the brain. In order to test his theory, he measured reaction time in subjects under varying degrees of visual and cutaneous distraction. The increase in reaction time on a standard task after exposure to a distractor was considered to be a measure of the intensity of the subject's attention. In a series of experiments on insane subjects, using reaction time as a measure of resistance to distraction, Obersteiner demonstrated a "weakness" in attention which he attributed to organic degeneration of the brain. At the same time, other researchers (Fechnerl, 1854; Geissler, 1909; Kulpe, 1895; Lipps, 1883 and Stumpf, 1890) of an introspectionist orientation sought to measure attention in terms of the degrees to which a stimulus object appeared "clearly" in the consciousness of a subject. Equating the term *clearness* with *attention*, these investigators undertook studies to determine the factors affecting the clarity of stimulus perceptions along a theoretical continuum. The subjects were asked to increase the clearness of their perception of an idea or stimulus object by equal, successive degrees of clearness. Needless to say, the results were difficult to interpret. In one such study, Geissler (1909) attempted to correlate clearness of the subject's perception of a stimulus object with reaction time and muscle tension. The subjects were given cognitive tasks of varying difficulty while being exposed to various distractors. In addition, subjects were required to grip a device which measured muscle tension, and to react periodically to the ringing of a bell by flicking a switch. Geissler concluded that there was a significant positive correlation between these variables. That is, reaction time was shortest when stimulus "clarity" was rated as highest and muscles were flexed.

Other early authors have studied the effects of stimulus intensity, activity level (Sully, 1885) and difference limens (Titchner, 1908) on the activity of clearness. In a survey of the literature, Burnham (1908) concluded that it was not possible to separate physiological (visceral, circulatory, vasal motor) factors from cognitive factors in the study of attention. Woodrow's (1914) monograph on attention criticized studies which defined attention as the "clearness of thought." Citing the fact that not all tasks were of equal interest nor all distractors equally effective with different subjects, Woodrow questioned the value of the clearness approach. In addition, no clearness study had controlled for the effects of habituation. In an allusion to studies by Mentz (1893), Pillsbury (1896) and Wunt (1892), Woodrow equated attention to muscle tension. Following Woodrow's lead, Johnson (1925) and Dashiell (1928) used the term *set* to describe the behavior in which a subject took up an attitude that facilitated his response to a stimulus, i.e. attention. The components of this response were later specified by Hebb (1948) as both neural and muscular. In a more recent study, Allport (1955) equated attention to a neural state in which pathways, still excited from a previous response, reacted more quickly than pathways not previously excited.

All of these studies confounded the theory of assessing attention with distractibility. They seem to have little relevance for the average classroom teacher.

There is a need to understand the more practical aspects of attention-distractibility. The common concept of attention is that it is a unitary process; that is, it has come to be thought of as a mental faculty. A child is considered to have either "good attention" or to be "highly distractible." This concept primarily stems from the commonly held practice of equating attention with attention span. That is, attention, is commonly thought of as the length of time that a person can spend at a given task, i.e. span. Distractibility has also come to be viewed as the unitary process. The "easily distractible" child is one who is described as being stimulus-bound. He is described as a youngster who is unable to resist responding to the lure of distracters in a classroom setting. Actually, the concept of attention and distractibility as unitary processes is far from accurate. A review of the recent literature on attention alone indicates that attention refers to three separate cognitive processes (Alabiso, 1972). These processes involve attention span (length of time that a subject can spend at a given task), focus of attention (the ability to respond to relevant characteristics of stimuli) and selective attention (ability to make accurate two-stage stimulus discriminations). It is very difficult to operationally define the differences between attention and distractibility. Actually, attention-distractibility may represent points on a continuum of span, focus and selectivity. In this chapter, attention and distractibility are treated in this manner.

Research which supports this continuum concept of attention-distractibility shows that the same variables affect attention and distractibility. Such variables as age, sex, intelligence, developmental level, presence of minimal cerebral dysfunction and the introduction of competing stimuli seem to have nearly the same effect on distractibility as they do on attention. The research of Martin and Powers (1967) led them to conclude that the behavioral differences between short attention span, distractibility and hyperactivity are negligible.

In this chapter the concepts of attention span, focus of attention, and selective attention will be reviewed in depth. The theoretical concept of distractibility and the variables affecting it will also be evaluated. Psychological approaches to the study of attention-distractibility will be reviewed with emphasis on viewing attention-distractibility as learned responses which are subject to both stimulus control and conditioning. Finally, classroom strategies will be reviewed and the chapter will be summarized.

CONCEPTS OF ATTENTION

Attention Span

Perhaps the most researched concept of attention is that of span. Span is best understood in terms of the variables which affect it. In other words, the child's ability to remain at a given task for a specified length of time depends on the task, the environmental circumstances and the abilities of the individual child.

DEVELOPMENTAL LEVEL. Perhaps the most important variable affecting span, as well as the other types of attention, is that of developmental level. Herring and Koch (1930) observed that when the environmental conditions were held constant, the length of time that preschool subjects could spend on a given task varied according to age. Generally, the higher the developmental level, the greater the ability to remain at a task for a specified length of time. The importance of developmental level was pointed out by the research of Brown (1930) who reported that the effects of the environment on attention span could not be meaningfully researched unless developmental level was held constant.

After studying the attention span characteristics of a large group of preschool children, Leontiev (1932) proposed that the ability to remain at a given task for a specified interval undergoes three main stages corresponding to various developmental levels. Each of these stages is associated with a successive level of development. During the first stage, which Leontiev described as the First Order of Attention, the length of time that the child could spend at a given task was described as being determined by the characteristics of the task itself. That is, attention span was completely subject to the ability of the stimulus to maintain the child's interest. Such variables as the complexity of a task, the interest value of the task and the intensity of the stimulus were considered to determine the length of time the child spent at a task. At this stage of development, the child was credited with little ability to remain at a task independent of the task's characteristics. Span could be increased or decreased at this stage by altering the characteristics of the test stimulus. During stage two (Second Order of Attention), the child is able to extend the length of time spent at a given task by the introduction of a future reward. In other words, the child was able to remain at the task longer in an attempt to earn a reward. The Third Order of Attention is one in which the individual directs his own attention. That is, during this highest form of attention, the child is capable of increasing the length of time spent at a given task by observing his own distraction responses and using them as cues to spend added time at the task. This form of attention was termed Voluntary Attention and was thought to be the highest level of attention. Leontiev's research indicated that the First Order of Attention was present in preschool children, while the Second Order of Attention did not appear until school age. Finally, the First through the Third Orders of Attention were present in adults. In other words, each Order of Attention was acquired at successive developmental levels. From a behavioral point of view, Leontievs' theory parallels the processes of stimulus control over attention behaviors, as well as the maintenance of these behaviors through the use of delayed reinforcement and self-reinforcement.

The predominant role played by developmental level in the concept of span has led several researchers to attempt to develop tests of attention span. Such tests have been designed to differentiate between subjects at various developmental levels by measuring the length of time that a subject could spend engaged in a standardized task. Schrater (1933) reviewed the literature on attention in order to develop a readily scorable measure of attention span for young children. In keeping with the long-held definition of attention as span, a child's attention score was rated in terms of minutes and seconds devoted to a certain task. Schrater tabulated the average amount of time that groups of subjects, representing various developmental levels, devoted to a given task. He published a table of attention span levels for various groups between the ages of three and five years. Due to the small sample size (twelve subjects in each group) and the lack of control for other variables such as IQ and sex, the value of Schrater's work lies primarily in his conceptualization of attention as a measurable behavior.

More recently, Kassinove (1968) sought to establish an objective, reliable, age-differentiating measure of the ability to attend. These authors standardized a measure of attention which differentiated between youngsters at various developmental levels (The Developmental Attention Test). One hundred and seventy-one elementary school children, ranging in age from six to twelve years, were studied. This sample included one hundred and five males and sixty-six females. Children at each developmental level were grouped and presented with a stimulus card, on which six rows of numbers were printed in random order. The numbers ranged from the digits 10 to 33. Each row was printed in one of three colors (Form A). A second form of the test (Form B) presented essentially the same arrangement of stimuli except that the colors were varied in order to provide an alternate form of the test to be used in establishing reliability. The child's task was to read each number in order and to state its color. Each child earned a score based on the time in seconds for each response, the number of omissions, the number of repetitions and the number of primary, secondary, tertiary and ulterior responses. Test results indicated that this test accurately differentiated between children at each of the six developmental levels between six and twelve years of age. In addition, reliability coefficients were significantly high for both forms of the test. The groups in each developmental level were matched for sex and IQ. There was no correlation between performance on the Developmental Attention Test and sex of the subjects. Test performance did seem to be associated with IQ for the younger children. In this group, high developmental attention scores correlated significantly with high intelligence. However, with increases in mental age and developmental level, this relationship tended to disappear.

PERSONAL VARIABLES. In addition to developmental level, other subject variables have been studied. The early work of Strauss and Lehtinen (1947) and the research of Strauss and Kephart (1955) suggested that mental retardation acted to decrease attention span. It was further hypothesized that brain-injured, retarded persons were more distractible and more subject to shorter attention span than familial retarded individuals. Bestor's (1934) early research sought to investigate the relationship between developmental level, sex and IQ for matched groups of two, three- and four-year-old children on tests of auditory and visual attention span. In a series of three experiments, matched groups of two-, three-, and four-year-old children were exposed to auditory stimuli, visual stimuli and simultaneous auditory and visual stimuli. The overriding conclusion of this study was that developmental level alone significantly discriminated between the groups' performances on the three experiments. Attention behavior patterns seemed to exist irrespective of the subject's chronological age, sex, IQ or previous educational experiences. In addition, Bestor observed that attention span ability varies depending on the type of stimuli being attended to. In other words, he observed that a child's attention span for visual stimuli is greater, at each developmental level than is his span for auditory stimuli. An important conclusion of this finding was that attention span may not be a unitary process. That is, it may vary with the sense organ that is called into focus. These findings support a general theory which views attention as a series of distinct behaviors rather than as a single mental faculty.

EXTERNAL STIMULI. External variables also play a critical role in attention span. Indeed, the characteristics of the stimulus attended to, as well as the environment in which attention is being observed, are an integral part of attention span. It is literally impossible to conceptualize a faculty of attention span independent of the characteristics of the test stimulus and the test environment.

In a discussion of attention span, Skinner (1965) described the process of attention as a ". . . controlling relation . . . the relation between a response and a discriminative stimulus. . . . When someone is paying attention he is under special control of a stimulus" (p. 123). In other words, Skinner equated attention span to the control that a stimulus exerts over looking behaviors. Other researchers have also referred to the relationship between the characteristics of the stimulus and the subject's ability to attend to it.

Span was thought to be highly influenced by the characteristics of the stimulus object observed. Theoretically, a more interesting stimulus object held attention span for a greater length of time. Early research in this area by Moyer and Gilmer (1954, 1955) indicated that the characteristics of the stimuli do indeed significantly affect attention span. These researchers attempted to measure the affects of this variable on attention span by experimentally designing toys that would maintain increased attention span in preschool and school-age children. Using the term *maximum holding power* to describe what Skinner (1965) called stimulus control over attention behavior, these authors constructed a number of toys that varied in complexity. Six hundred and eighty-one subjects (335 male and 346 female) ranging in age from eighteen months to seven years, of normal intelligence, from middle socio-economic class families were divided into groups according to their developmental levels. Attention span was measured in terms of the length of time the child played with a specified toy. A child's attention score was equal to the mean number of minutes spent on a standard stimulus object. Moyer and Gilmer observed that the length of attention span not only varied with the child's developmental level but also with the distractors present in the room and the characteristics of the stimulus itself. They concluded that certain stimuli held attention longer at each age level. The adequacy of attention span varied with age in that attention span increased with increments in age. However, the increments in attention span by age were not fixed. That is, attention span during certain twelve-month periods appeared to increase dramatically, while during other twelve-month periods it appeared to progress at a much slower rate. There were no significant relationships found between sex of the subject, social class and attention span. The most important observation in helping to understand the relationship between attention span and the stimulus object was the observation that span was functionally related to the characteristics of the stimulus object. For example, these authors found that attention span for a four-year-old ranged from five minutes for a red car, to thirty-nine minutes for a take-apart airplane. Children at the age of five or older spent twice as much time with a complex toy like the take-apart airplane than did the younger children.

Still other stimulus characteristics affect the duration of attention span. Berlyne (1950) investigated the effects of stimulus intensity on attention span. In a series of three experiments, he was able to demonstrate that the greater the intensity of the stimulus, the greater the likelihood that the stimulus will hold a subject's attention. In these studies, Berlyne presented the subjects with several stimuli which were matched for size and brightness. On each trial the test stimulus varied on one of these dimensions. That is, on each trial the tested stimulus was either larger or brighter than the other stimuli presented to the subject. Berlyne's observations indicated that brighter and larger visual stimuli maintain attention span for significantly greater periods of time. In a later study, Berlyne (1951) proposed that attention span be measured in terms of the subject's ability to recall a test stimulus as well as in terms of the resistance of the attention response to extinction. In other words, Berlyne proposed that the study of attention should involve an investigation of the relationship between attention behavior and learning theory.

INTERACTION OF PERSONAL AND EXTERNAL VARIABLES. Taking into consideration the fact that attention span is subject to both subject variables and stimulus variables, Ellis, Hawkins and Jones (1963) designed a study to investigate the interactions between these two types of variables. The performances of three groups of mentally retarded, average and above-average intelligence subjects were compared with the performances of three groups of moderately retarded subjects in an experimental task which measured duration of attention span. For all groups of subjects, the duration of attention span was observed under two stimulus conditions. The groups were observed while being exposed to highly distracting visual stimuli as well as being rated for duration of attention span for low-distracting visual stimuli. A four-way analysis of variance indicated that the nonretarded subjects performed at a significantly higher level under both conditions. In addition, the groups were rated on their degree of distractibility during the period of time when the high- and low-distracting stimuli were introduced. Interestingly enough, there were no significant differences between the groups with respect to their distractibility. While no generalization about the process of distractibility could be made from this finding, Ellis, Hawkins and Jones did conclude that subjects of average intelligence do maintain a significantly greater degree of attention span than mentally retarded subjects, but that both groups of subjects are equally susceptible to distractors when mental ages are held constant. In other words, at least for the population sample studied, intelligence seems to be related to attention span but not to distractibility.

In another study which evaluated the interaction between subject variables and stimulus variables, Gardner, Cromwell and Foshee (1959) studied the effects of varying amounts of distal stimulation on groups of institutionalized brain-injured and non-brain-injured mentally retarded subjects. The groups were matched on mental age and chronological age as well as on IQ score. Both groups were observed to be significantly more attentive under conditions of increased distal stimulation. Activity level was observed to increase significantly as the amount of stimulation was decreased. The researchers concluded that retarded subjects who are not adequately stimulated by the environment may compensate for the lack of stimulation by increasing activity level, and in turn reducing attention span. The observations of other investigators seem to support these findings (Hermelin and O'Connor, 1963; Tizard, 1968a, b).

Fisher (1969) compared the performances of matched groups of brain-damaged and non-brain-damaged children of below-average intelligence on seven measures of attention. Group A consisted of mentally retarded subjects who were known to have organic brain syndrome. Group B consisted of inorganic retardates, and Group C contained mentally retarded subjects whose IQ scores were determined to be significantly higher than those of the subjects in the other two groups. All the subjects had mental ages between three years and four years six months. The performances of the three groups of subjects on measures of attention span for auditory and visual stimuli were compared. No significant differences were found between the performances of the organic and the inorganic mentally retarded subjects. Sex was found to be an insignificant variable. Intelligence did seem to play an important role since there was a positive significant correlation between IQ and performance on the measures of attention span. The performances of all three experimental groups were generally lower on the seven measures of auditory and visual attention span than were the performances of the control groups of normal non-brain-damaged subjects. Fisher concluded that on measures of attention span, there is a significant difference between average IQ children and mentally retarded children. More importantly, he reported no significant differences between brain-damaged and non-brain-damaged subjects on measures of auditory and visual attention span.

SUMMARY. In his review of the literature on attention span, Alabiso (1972) concluded that studies on the effects of stimulus variables on visual attention span had demonstrated that certain stimulus characteristics such as intensity and complexity acted to prolong the length of time that a subject could remain at a specified task. He also reported that, while there is a negative correlation between mental retardation and attention span, the type of retardation seemed to have little effect on the subject's ability to remain at a given task. These conclusions challenged the long-held assumption that brain-injured mentally retarded persons maintained poorer attention span abilities than non-brain-injured mentally retarded youngsters. Alabiso also concluded that studies which compared the performances of retarded subjects with those of nonretarded subjects suggested that when mental age is held constant, differences in attention span seem negligible. In other words, the most important variable in determining attention span is developmental level rather than intelligence. Other varaibles, such as sex and social class, do not seem to play a significant role in the development of attention span abilities.

Little is known about auditory attention span. Most of the research that has been done in this area has been limited to investigations of visual attention span. The preliminary research comparing auditory attention span with visual attention span seems to suggest that these may be two distinct processes.

In recent years, there has been little current research on attention span concerning its role of importance as one of the primary characteristics associated with hyperactivity. Few studies have addressed themselves to a thorough evaluation of the stimulus characteristics which affect attention span. Other than intensity and complexity, little is known about such variables as novelty, familiarity and social value of the test stimulus. Much work needs to be done in order to establish a reliable, valid, measure of attention span, which is able to differentiate the degree of attention span at various age levels from infancy to adulthood.

One important conclusion which does emerge from the current research is that attention span does not seem to fit the stereotyped concept of a unitary process or mental faculty. A child's attention span is clearly subject to many variables, not the least of which are the characteristics of the stimulus itself. Furthermore, the definition of attention as being the length of time that a subject is able to spend at a given task does not seem to adequately fill all of the requirements of a broad concept of attention. In other words, span alone does not adequately account for all of the behaviors which are taken into consideration in determining a child's degreee of attention skills. Recent reviews of the literature (Alabiso, 1972; Reeves, 1973) have shown the concept of attention to include attention span, focus of attention and selective attention. In other words, a child with unimpaired attention is one who is not only able to spend an adequate amount of time on tasks, but is also able to focus on the relevant characteristics of the stimulus observed and is able to make complex stimulus discriminations.

Selective Attention

Selective attention is the most complex of the three attention behaviors. In an attempt to explain the process of selective attention, Broadbent (1957) developed a mechanical model of attention to describe the activity of selective responsiveness. In essence, he described selective attention as a "filtering system." According to Broadbent's theory, all sensory input stimuli arrive at a single location for processing. This location was termed the *central analyzing mechanism.* The order in which sensory inputs were processed by the "central analyzing mechanism" depended on the characteristics of the external stimuli about which information was being carried, the amount of information transported to the central analyzing mechanism and the temporal relationship between sensory inputs. According to Broadbent's theory, stimulus inputs carrying smaller bits of information were able to be processed but at a slower rate. Those sensory inputs which carried larger units of information were processed more readily. Several inputs arriving at the central analyzing mechanism simultaneously were processed according to the amount of information that they carried. This process of responding selectively to one of several sensory inputs received at the same time was termed *the process of selective attention.* Although Broadbent strongly cautioned other researchers that the model which he had described was not intended to explain the physiology of sensory discrimination, it is interesting to note the similarity between this mechanical model of the "central analyzing mechanism" and the role of the thalamus in regulating sensory input. The thalamus, much like the hypothetical central analyzing mechanism, serves just such a function. It is also interesting to note that the thalamus is one of the major subcortical centers located in the reticular activating system.

Deutsch and Deutsch (1963) used Broadbent's mechanical model of selective attention to study the relationship between selective attention and arousal (activity level). The child who was usually thought of as paying attention to everything, but giving selective attention to nothing, was described as having a central analyzing mechanism which was receiving but not processing sensory inputs. The results of this study clearly pointed out that selective attention decreased as activity level increased. In other words, the faster sensory inputs came into the central analyzing mechanism, the longer it took the subject to make a discriminative response.

The central concept to any theory of selective attention is that of discrimination learning. Indeed, selective attention may be defined as a discriminative learning task involving selective responsiveness to more than one characteristic of the test stimulus. Egeth (1967) saw this form of attention as being the most complex of all attention behaviors. Indeed, selective attention was thought to be an integrated process involving perceptual mechanisms, memory and response readiness.

In earlier attempts to define the process of selective attention, Sullwold (1954) factor-analyzed ten tests of attention. The factor analysis of these tests showed that they contained measures of span, preparatory set and stimulus discrimination. Based on these findings, Sullwold developed a test of selective attention which yielded a selective attention score based on the number of correct responses and the length of time it took to complete the test tasks.

Perhaps the clearest explanation of the process of selective attention was put forth by Zeaman and House (1963). These authors combined the research on attention with research on discriminative learning, in order to produce a testable theory of selective attention. According to Zeaman and House's definition, selective attention is a two-stage discrimination learning task. During the first stage, the subject is required to respond to the relative stimulus dimension, e.g. form. The second stage required the subject to respond to the correct stimulus cue on the dimension, e.g. size. This two-stage discrimination learning process differed from the concept of focus of attention which involves a simple discrimination learning task of responding to a relevant stimulus characteristic. According to their definition of selective attention, the subject is faced with a task in which he has an opportunity to observe the test stimulus. After the stimulus is removed, he is asked to select that stimulus from a display panel containing the test stimulus along with a number of other stimuli which vary in size and shape. A correct response requires the subject to, first, discriminate the proper dimension, e.g. shape, and then the correct cue, e.g. size. Subjects suffering from a deficit in selective attention, when shown a test stimulus of a small circle, would be expected to have difficulty finding that test stimulus in an array of other stimuli containing small, medium and large circles, squares and triangles. Close evaluation of the performances of subjects, who suffer from deficits in selective attention, indicated that they have difficulty selecting the correct stimulus dimension. In layman's terms, they have difficulty picking out the important characteristics of the test stimulus. Once they have mastered this task, they seem to have little difficulty in identifying the correct stimulus cue. This means that if the subject is able to select the important dimensions of stimuli, he should have little difficulty identifying the important stimulus cue. Zeaman and House believed that selective attention was subject to the principals of learning theory. Reinforcements for selecting the correct stimulus dimension and the correct stimulus cue was thought to strengthen both the instrumental response and whichever observing response immediately proceeded it.

In earlier research, Harlow (1959) described four major types of errors which may occur in the selective attention process. These errors provide a convenient means of analyzing a child's deficits in two-stage discrimination learning tasks. The first error, referred to as *stimulus perservation,* refers to a tendency to repeat incorrect responses on subsequent trials of the same problem. The second type of error, called *position preference errors,* refers to the tendency to consistently respond to the left or the right stimulus position in the discrimination learning task. *Response shift errors* are defined as those errors in which the subject explores stimulus objects regardless of their correctness. Finally, *differential cue errors* may be a source of faculty selective attention. These errors refer to the greater frequency in which errors occur when the correct stimulus object changes position from the previous trial, when compared with the frequency of errors which occur when the test stimulus remains in the same position over successive trials. These four types of errors are particularly important in helping the classroom teacher understand defiicits in selective attention. Being able to identify the four types of errors, for example, will greatly help the classroom teacher to develop a strategy for reinforcing correct selective attention responses.

Research in the area of response errors by Ellis, Giardeau and Prior (1962) indicated that position preferences accounted for the majority of errors in two-stage stimulus discrimination problems. In other words, the child having difficulty with selective attention is most likely to err by responding to the position of the stimulus rather than its dimension. Stimulus perseveration errors were found to occur more frequently among slow learners than among normal subjects (Kaufman and Peterson, 1958). These errors are ones in which the subject repeats incorrect responses regardless of whether their response is reinforced or extinguished. In an updating of this research, Harter, Brown and Zigler (1971) confirmed that subjects who show deficits in two-stage stimulus discrimination tasks generally tend to make the error of responding to the position of the stimulus rather than to the dimension or cue. Reeves (1973) concluded his review of the literature in this area by stating that ". . . an appropriate remediation tactic is generally found in the systematic application of reinforcement" (p. 13).

PERSONAL VARIABLES. As with attention span, selective attention should not be considered as a unitary process or mental faculty, but rather as a behavioral phenomenan. This complex stimulus discrimination task has been shown to be strongly affected by subject as well as environmental variables. Reeves (1973), for instance, demonstrated that mental retardation significantly affects selective attention. In his review of the literature in this area, Reeves summarized studies on the relationship between mental retardation and selective attention by noting that mental retardation significantly decreases the likelihood that the child will be able to select the correct dimension. In other words, his review of the literature pointed out that retardates have significant deficits in their ability to discriminate between form, size, color, etc. Reeves further pointed out that once the mentally retarded child learns the correct dimension, he seems quite capable of responding to the proper cue.

As with the other primary characteristics of hyperactivity, the effects of brain damage on selective attention is an important research variable. Cromwell and Foschee (1960) studied the selective attention responses of two groups of mentally retarded subjects. The experimental group contained brain-injured mental retardates, while the control group was composed of familial retardates. The groups were matched for chronological age, sex, IQ and mental age. The performances of the two groups on a selective attention task under conditions of visual distraction were studied. No significant differences were found between the performances of the two groups. In other words, in their study, Cromwell and Foshee concluded that for mentally retarded subjects, presence of organic brain injury was not found to affect selective attention behaviors. These results seem to be valid when the brain damage is minimal. There is no question that severe organic brain damage affects all forms of complex cognitive behaviors.

In an earlier study, Foshee (1958) studied the relationship betwen activity level and selective attention. Foshee used balistograph scores to assign mentally retarded, institutionalized subjects matched on age, sex and IQ into high and low activity groups. He has hypothesized that low activity subjects would perform better on simple discrimination learning tasks while highly active subjects would perform best on complex discrimination tasks. In other words, Foshee predicted that there would be a positive correlation between high activity level and selective attention behaviors. The results of this study forced Foshee to conclude that activity level was unrelated to selective attention. There were no significant differences between high and low activity groups for two-stage discrimination learning. This finding also seems to support Kaspar and Schulman's (1972) conclusion that the primary characteristics of hyperactivity probably represent parallel but separate biosocial processes.

REINFORCEMENT VARIABLES. Sirvastava (1968) examined the inneractions between intelligence, primary and secondary reinforcement and selective attention. Mentally retarded subjects were divided into low and high IQ groups, and subject to either primary or secondary reinforcement while performing a selective attention task. During acquisition training, one of the experimental groups received primary reinforcement (candy), while the other experimental group received secondary reinforcement (praise) for correct responses to a two-stage stimulus discrimination task. The control group received no reinforcement during the acquisition training. The control subjects (nonreinforcement group) showed no significant improvement in selective attention learning, while both experimental groups did show positive gains. IQ did not appear to be an important factor within the IQ ranges studied (mean mental ages ranging from four years five months to eight years nine months). Primary reinforcement significantly increased the rate of selective attention learning. These findings also tend to support the concept that selective attention is not convergent with the other characteristics of hyperactivity.

Ellis and Pryer (1958) also studied the effects of primary and secondary reinforcement on selective attention learning in mentally retarded subjects. These researchers used an experimental design similar to the one described by Sirvastava (1968) to study the relationship between type of reinforcement and selective attention learning. Two groups of institutionalized mentally retarded subjects, matched on mental age and chronological age, were given a selective attention learning task. One group received secondary reinforcement for correct responses while the other groups' responses were followed by candy reinforcement. No significance between group differences were established. This finding would seem to discount the later work of Sirvastava. However, the subjects in this study were trained for only fifty acquisition trials followed by thirty extinction trials. It seems likely that, had the study been carried out further, different results may have occurred.

STIMULUS VARIABLES. The characteristics of the stimuli to be discriminated also represent an important factor in successful selective attention learning. Ross (1967) studied the effects of various stimulus dimensions on selective attention learning in retarded subjects. Subjects matched on age, sex and IQ were required to press a button representing one of three stimulus dimensions corresponding to the stimuli presented to them on a screen. In the first study, Ross studied the differential responses of subjects to the dimensions of form, size and brightness. The results of this study indicated that brightness was significantly easier for the subjects to discriminate than size and form. No significant differences in selective attention learning were found between size and form. In other words, selective attention learning was significantly facilitated when the correct stimulus dimension was brightness. In a second study, Ross compared the performances of normal IQ subjects with those of mentally retarded subjects. He repeated the first part of the experiment in which the subject was faced with the task of learning the correct stimulus dimension (form, size or brightness). His findings demonstrated that brightness was significantly easier for both groups to discriminate, although normal IQ subjects had fewer errors in all categories. Evidently subjects with normal intelligence perform higher than retarded subjects at all levels, but are still subject to the same learning processes as mentally retarded subjects.

SUMMARY. Selective attention represents a two-stage stimulus discrimination task requiring the subject to correctly identify the dimension of a stimulus as well as the stimulus cue. Errors in selective attention may be conveniently categorized into one of four types. Position errors, errors of perseveration, errors caused merely by an inability to shift one's response, and errors which primarily represent a subject's failure to respond to differential cues. The primary error associated with selective attention appears to be that of position preference errors followed by perseverative errors. As with the other forms of attention, selective attention is neither a mental faculty nor a unitary cognitive process, but rather it reflects an interaction between subject variables, stimulus variables and reinforcement variables.

Our review of the literature in the area of subject variables revealed that mental retardation does seem to affect selective attention performance since mentally retarded subjects are less likly to discriminate the proper dimension of a stimulus. Interestingly enough, brain damage was not found to play a significant role in determining selective attention performance between various groups of mentally retarded subjects. However, it was evident from the studies reviewed that subjects of normal intelligence clearly have the advantage in selective attention learning. The subject's activity level seems to be an insignificant variable.

Stimulus variables also seem to play an important role. Studies comparing various stimulus characteristics such as form, brightness and size revealed that the correct selective attention response is more likely to occur when the test stimulus is brighter than the other comparison stimuli.

The literature surrounding reinforcement variables has yielded contradictory findings. There is a general trend suggesting that primary reinforcement is more effective than secondary reinforcemest in increasing the probability of correct selective attention responses.

The concept of attention contains still another aspect, that of focus of attention. In his review of the literature, Alabiso (1972) described focus of attention as one of the three basic components of human attention.

Focus of Attention

The length of time that a subject spends both at a given task (span) and the ability to make complex two-stage discriminations (selectivity) do not account for all of the behaviors normally associated with attention. Certain children are able to remain at a given task for long periods of time without ever demonstrating progress in mastering it. These same children may be capable of making complex two-stage stimulus discriminations necessary for selective attention, and yet their ability to respond correctly on less complex tasks may be impaired. Studies on focus of attention have concerned themselves with the process by which a subject comes to master a task by learning to respond correctly to relevant stimulus characteristics. In developing a concept of focus of attention, Wachtel (1967) likened the focusing process to a beam of light. Using the terms "broad and narrow" attention he described the process of focusing attention as one in which the subject scans the perceptual field. Following this analogy, Wachtel hypothesized that focus of attention, like a beam of light, would be more intense at the center of the perceptual field and become weaker at its periphery. Accordingly, the likelihood of identifying relevant stimulus characteristics was greatest for those stimuli which were located in the center of the subject's visual field. The further the stimuli were located from the center of field, the less likely the subject was able to pick out important stimulus characteristics. Using the concept of broad attention to describe perceptual scanning, Wachtel predicted that the subject would scan the entire perceptual field during this phase of focus of attention behavior. During narrow attention, the scanning activity was limited to the center of the visual field. In effect, Wachtel defined focus of attention as a perceptual behavior which involved the identification of important stimulus characteristics as well as screening out those characteristics which are irrelevant.

Using overt observing responses to measure focus of attention, White and Plum (1964) recorded the eye movements of children during visual discrimination learning. They found a significant positive correlation between the amount of perceptual scanning of the stimulus field and the rapidity with which discrimination learning occurred. In a related study, Wright and Dahler (1966) found that reinforcement of overt observing responses in school age children significantly improved their performance on visual discrimination tasks. Wright and Dahler concluded that training the child to observe relevant stimulus characteristics did generalize from one test situation to another. This finding was important in that it suggested that what was being reinforced was the child's ability to focus his attention on relevant stimulus characteristics. In a later study, Wright and Smothergill (1967) made focus of attention measurable by reinforcing correct overt observing responses. In this study, the subject was faced with the task of pressing a lever which brought a visual stimulus into focus. The subject received reinforcement as long as the operation of the lever caused the picture on the screen to become clearer. Reinforcement was withheld whenever the subject did not manipulate the lever in such a way as to produce a clear image on the screen. In this manner, subjects were reinforced for continually observing the test stimulus.

Kagan and Huntsman (1971) further defined the measurement of focus of attention by not only including the measure of a child's ability to select the correct stimulus characteristic, but also by including the measure of his ability to select and disregard irrelevant characteristics of the stimulus. In this study, Kagan and Huntsman presented subjects with a test stimulus which contained a central figure as well as an incidental figure. After removal of the stimulus cards, the subjects were required to identify both the relevant (central) stimulus characteristics as well as the irrelevant (incidental) stimulus characteristics. The mentally retarded subjects in the study had significantly greater difficulty in identifying the relevant stimulus characteristics than did the normal subjects. Kagan and Huntsman concluded that mental retardation seriously handicaps the child's ability to focus his attention on the relevant stimulus characteristics.

PERSONAL VARIABLES. As with the other forms of attention, focus of attention should not be viewed as a unitary mental faculty which operates independent of environmental factors and the individual's characteristics. Subject variables have been found to be an important factor in determining the subject's ability to focus his attention. Jensen (1963) researched the relationship between intellectual development and focus of attention ability. In this study, Jensen compared the learning rates for groups of mentally retarded, intellectually average and intellectually above-average children on three focus of attention tasks. Jensen found a significant relationship between intellectual ability and the ability to focus attention. Focus of attention ability improved with increments in intellectual ability. Jensen did caution, however, that his results could be misinterpreted. He noted that the fastest-learning mentally retarded subjects were able to produce learning scores on par with those produced by children of average intelligence.

O'Donnell (1969) studied the relationship between intellectual ability and pretraining on a focus of attention task. The performances of groups of intellectually normal children with and without pretraining in observing responses were compared with the performances of groups of mentally retarded children. As was the case for the normal children, one group of mentally retarded subjects received pretraining in observing responses, while the other group did not. Both the mentally retarded subjects and the subjects of normal intelligence were rewarded with candy reinforcement. For each observing response made during the pretraining sessions, an analysis of the data verified that both mentally retarded subjects and subjects of normal intelligence performed at a significantly better level as a result of pretraining. In addition, the results of the study also indicated that subjects of normal intelligence performed significantly better than mentally retarded subjects when comparing both the normal subject pretrained and not pretrained groups with the mentally retarded subjects' pretrained and not pretrained groups. O'Donnell concluded that pretaining as well as level of intelligence were significant factors influencing focus of attention behaviors. As with the other forms of attention, the relationship between brain damage and focus of attention behaviors has been researched. Using vigilance tasks as a measure of both auditory and visual focus of attention, Fisher (1969) compared the performances of brain-injured and non-brain-injured, high IQ mental retardates with low IQ mental retardates. He also compared the performances of subjects of normal intelligence with high IQ mental retardates and low IQ mental retardates. Subjects were matched for age and sex, and differed only on the variables of level of intelligence and presence or absence of brain damage. Fisher's findings suggested that the presence of brain damage does not play a significant role in focus of attention behavior for the samples studied. No significant differences in visual focus of attention performances were found between the brain injured and the non-brain-injured, mentally retarded groups. Fisher did find a significant relationship between performance and level of intelligence in the mentally retarded groups. His findings in this area suggested that intelligence plays a significant role in focus of attention ability.

Unfortunately, there has been no study to date which reports on the relationship between mental age, i.e., developmental level, and focus of attention ability. Until such a study is undertaken, it is not possible to be completely assured that level of intelligence plays the significant role that the studies of Jensen (1963), O'Donnell (1969) and Fisher (1969) suggest.

EXTERNAL VARIABLES. The relationship between focus of attention and behavior, and the actual characteristics of the observed stimulus, needs further investigation. It is probably safe to assume, however, that the intensity of the relevant stimulus characteristics and their location in the subject's perceptual field are likely to be significant variables. The nature of the irrelevant stimulus characteristics probably plays an important role in focus of attention behavior. Reeves (1973) reviewed the literature in the area of focus of attention and concluded that focus of attention represents an overt observing response which is subject to the laws of learning. That is, focus of attention behaviors conform to reinforcement theory. In addition, Reeves concluded that developmental level significantly affected the subject's ability to focus his attention.

SUMMARY. It is clear from the review of literature in this area that focus of attention calls for the identification of and response to relevant stimulus characteristics. Research in this area of attention has been concentrated primarily on subject variables. As with the other forms of attention, mental retardation significantly inhibits focus of attention ability. Children of normal intelligence have a decided advantage in the ability to focus their attention. However, pretraining in focus of attention responses seems to help both subjects of normal intelligence and mentally retarded subjects to acquire, maintain and generalize focus of attention behaviors. As with the other forms of attention, brain damage seems to have little effect on the performances of subjects matched for level of intelligence. Of all of the areas of attention, the area of focus of attention is the most obviously lacking in research on the effects of developmental level. A great deal more research on this variable is needed to complete our knowledge of its effect on focus of attention.

Unfortunately, there is little information on the effects of certain stimulus characteristics such as intensity and position in the perceptual field. It is probably safe to assume that, with respect to these variables, focus of attention conforms to the same findings as did selective attention and attention span. It would be particularly important, however, to study the relationship between the position of the relevant stimulus characteristic in the subject's perceptual field and the accuracy of focus of attention responses.

Conclusion

Subject variables such as social class, chronological age and sex of the subject do not seem to significantly affect focus behaviors. In addition, such subject variables as organic brain syndrome seem to have little direct affect on focus behaviors. The relationship between level of intelligence and attention behaviors can only be understood in terms of developmental level. It would seem that mental age serves as a better predictor of attention behaviors than does IQ. A review of the literature in this area points to a general conclusion that, regardless of presence or absence of mental retardation, the subjects of the same mental age tend to do equally well on measures of attention. One very important conclusion is that attention cannot be considered as a mental faculty which operates irrespective of the environment in which the subject finds himself. Such factors as the intensity and location of the test stimulus significantly influence attention behaviors.

Alabiso (1972) reviewed the literature on all three forms of attention. He concluded that span, focus and selectivity represented three separate and possibly unrelated aspects of attention. Span was defined as the length of time that a subject could spend at a given task. By definition, measures of attention span involve recording the duration of time spent on tasks. Selective attention was defined as the execution of a two-stage stimulus discrimination in which the subject first had to identify relevant stimulus dimension and then complete the response by identifying the relevant stimulus cue. Selective attention behaviors were measured in terms of the subject's ability to correctly make both of these responses. Focus of attention was defined in terms of the subject's ability to identify relevant stimulus characteristics. This ability was measured in terms of the correct number of responses to relevant stimuli. In other words, focus of attention was measured according to the subject's rate of acquisition. However, Alabiso cautioned that the use of the number of correct responses as a criteria for measuring focus of attention may tend to obscure the observation that any such measure must consider the subject's ability to inhibit responses to irrelevant stimuli. This inhibitory ability lies at the base of research on distractibility. In other words, the inability to restrict responses to irrelevant stimuli may be equated to distractibility. The concepts of distractibility are so closely linked to attention that they warrant a special section in this chapter.

CONCEPTS OF DISTRACTIBILITY

Attempting to define the difference between poor attention and high distractibility is something like trying to determine whether a water glass filled to the midway point is half full or half empty. Actually, we know little about distractibility, and so it is important to caution that at this point in the text, distractibility is being discussed conceptually. Its tenuous theoretical status, however, makes it no less a critical factor in our study of attention. Indeed, Kaspar (1974) noted that "the consequences of faculty attention, i.e. distractibility, are much more ubiquitous and devastating than the consequences of deviations in activity level" (p. 1).

Perspective

For many years the term *distractibility* has been used freely as if an agreed-upon definition has been common knowledge.

Nothing could be further from the truth. Until recently (Kaspar, 1974) the definitions of distractibility have been varied, and even though they have been used as such, they have not been interchangeable.

Confusion in terminology is evident; many references describe distractibility as inattention. The implication is, of course, that the child who is not attentive is distracted, and therefore, all inattentive behaviors would be classified as distraction responses. In view of our understanding of attention as constituting three distinctive behaviors, one wonders if defining distractibility as inattention is adequate. For example, take the case of a child who demonstrates adequate attention span while failing to make the complex two-stage stimulus discrimination response called for by selective attention. Such a child could hardly be called distractible although his performance at a selective attention task might be poor. Other definitions of distractibility have referred to this phenomenan as a response to irrelevant stimuli. Once again, this concept of distractibility competes with our concept of focus of attention.

Early research regarding distractibility contributed to a confusing definition. In some early studies, the subject's attention ability was tested by measuring reaction time while he was exposed to varying degrees of visual and cutaneous stimuli which were referred to as distractors. One problem with this approach is that it does not differentiate between the physiological process of distractibility and the effects of the particular types of distractors. For example, questions such as whether the subject's reaction time would decrease markedly with the introduction of visual stimuli, as opposed to the introduction of auditory stimuli, have gone unanswered.

More recently, the research of Turnure and Zigler (1964) and Turnure (1966) have pointed out the complex relationship between distractibility, distracting stimuli and attention. In his first study, Turnure and Zigler (1964) established that high distractibility and focus of attention were distinct phenomena which could occur simultaneously. In this study, groups of mentally retarded subjects were matched according to mental age with a group of normal subjects. Both groups were required to perform three standardized tasks. The experimenter served as a distractor while each of the subjects worked on the first task. The experiment was designed in such a way that focusing attention on the experimenter during the first task would give the subject an opportunity to observe the procedure for solving the second task. The performance of the normal subjects on the first task was significantly better than the performance of the retarded subjects. Interestingly enough, the retarded subjects performed significantly better on the second task than did the normal subjects. Turnure and Zigler concluded that the retarded subjects exhibited more distractibility than the normal subjects. According to them, their distractibility in focusing their attention on the experimenter during the first task accounted for the significantly better performance on the second and third tasks. They concluded that, while mentally retarded subjects are more distractible than normal subjects, their distractibility did not impair their ability to focus their attention. Indeed, Turnure's (1966) observation that certain distractors served to mobilize attention led him to predict that the introduction of distracting stimuli could facilitate the focus of attention behaviors in younger subjects. The data supported this hypothesis. Turnure concluded that at successive developmental levels the child learns to resist distractors. At lower developmental levels the child responds readily to the introduction of distraction stimuli. However, as development level increases, the introduction of a distracting stimuli becomes a cue to mobilize focus of attention responses to the task at hand. At the higher developmental levels, the introduction of the distracting stimuli actually serves as a cue for improving focus behaviors. It is not difficult to see that the interaction between distractibility, distracting stimuli and attention behavior is a highly complex one.

Fortunately, much of the confusion regarding distractibility has been clarified by the work of Kaspar and his colleagues (Kaspar, 1968; Kaspar, Millichap, Backus, Child and Schulman, 1971; Kaspar and Schulman, 1972; Kaspar, 1973, 1974; Kaspar and Kashaba, 1975). In his review of the literature, Kaspar

(1972) clearly pointed out the difference between distractibility and activity level, and between distractibility and impulsivity, thus freeing the concept of distractibility from being confused with two of the other characteristics of hyperactivity. In a more recent work, Kaspar (1974) described distractibility as a biosocial phenomena. In doing so, he pointed out that distractibility involves an interaction between the child's ability to attend and the characteristics of the environment: "A distractible child is one whose ability to, at least, fane attention does not meet his teacher's level of acceptable attention. To reiterate, we are in a social or at least biosocial area of definition" (p. 4). Over the past several years, Kaspar and colleagues have worked to develop an operational definition of distractibility which is not dependent on the introduction of distracting stimuli. Recently, Kaspar and Kashaba (1975) have summarized several years of research on distractibility.

STANDARDIZED PERFORMANCE TESTS. As a result of a series of successive studies, Kaspar redefined distractibility in terms of the subject's performance on four standardized tasks. Citing the work of Schulman et al. (1965), Kaspar et al. (1971) identified four measures of distractibility. Each of the four measures involve a stimulus discrimination task. The measures differed according to the type of sensory input and sensory output required by the task. The measures were constructed in such a way as to be able to measure distractibility stemming from deficits in either visual or auditory reception or in either verbal or motor expression. The measures were constructed in such a way as to appeal to children.

The first test, called the Cards Test, was a continuous performance, stimulus discrimination task in which the child was exposed to visual sensory input. He was expected to respond with a verbal output. Essentially, this test required the child to observe a series of cards as they are turned over, one at a time. Nearly all of the cards have identical images of rabbits on them. Several cards containing pictures of babies were randomly interspersed throughout the deck. The child's task is to say the word "baby" when the baby card appears.

The Tones Test represented a stimulus discrimination task with auditory sensory input, requiring a motor output response. This test requires the child to listen to a tape recording of the words "up" and "down." The output task is for the child to raise his hand when he hears the word "up."

The remaining two tests are similar in that they both are "wait-go" tasks. The subject is required to be vigilant for a specified interval before a correct response can be made. If the response is made before the interval is up or after it is over, the response is considered incorrect.

The first of the two tests of this type is the Clock Test. This test is also a continuous performance, stimulus discrimination task with a verbal sensory input and a motor sensory output. In this task, a stop clock had been adapted in such a way that a mouse was affixed to the second hand and a picture of a piece of cheese was pasted to the face of the clock covering the area from approximately eighteen seconds to twenty-one seconds. A mouse's cage was also affixed to the clock at the twenty-eight second mark. The child is advised that his job is to allow the mouse to get the cheese but to return him to the starting point before he enters the cage. Returning the mouse to the starting point before eighteen seconds or after twenty-eight seconds results in an error.

The final distractibility task was a stimulus discrimination task known as the Jack-In-The-Box Test. This test required auditory sensory input and verbal sensory output. In this test the child was required to help the jack-in-the-box "go into outer space." He is instructed that the experimenter will count down from ten to zero at one-second intervals. The subject's task is to say "fire" at the precise moment that the experimenter says "zero" and pulls the cord allowing the jack-in-the-box to spring out.

Using these four measures of distractibility, Kaspar, Millichap, Backus, Child and Schulman (1971) studied the relationship between neurological evidence of brain damage, activity level and distractibility in children. In this study, twenty-four males and twelve females ranging in age between five and eight years, with a diagnosis of minimal brain dysfunction, were compared to a control group of normal subjects matched for age and sex on measures of activity level and distractibility. The mean IQ for both groups was within the normal range, though control subjects were significantly more intelligent. The study was designed to investigate the possibility of a relationship between brain dysfunction, activity level and distractibility. Actometers attached to the children's wrists and ankles were used to measure the amount of activity occurring under conditions of free play and during a standardized testing situation. The mean amount of activity per minute under each of the two testing conditions was recorded for both the groups. During the free play situation, the children's activity levels were monitored in the playroom in which toys were available for their use. During the structured activity time, the children were involved in the distractibility testing. The data were analyzed in order to determine both the level of activity under structured testing conditions and under free play conditions. The differences in performances between the two groups on the four measures of distractibility were also analyzed. As reported earlier in the chapter on activity level, the brain-damaged children were significantly more active during the structured task condition. There were no significant differences between the groups in the amount of activity level during free play.

Most important, for purposes of this section, were the findings with respect to distractibility. Three of the four distractibility measures differentiated between normals and controls and between males and females. Only the Jack-In-The-Box test (auditory input-verbal output) did not differentiate between the two groups. The difference between male and female subjects and between normal and control subjects was found to be significant at the .001 level for the Cards Test (visual input-auditory output), the Clock Test (visual input-motor output) and the Tones Test (auditory input-motor output). The authors also reported a positive significant correlation between intelligence and the visual input-verbal output measure of distractibility (Cards Test). However, it should be remembered in evaluating this conclusion that the measure used to assess intelligence was the Peabody Picture Vocabulary Test which in itself is a visual input-verbal output task. It is quite likely that the high positive correlation between the cards test and IQ is due to the fact that they are essentially the same task.

The primary value of this study was that it yielded much information about a subject about which little had formerly been known. For instance, the overall analysis of the data strongly suggested that the concept of distractibility as a syndrome could not be ruled out. There was enough data to suggest the possibility that distractibility may be present as a syndrome in brain-injured children. The all-important variable is the nature of the input stimulus. The clearest finding along these lines was the significant correlation between brain damage and visual input stimulus material. Another important finding was that auditory distractibility tends to decrease with age, while visual distractibility seems to not be significantly influenced by age. Apparently, auditory distractibility and visual distractibility do not respond in the same way to certain other variables. For instance, there was no significant correlation between activity level and distractibility in the free play situation on either auditory or visual input measures of distractibility. However, for the structured testing situation there was a significant positive correlation between brain damage and auditory input measures of distractibility, but no significant correlation between brain damage and visual input measures of distractibility. This finding, along with several others, forced the authors to conclude that the only meaningful construct of distractibility was one which viewed auditory distractibility and visual distractibility as separate entities. While the auditory distractibility measure (Tones Test) seems to have its place in the evaluation of distractibility, the one test which yielded the most information about distractibility was the visual input-verbal output measure, the Cards Test. This test correlated significantly with all three other measures of distractibility. This correlation seemed to be a combination of two factors. First, the nature of the task as a visual input task seems to be a crucial factor. Second, it is the only one of the four measures of distractibility that is a continuous performance task.

In a more recent article, Kaspar and Kashaba (1975) integrated the findings of the Kaspar et al. (1971) study with the results of three subsequent studies. Their summarization of these research findings was prefaced by a discussion of the measurement of distractibility. In this discussion, Kaspar defined distractibility as ". . . the child's internal ability to control his immediate interactions with the environment . . ." (p. 8). This distinction is an important one, because it helps us understand the difference between distractibility as a biosocial phenomenon and the child's performance on measures of distractibility. Kaspar further points out that the importance of social environmental factors on distractibility should not be minimized. ". . . a child is considered distractible when he does not attend to the stimuli that the adult who is in controlling relationship to him feels he should attend to . . ." (p. 8).

One interesting finding reported in the study was that the introduction of a distracter effects the subject's performance on the various measures of distractibility in different ways. For example, in the first study, the visual input-verbal output measure, the auditory input-motor output measure and the visual input-motor output measure were found to be reliable when tested without the presence of a distracter. The same three tests were readministered to the same subjects in the presence of an auditory distractor. Only the auditory input-motor output test retained its reliability under these conditions. It seems strange that the auditory test was the least affected by the presence of an auditory distractor. In addition, the authors observed that the presence of the auditory distractor affected different subjects in different ways. Many of the subjects actually improved their performance on all three of the tests when an auditory distracter was present. This finding in itself was invaluable in that it forwarned of the importance of distinguishing between distractibility and a response to a distracting stimuli. As mentioned earlier, the work of Turnure and Zigler (1964) suggested that the introduction of distracting stimuli may actually act to reduce distractibility by serving as a cue for mobilizing attention in older subjects. This would be one explanation to Kaspar's findings with respect to the introduction of an auditory distracter.

Another important finding of the study resulted from the correlations among three measures of distractibility. The data revealed that in reality there was a poor correlation between each of the measures of distractibility. It was only the visual input-verbal output measure of the Cards Test which was able to demonstrate a significant relationship between test performance and minimal brain dysfunction. This finding is a most interesting one. If we assume that all three of the measures are valid as well as reliable, it is quite likely that there is actually more than one type of distractibility. Type of distractibility may vary according to the type of stimulus material used in the testing and the sensory input system utilized by the subject. In other words, visual and auditory distractibility may be separate processes which respond to input stimuli in different ways.

The findings in the studies also provided information about the relationship of subject variables to performance on measures of distractibility. While there is no clear-cut relationship between age and distractibility at the lower age levels, there does seem to be a trend for older children to be less distractible. No significant relationship was discovered between sex of the subject and distractibility in any of the studies reported. However, there was a trend for brain-damaged females to be less distractible than brain-damaged males. A significant correlation was found to exist between performance and distractibility measures in the presence of a diagnosable form of brain dysfunction (phenylketonuria).

The relationship between intelligence and distractibility is a complex one and seems to vary according to certain subject variables. For instance, there seems to be no significant relationship between IQ and distractibility for subjects of average or above intelligence. However, when studying performances of subjects known to be suffering from some form of brain damage, a positive significant interaction was found to exist between distractibility, IQ and minimal brain dysfunction.

The relationship between distractibility and brain dysfunction itself remains unclear. For instance, there was no significant correlation between three of the measures of distractibility and brain dysfunction as rated by an EEG and a neurological examination. Other aspects of the study did suggest a relationship between distractibility and brain dysfunction. These results taken together suggest that distractibility tests seem to measure a different aspect of brain dysfunction than does the EEG or the neurological examination.

A final study was undertaken in order to resolve the ambiguity in the previous research findings regarding the relationship between distractibility and age, and between distractibility and intelligence. The results of this study show brain-damaged subjects to be more distractible than control subjects, and younger subjects to be more distractible than older subjects. This finding suggests that there is a relationship not only between brain damage and distractibility but between age and distractibility. Children with a mental age of six years or above were noticeably less distractible than younger subjects. This finding, taken together with the other reported findings related to the relationship between intelligence and distractibility, suggests that the critical factor in this relationship is not IQ itself, but rather the mental age or developmental level of the subject being tested. This study clearly pointed to the Cards Test (visual input-verbal output) and the Tones Test (auditory input-motor output) as the most discriminating measures of distractibility. These findings indicate that the most accurate measures of distractibility are measures of stimulus discrimination. The modality of sensory input also seems to be a critical factor. The results point to a general conclusion that there are probably several types of distractibility.

One critical research area which remains to be investigated is the relationship between distractibility as Kaspar has defined it and response inhibition. It is likely that many of the unanswered questions about the nature of distractibility will be found in this area of investigation.

MODIFICATION OF ATTENTION BEHAVIORS

The reconceptualization of attention-distractibility as a biosocial response rather than a fixed process or mental faculty has opened this characteristic of hyperactivity to learning theory research. Crosby and Blatt (1968) summarized this change in thinking in their statement that ". . . the crucial point for education is that attention as stimulus selection is, at least within rather broad limits, a learned response and therefore susceptible to manipulation by the teacher" (p. 33).

Attention Span

Although their research was not done with hyperactive children, Brooks, Morrow and Gray (1968) utilized positive reinforcement to increase visual attention span with an institutionalized autistic child. Prior to treatment, the child refused eye contact with any other human being. Within twenty-six days of making visual attention span for looking at other human beings contingent on positive reinforcement, the child was able to look at another person for twenty consecutive minutes. One other important observation from this study was that visual attention span for looking reverted to its baseline level when positive reinforcement was withheld.

Kennedy and Thompson (1967) did attempt to increase attention span for looking in a first grade hyperactive boy of average intelligence. The youngster had received counseling from both the school psychologist and his classroom teacher on the importance of looking at the teacher, completing assignments and following instructions. The counseling sessions did not affect attention span. During the reinforcement phase of the study the youngster received positive reinforcement for each sixty-second interval during which he looked at the experimenter. When the attention span for looking at the experimenter had reached a predetermined criteria, the child was returned to the classroom. A significant improvement was reported in his attention span for looking at the teacher.

Quay, Spague, Werry and McQueen (1967) also studied the increase of visual attention span in hyperactive youngsters. Their study differed from the others reported above in that they attempted to work with a group of five hyperactive children in an actual classroom setting. In addition, they compared the effectiveness of positive primary reinforcement with that of social reinforcement in increasing attention span for observing the teacher. Children's desks were arranged in a semicircle in order that they might all be observed and have equal opportunity for observing the teacher. The children's task was to watch the teacher as she read a story to them. A light was mounted on each child's desk, and flashed for every ten seconds in which the child was observed to be looking at the teacher. At the end of the story, each child received candy reinforcement and praise for each flash of light that he had received. The visual attention span for each member of the group increased significantly. In order to compare the effectiveness of social reinforcement in increasing attention span, the process was repeated using only social reinforcement as a reward. The response rates decreased initially, then gradually began to increase, although they never reached the level attained when visual attention span was contingent on candy reinforcement. To date, the research on attention span indicates that span is responsive to reinforcement, particularly if the reinforcer is a primary one. A more detailed description of this study is given in the section on Reinforcement Strategies.

Focus of Attention

A few researchers have attempted to modify focus of attention behavior in hyperactive children. In one such study, Knowles and Prutsman (1968) developed a two-part reinforcement program in order to bring focus of attention behavior for correctly copying numbers and letters under the control of a positive reinforcer. The youngster being treated was reported to have a history of excessive out-of-seat behaviors as well as having been reported to reverse every number and letter that he copied. In the first part of the study, Knowles and Prutsman used positive reinforcement to increase the child's span for sitting. Out-of-seat behaviors were ignored while positive reinforcement was given for remaining seated. Once attention span for sitting had increased to a level which allowed for reinforcement of focus behaviors, Knowles and Prutsman made positive reinforcement contingent on correctly forming letters. This was truly a focus of attention task because the reinforcement contingency required the child to discriminate between the stimuli which he was to copy. The child's task required him to identify the relevant characteristics of the stimulus to be copied and to reproduce those characteristics in the correct manner. For instance, he had to discriminate between the letter "D" and the letter "B" in order to receive reinforcement. Continuous reinforcement and variable ratio reinforcement were received for the correct formation of numbers and letters. Not only did the focus of attention responses increase significantly during the testing period, but the high rate of correct focus responses maintained itself over a six-week period even though positive primary reinforcement had been discontinued at the end of the reinforcement stage of the study. In addition to the reported increases in focus of attention responses, an important conclusion for this study was that attention span training was a prerequisite to reinforcement of focus behavior. Indeed, it is unlikely that the subject's focus of attention would have improved significantly had the authors not addressed themselves to the need to increase attention span for sitting behaviors.

Brown (1968) reported a study which clearly demonstrated the relationship between positive reinforcement and focus of attention. In this particular study, four mentally retarded, hyperactive, deaf youngsters received positive reinforcement for correctly imitating the vowel and consonant sounds made by a speech therapist. This study clearly related to focus of attention behaviors because it required the subjects to identify and reproduce the relevant characteristics of lip and tongue movements in order to produce the desired sound. During the training period, correct imitative responses were followed by primary reinforcement. Incorrect responses were ignored. The result was a significant improvement in the children's ability to focus their attention on the relevant characteristics of speech behaviors.

Selective Attention

The number of studies reporting the use of learning theory to increase selective attention responses has been limited. Nelson (1969) used positive reinforcement with a group of hyperactive subjects of average intelligence, in the hope of increasing the frequency of correct responses to a two-stage stimulus discrimination task. In this study, subjects were required to discriminate the relevant characteristics of the test stimulus, i.e., dimension. The second stage of the discrimination task required them to compare the dimensions of several test stimuli in order to differentiate between them on the basis of their cues. In other words, the task of the subject was to observe the test stimulus in order to identify which of its characteristics matched those of several other stimuli presented after the observation period. The task was a two-stage stimulus discrimination task in that it required the subject first to respond to the correct dimension of the test stimulus and then to discover the specific stimulus characteristics of that dimension which made it appear different from the other nearly identical stimuli. Prior to training, the performances of the experimental subjects and a matched group of control subjects were compared. The control subjects, as would be expected, performed significantly better at this stage of the experiment. During the training phase of the study, experimental subjects received positive reinforcement for correct two-stage stimulus discrimination responses. These subjects were observed to have made gains in increasing the frequency of observing responses, in canvassing the array of alternatives more equitably and in taking into account a greater amount of information before making a response. A comparison between the performances of the two groups after training revealed that there were no significant differences. In other words, positive reinforcement was a significant factor in increasing selective attention behaviors in hyperactive subjects.

Combined Dimensions

To date, two studies have been reported in which there has been an attempt made to increase the attention span, focus of attention and selective attention behaviors in the same group of subjects. Alabiso (1975) used positive reinforcement to increase attention span, focus of attention and selective attention behaviors in a group of mentally retarded, institutionalized, hyperactive youngsters. Positive token reinforcement was made contingent upon attention span for sitting behaviors. This phase of the training program was enforced for ten 30-minute training sessions. Following a thirty-minute extinction session, training for focus of attention was begun. During this phase of the study, the subjects received token and social reinforcement for correct responses on an eye-hand coordination task. In addition, the subjects continued to receive concurrent token reinforcement for attention span for sitting behavior during this phase of the study. In other words, the subjects were simultaneously rewarded for both attention span behaviors and correct focus of attention responses during this phase of the study. During the third phase of the study, subjects received token and social reinforcement for correct two-stage stimulus discrimination responses. The response-reinforcement ratio for attention span training also remained in effect. At this point, the subjects received positive reinforcement for attention span behaviors while being reinforced for making correct selective attention responses. Each of the reinforcement phases for attention span, focus of attention, and selective attention behaviors were followed by periods in which no reinforcement was available. Several days later, subjects were observed in their home classrooms. Attention span for sitting, focus of attention for eye-hand coordination tasks similar to the one used during training, and selective attention responses were recorded during a generalization period. All three forms of attention responses were reported to have increased as a result of the training sessions. In addition, the high rate of attention responses decreased little during the extinction periods. Finally, trends towards improved attention span, selective attention and focus of attention behaviors maintained themselves throughout the generalization period. Alabiso concluded that attention span, focus of attention and selective attention behaviors could safely be identified as learned responses which were subject to modification. A more detailed description of this project is provided, in the section on Reinforcement Strategies, as a suggested guide for classroom application.

In another study devoted to increasing all three forms of attention behaviors, Reeves (1973) sought to measure the effectiveness of various types of reinforcement on increasing attention behaviors. The performances of three groups of moderately retarded hyperactive youngsters, matched on age, sex and IQ, were compared. The first group received training under a reinforcement-punishment response contingency. These subjects received positive reinforcement for correct responses while also receiving punishment, i.e. negative reinforcement, for incorrect responses. The second group received positive reinforcement only for correct responses. Incorrect responses were followed by non-reinforcement. The third group received punishment for incorrect responses and non-reinforcement for correct responses. Standardized tasks of attention span, focus of attention and selective attention behaviors were performed by all three groups. Based on the research findings of Meyer and Offenbach (1962) and Harter, Brown and Zigler (1971), Reeves predicted that the group which received punishment would show the greatest gain in selective attention. Reeves further predicted that punishment and reinforcement would differentially affect the subjects' performance on measures of attention span, focus of attention and selective attention. This prediction in itself was important in that it pointed to a general theory which viewed the three attention responses as separate behaviors which would respond differentially to various types of reinforcement. The outcome of this study clearly pointed out that neither punishment alone nor punishment combined without reinforcement significantly increased attention span. Furthermore, no significant differences were found between the three groups for focus of attention behaviors. Although focus of attention was affected by reinforcement, punishment alone was not a sufficiently potent reinforcer to produce the response rate necessary to differentiate this method of reinforcement from either positive reinforcement or the combination of positive and negative reinforcement. With respect to selective attention, there was a general trend for the reinforcement-punishment group to produce a greater number of correct responses than the punishment group. The reinforcement group yielded a response rate midway between the reinforcement-punishment group and the punishment group. The importance of this study lies in the fact that it attempted to alter three different types of attention behaviors by using operant techniques. As can be seen from the differential effects of the various types of reinforcement on each of these attention behaviors, much work needs to be done before we will fully understand each of the different types of attention and how they respond to various stimulus variables, reinforcement variables and subject variables.

Distractibility

Research in the area of distractibility as such has been minimal. Indeed, the concept of distractibility is so linked to the concept of attention that most studies refer to the measurement of reduction of distractibility in terms of increased performance on attention tasks. It does appear that the concept of attention includes distractibility, because these behaviors are usually considered to be reciprocal inhibitors of one another. Learning theory studies on distractibility for this reason are confounded with research on attention. Unfortunately, no research study on the relationship of learning theory to distractibility has provided a direct measure of this response. On the contrary, the few studies that have been completed measure distractibility in terms of increases or decreases in attention behaviors.

As the body of knowledge and the technology surrounding research in attention-distraction increase, we may expect to develop a direct measure of distractibility. For the present, we are forced to content ourselves with indirect measures of distractibility. In one such study, Martin and Powers (1967) sought to measure the effectiveness of positive reinforcement in increasing attention span for lever-pressing in a mentally retarded subject. Using the traditional distraction method, a distracter was instructed to sit across the table from a mentally retarded subject who was being reinforced for pressing a lever. Both subjects were instructed that the task was to continue lever pressing, with the distractor having been previously instructed to attempt to divert the experimental subject's attention. As might be expected, the experimental subject's response rate initially decreased greatly as a result of the instruction of the distractor. However, as the loss of reinforcement resulting from the reduction of lever pressing increased, the experimental subject's response rate returned to the predistraction level. As mentioned above, distractibility in this study was measured in terms of attention span for lever pressing.

In another study, Walker and Buckley (1968) sought to reduce distractibility in a hyperactive boy of average intelligence by reinforcing attention span for observing and operating a teaching machine. Prior attempts at reducing distractibility in this particular child included placement in special education classes as well as involvement in a token economy program. In their study, Walker and Buckley attempted to reduce distractibility by rewarding the subject with a checkmark for every ten seconds that he continued to look at and operate a teaching machine. Checkmarks were exchangeable for toys. The authors reported significant increases in visual attention span in the testing situation. Furthermore, visual attention span responses generalized to the classroom setting. Perhaps the most important observation regarding this study was that the authors attempted to reduce distractibility by reinforcing those attention behaviors which were thought to be incompatible with high rates of distraction responses.

Conclusion

Unfortunately, there have been no other major studies which have investigated the interaction between attention and distractibility. At this point in the development of research in this area, we are forced to look at these two behaviors as dimensions along a continuum. Hopefully, as our understanding of these behaviors and our technology of measurement improves, we will be able to view them more clearly as separate, interdependent processes. In the next section, four reinforcement strategies, adaptable to classroom use, will be presented. While the strategies presented are representative of research in the area of attention and distractibility, no one of the strategies presents a comprehensive treatment approach that works simultaneously with attention deficits and distractibility. This is representative of our current level of research knowledge in these areas. Hopefully, future research will produce studies which measure the behavioral parameters of each of these responses along with their physiological correlation and the interaction between them.

REINFORCEMENT STRATEGIES

The simultaneous acceleration of attention behavior along with extinction of distraction responses usually calls for a reciprocal inhibition learning model. That is, in such strategies, positive reinforcement is used to increase attention behavior. The increase in attention behavior becomes inhibitory of distraction responses due to the fact that the performance of attention behaviors is incompatible with distraction responses.

Reinforcement

Studies which modify attention span behaviors use the length of time that a child spends at a given task as the measure of behavior change. Such studies are usually characterized by the use of interval schedules or reinforcements. In other words, the frequency of reinforcement is contingent on the length of time that the child spends engaged in a given behavior. Fixed reinforcement schedules are those in which the subject is reinforced after a preset interval of continuous responding. Such schedules of reinforcement can be expected to initially produce brief periods of attention span behavior followed by short intervals of distractibility. As the child continues to be rewarded under this schedule, it can be expected that the length of time between distraction responses will increase steadily until engaged in a given behavior. Fixed interval reinforcement schedules are those in which the subject is reinforced after a preset interval of continuous responding. Such schedules of reinforcement can be expected to initially produce brief periods of attention span behavior followed by short intervals of distractibility. As the child continues to be rewarded under this schedule, it can be expected that the length of time between distraction responses will increase steadily until he has reached the point where he is responding continuously between the specified intervals of reinforcement. This "time-telling ability" is characteristic of this schedule reinforcement, and as such usually produces good attention span behaviors but only for the specified interval.

Generally speaking, variable interval schedules of reinforcement produce more consistent continuous response rates. The variable interval or intermittent interval schedule of reinforcement is one in which the period of time between the last response and the next reinforcement varies from trial to trial. The time between reinforcements approximates an average time interval. However, the subject never knows on any given trial when the reinforcement will occur. Although the rate of learning attention span behaviors is not quite as rapid as it would be on a fixed interval schedule, a variable intermittent interval of reinforcement produces a rather steady rate of attention span behaviors over a long period of time. Furthermore, attention span behaviors learned under this schedule of reinforcement maintain themselves for a longer period of time after the reinforcement is withdrawn completely.

In the strategies which are presented below, schedules of reinforcement play an important role in attention span behaviors. Likewise, schedules of reinforcement play an important role in the acceleration of other forms of attention behaviors. Both focus of attention responses and selective attention responses are measured in terms of the frequency of correct responses. As was the case with attention span behaviors, focus of attention behaviors and selective attention behaviors may be increased directly, according to the schedule of reinforcement used. A fixed ratio of reinforcement schedules is one in which reinforcement is made contingent upon producing a prespecified number of correct responses. On this reinforcement schedule, we can expect the child to gradually make an increasing number of correct responses. Eventually, once the child has "learned" the relationship between the number of responses and the reinforcement, we can expect to see consistent high rates of correct responses.

The variable ratio schedule of reinforcement is one in which the number of correct responses necessary to produce a reinforcement varies from one trial to the next. In other words, the number of responses necessary to produce a reinforcement changes from trial to trial. This schedule usually produces an initial high frequency of correct responses. Once the response has been learned, we can expect selective attention and focus of attention responses to be retained with a high frequency when the reinforcement varies from trial to trial.

Unfortunately, we have no such clear-cut measures of learning when it comes to distractibility. This is primarily due to the fact that, other than the work of Kaspar, distractibility has mainly been defined in terms of a decrease in frequency of attention responses. Thus, the degree of distractibility has been inferred by the degree of attention responses present. Although the research of Kaspar and his associates has moved the measurability of distractibility in the proper direction, the unit of response for the measurement of distractibility has not been defined clearly enough to allow for a separate measure of distractibility. In the studies presented below, distractibility will be most commonly measured in terms of the decrease in the frequency and number of correct attention responses.

STRATEGY I: REINFORCEMENT OF ATTENTION SPAN BEHAVIORS ACCOMPANIED BY NON-REINFORCEMENT OF DISTRACTION RESPONSES —A RECIPROCAL INHIBITION MODEL. Quay, Spague, Werry and McQueen (1967) sought to increase the duration of visual attention span in a group of five hyperactive youngsters of average intelligence who were enrolled in a special class for children with behavior disorders. The subjects ranged in age from six years one month to nine years three months. All had been diagnosed as being hyperactive. The experiment took place over a period of 130 days. During the baseline phase, all subjects were seated at their desks in a semicircle around the teacher who read a story. Each desk was equipped with a green light which was controlled by a remote switch operated by the experimenter who sat in the back of the classroom. During the reinforcement period, the experimenter operated the lever, which flashed the green light for each interval of ten continuous seconds that the subject observed the teacher as she read. In other words, each of the children was reinforced for visual attention span. The number of light flashes were recorded, and at the end of the reading session each child received candy reinforcement for each flash of light earned. At the end of each experimental session, the child was told his score and given praise as well as candy reinforcement. As soon as each of the children was making consistent, ten-second attention span responses, the next interval of reinforcement was increased by five seconds. During this phase of the study, each of the children had to exhibit fifteen seconds of visual attention span in order to receive reinforcement. At the end of forty-five such sessions, candy reinforcement and the flash of light were withdrawn. During the remaining reinforcement sessions, only the social reinforcement (praise) was offered for correct attention span responses. During the final phase of the study, all forms of primary and secondary reinforcements were withheld.

The results of this study indicated that all of the subjects demonstrated a significant increase in attention span behaviors when candy and social reinforcement were made contingent on attention responses. The results also indicated that the duration of attention span responses decreased slightly when social reinforcement was the only reward offered. While the duration of attention span responses increased overtime during this phase of the study, the overall level of correct responses never reached the level which was attained when both candy and social reinforcements were available. Nevertheless, the duration of visual attention span responses was significantly better during this stage than it was during the baseline period. During the extinction phase of the study, the duration of attention span responses increased gradually at first even though no reinforcement was available. However, over the last two experimental sessions of this phase of the study, the duration of attention span behaviors decreased markedly. It is significant that even during the final stages of extinction, the overall duration of visual attention span responses was significantly higher than the duration of these responses during the baseline period. While there was no direct measure of distractibility in this study, it can be inferred from the authors' comments that the frequency of distractibility responses decreased with increases in the duration of attention span.

STRATEGY II: EXTINCTION OF DISTRACTIBILITY RESPONSES

THROUGH POSITIVE REINFORCEMENT OF ATTENTION SPAN BEHAVIORS WITH PRIMARY AND SECONDARY REINFORCEMENT AND FIXED INTERVAL AND VARIABLE INTERVAL SCHEDULES OF REINFORCEMENT. The research of Walker and Buckley (1968) aptly demonstrated the extinction of distractibility responses by treating attention span behaviors as reciprocal inhibitors of these responses. The subject of this study was a nine-year-old hyperactive boy of bright-normal intelligence. This youngster had been described as exhibiting frequent disruptive classroom behaviors and was observed to attend to classroom assignments only 42 percent of the time. The child had been placed in a special class for children with behavioral problems. During the course of his enrollment in the special class, his social skills and academic achievement improved satisfactorily. However, the high frequency of distractibility responses which he had emitted had not been reduced in spite of the fact that he was maintained on a token reinforcement program for appropriate classroom behaviors.

During the first phase of the study, the child left his classroom each day for reinforcement sessions which took place in a smaller room in which the number of social distractors was significantly decreased. During the reinforcement sessions, the child received fixed interval reinforcement for the length of time that he spent using a teaching machine to work on math problems. Throughout this stage of the training, the child received token reinforcement for every ten seconds during which no distraction responses were emitted. Tokens were exchanged for trinkets at the end of the session. Each time the child reached a criterion of twenty reinforcements, the interval between reinforcements was increased thirty seconds. Finally, during the last phase of the study, only attention span intervals of sixty seconds or more were reinforced. In this phase, the average length of time of distraction-free responding approximated sixty seconds. The reinforcement during this phase of the study was offered on a variable interval schedule such that there were times when the subject was required to respond for several minutes between reinforcements.

The results of this study indicated that the child made significant decreases in the number of distraction responses. Indeed, the duration of attention responses increased from a baseline of 42 percent of total attending time to a high of 93 percent total attending time. During the extinction phase, the duration of attention span responses decreased from the reinforcement phase high of 93 percent to an average of 44 percent. The effectiveness of attention behaviors reinforcement in decreasing distractibility responses speaks for itself.

Walker and Buckley continued to reinforce the child for attention span responses after he returned to the classroom. During the follow-up phase, the child received variable interval reinforcement for attention span responses. After only ten minutes of reinforcement on this schedule, the duration of attention span behaviors attained during the reinforcement phase of the study returned. Walker and Buckley noted that this rate maintained itself even though the classroom setting included many more distractors than the child had encountered in the experimental room.

Their research has practical applications for the classroom teacher. Reinforcement of the length of time that the hyperactive child spends at a given task for either specified or varying intervals would act to increase attention span while decreasing distractibility.

STRATEGY III. CONCURRENT POSITIVE REINFORCEMENT OF FOCUS OF ATTENTION BEHAVIORS AND ATTENTION SPAN BEHAVIORS. Packard (1970) sought to simultaneously increase the duration of attention span and the frequency of correct focus of attention responses in the same group of subjects. Packard worked with groups of normal youngsters who were enrolled in kindergarten, third, fifth and sixth grade classes. Although he did not state it as such, Packard defined attention responses in such a way that called for the simultaneous reinforcement of attention span behaviors and focus of attention behaviors. He defined attention as occurring when the students' bodily position was appropriate to and directed towards the designated academic stimuli, i.e. the child was to be properly seated and looking at the teacher.

Additionally, he defined attention as responding appropriately to instructions. In other words, attention was defined as the length of time that each child spent properly seated looking at the teacher, and as the correct number of responses the child made in following instructions.

The study was set up in such a way that the teacher placed a kitchen timer at the front of the classroom. The time was turned on only when all children met the criteria for attention. That is, when all were properly seated, looking at the teacher and correctly following instructions. If one or more of the children was not engaged in both these forms of attention, the timer was turned off. After the baseline period, the timer was set for a specified fixed interval. During this phase of the study, the entire class was reinforced if the timer went off. In other words, all children had to be properly seated, looking at the teacher and correctly completing instructions for a specified fixed interval in order to be reinforced. Packard measured the effectiveness of reinforcement in terms of the amount of time spent in both forms of attention over the total amount of class time. Cumulative attention time was tallied from the timers in order to determine the percentage of attention time. During the reinforcement phase of the study, children in all the classes were instructed that they had to attend by being properly seated, looking at the teacher and correctly following instructions for a specified percentage of class time. When the criterion was reached for three successive trials, the interval was increased by 5 percent. Reinforcement was given at the end of the classroom period. The fifth and sixth grade children underwent a third phase of training. During extinction, these youngsters received no reinforcement for correct responses. Following this phase, the reinforcement was reinstated along with a negative reinforcement contingency. This contingency called for a fine of three tokens for each child who was not exhibiting the attention behaviors.

As might be expected from the other studies reviewed, the children as a group demonstrated a significant increase in attention span behaviors. The duration for being properly seated while looking at the teacher increased significantly. During the extinction phase, a noticeable decrease in attention behaviors was exhibited. Interestingly enough, the reinstatement of the reinforcement period which was experienced by the fifth and sixth graders resulted in a significant increase in attention behaviors. These youngsters exhibited an average increase of 90 percent in their behaviors during phase three. The overall gain for all groups of children was between 70 and 80 percent.

Unfortunately, Packard confounded the results of his study by using time length spent in attention behaviors as the unit of measure for both attention span and focus of attention responses. In other words, he attempted to measure the focus of attention responses (correctly following instructions) in terms of the length of time that these responses were in evidence, rather than in terms of the correct number of responses. Had the responses been measured as separate units, the results may have been even more clear-cut. While the results for focus of attention behaviors were not clear due to the lack of differentiation between span and focus responses, the results do suggest acquisition of attention behaviors in both studies. The value of this study rests primarily in the fact that it is one of the few attempts to reinforce both forms of attention simultaneously. Here again, the approach of bringing two types of attention behaviors simultaneously under control could be valuable for the classroom teacher. The use of the timer along with the system for reinforcing correct focus responses in an entire classroom of students has shown itself to significantly decrease both short attention span and errors in focus of attention responses.

STRATEGY IV: POSITIVE REINFORCEMENT OF ATTENTION SPAN, FOCUS OF ATTENTION AND SELECTIVE ATTENTION BEHAVIORS UTILIZING INCREASING FIXED INTERVAL REINFORCEMENT AND VARIABLE RATIO REINFORCEMENT. Alabiso (1975) sought to substantiate the hypothesis that attention span, focus of attention and selective attention behaviors could be brought under operant control in such a way as to reduce the high frequency of behaviors usually associated with hyperactivity.

Eight mentally retarded, institutionalized hyperactive youngsters ranging in age from eight years three months to twelve years four months, with a mean IQ of 44 and rated as the most hyperactive youngsters in their special education classes were selected for this study. Based on the teachers' requests that the study in some way reduce poor motor coordination, out-of-seat behaviors, and deficits in concept formation, attention span for sitting, focus of attention for correct eye-hand coordination responses, and selective attention for correct two-stage discrimination responses requiring the use of concepts of size, shape and color were targeted as objects of the study.

During the baseline period, all subjects were observed in the classroom. Attention span for sitting was recorded during six 10-minute observation periods. The mean length of sitting time and the average duration of out-of-seat behaviors was calculated at various times over a ten-day period. The baseline for focus of attention consisted of the correct number of responses produced by each child on twenty-five trials of an eye-hand coordination test in which the youngster was required to copy digits and symbols. This task essentially was a single-stage discrimination task. The baseline for selective attention responses consisted of the correct number of responses by all subjects on the last twenty-five trials of a two-stage stimulus discrimination task. This task required the subjects to discriminate between a test stimulus and an array of other stimuli on the basis of the test stimulus' dimension and its cue. Basically, it required the subjects to master the concepts of size, shape and color.

Training took place outside of the classroom in a room designed for the experiment. During attention span training, the experimenter sat across the desk from the subject. A panel containing a red light and a blue light was mounted on the desk slightly to the side of the subject. The blue light remained on for as long as the subject remained seated. The red light flashed, signaling token and social reinforcement whenever the subject had remained seated for a specified fixed interval. Whenever the child left his seat, the blue light was extinguished and not relighted until he was reseated. The subjects were reinforced according to an increased fixed interval schedule (Bijou, 1961). In this segment of the study, subjects were initially required to remain seated for a period approximating the average length of time that the group remained seated during the baseline period. Each time the subjects attained a criteria of five successful (reinforced) trials, the fixed interval was increased by thirty seconds. The training took place over ten 30-minute sessions, followed by one 30-minute extinction session.

Focus of attention training required the subjects to correctly copy digits and symbols in their proper order. This one-stage stimulus discrimination task was preceded by a "warm-up" period of ten reinforced responses. Subjects received continuous reinforcement during the first fifty trials of the training period. Over the next one hundred trials, subjects received fifty trials of fixed ratio three (FR3) reinforcement and fifty trials of fixed ratio five (FR5) reinforcement. In other words, on the first fifty trials of focus of attention training the subjects received a reinforcement for each correct response. Over the next fifty trials, one reinforcement was received for every three correct responses. Finally, over the last fifty trials, one reinforcement was received for every five correct responses. In addition, the subjects were concurrently being reinforced for attention span responses. The subjects received variable interval five-minute reinforcements for attention span for sitting behaviors throughout the focus of attention training. The blue light remained ignited while the red light was flashed on the average of one every five minutes. Subjects received social and token reinforcements for each flash of the red light. The training period was followed by fifty extinction trials.

During selective attention training, subjects were required to complete a two-stage stimulus discrimination task calling for the correct stimulus dimension and the stimulus cue. During this phase of training, the stimulus dimension and the stimulus cue were varied from trial to trial. The actual reinforcement training was preceded by a "warm-up" period in which the subjects received reinforcement for each of ten successful one-stage stimulus discrimination trials. Similar to the reinforcement ratio during the focus of attention training period, subjects underwent fifty continuous reinforcement trials followed by fifty FR3 trials and fifty FR5 trials. Also, the subjects underwent concurrent variable interval five-minute (VI5) reinforcement for attention span for sitting behaviors, similar to the focus of attention procedure. Finally, the training was followed by fifty extinction trials in which no reinforcement was available.

In order to measure the effectiveness of generalizing the reinforcement strategy to the classroom situation, the children were again observed in the classroom for each of the three attention behaviors several days following the training period. Baselines for attention span, focus of attention and selective attention responses were recorded using the method described in the original baseline period.

The results of this study clearly indicated that attention span, focus of attention and selective attention behaviors were dramatically influenced by positive reinforcement. All three of these attention behaviors accelerated rapidly during the reinforcement phase of the study. Only a slight decrease in the duration and frequency of these attention behaviors was noted during the extinction period. In addition, all three of the attention behaviors were observed to have occurred with a higher frequency during the generalization period than they did during the original baseline period. The author did caution, however, that, had the extinction period and the generalization period been of longer duration, the high response rates probably would have given way to the combination of non-reinforcement and the high frequency of competing distraction responses.

Unfortunately, this study made no attempt to study the interactions between the three attention behaviors and distractibility. Nevertheless, it did demonstrate that all the attention behaviors can be brought under operant control. Hopefully, future research in this area will introduce the concept of distractibility into the research design. While the scheduling of reinforcement and the research design for this study were more elaborate than is practical for the average classroom teacher to implement, it does point out that all of the attention behaviors would be treated in the classroom simply by reinforcing the length of time that a subject spends at a given task, while simultaneously reinforcing successful one-stage discrimination responses along with the reinforcement of two-stage discrimination tasks.

SUMMARY

Attention and distractibility may represent separate but associated processes which stand at either end of a theoretical continuum. In view of the fact that there has been a dearth of research in these two areas, we have been forced to assume that these two processes are in some way linked by some cognitive and physiological central process. This assumption will probably stand until disproven. However, it is equally likely that these two processes may be unrelated. Further research is needed to substantiate this hypothesis.

The review of the literature in this chapter has pointed clearly to the conceptualization of attention as a multi-behavioral process involving the length of time that a subject spends at a given task (span), the ability to make correct, simple visual discriminations (focus) and the ability to make complex two-stage stimulus discriminations (selectivity). While there has been much speculation about the interrelationship of these three forms of attention, there has been no firm data base to substantiate the hypothesis that these three behaviors are interdependent. It does seem likely, however that they form a hierarchy of attention. That is, it seems probable that average or above attention span behavior would facilitate the mastery of focus of attention behaviors. In a like manner, average or above attention span and focus of attention would in all likelihood facilitate the mastery of selective attention behaviors. It may be that these processes are not physiologically related, and therefore may act independently of one another. This would explain why some children have exceptionally short attention spans while being able to make the complex two-stage stimulus discriminations necessary for selective attention behaviors. Many important and interesting questions in this area remain unanswered.

In many respects the definition of distractibility has been unclear. It has commonly been thought of as "inattention." From a learning theory point of view, distractibility may be viewed as responses competing with attention, so they have been considered to be reciprocal inhibitors of one another (Alabiso, 1972; Reeves, 1973; Alabiso, 1975). Actually, very little is known about the behavioral and physiological correlations of distractibility. It would be tempting to infer that distractibility is part of a unitary process involving attention. However, the research of Kaspar and his colleagues (1968, 1971, 1972, 1973, 1974, 1975) cautions us against making such assumptions. It is interesting to note, however, that the covariance between attention and certain stimulus and subject variables parallels the covariance between distractibility and these same variables. A particularly important common variable is that of developmental level. This variable seems to underlie all of the primary characteristics associated with hyperactivity. Generally speaking, the higher the developmental level, the greater the degree of attention and the lesser the degree of distractibility.

Within the past several years, Kaspar's research has contributed greatly to our changing concept of distractibility. According to his definition, distractibility may be defined in terms of the efficiency of certain receptor-effector systems in processing incoming and outgoing visual, auditory and tactile stimuli. In other words, distractibility may be defined in terms of the child's ability to accurately perceive incoming stimuli from the world around him and in terms of his ability to accurately respond to these stimuli (Kaspar and Kashaba, 1975). At their present level of development these four measures of distractibility include a test of efficiency in visual input-motor output and auditory input-verbal output systems. While this research is in its early stages of development, the standardization of these tests by developmental level promises to provide much information about distractibility. Kaspar's research in this area is also valuable since it offers an alternative to conceptualizing distractibility as the opposite of attention. One important contribution which has arisen from this area of research has been the differentiation between the behavioral-physiological process of distractibility and the child's response to distracting stimuli. In other words, we must not only consider the process of distractibility itself in evaluating a child's proficiency in this area, but we must also take into consideration that certain stimuli have produced a variety of different distractibility responses. Actually, the introduction of certain distracting stimuli, especially at higher developmental levels, seems to decrease distractibility.

Our review of the literature has demonstrated that all three forms of attention are subject to learning theory and thus can be modified through the use of learning theory techniques. To date, there has been no research to demonstrate that distractibility is a learned behavior which is modifiable through the systematic application of reinforcement techniques. However, it seems likely that future research will confirm that distractibility is a learned response. While the research in these two areas has been rather complex, the use of behavior modification techniques in the classroom to increase various forms of attention while decreasing the high rate of distractibility behaviors should not be too encumbering. Basically, the reinforcement strategy calls for the systematic application of positive reinforcement and withholding of reinforcement, along with various schedules of interval and ratio reinforcement.

REFERENCES

Alabiso, F. P.: Inhibitory functions of attention in reducing hyperactive behavior. *American Journal of Mental Deficiency,* 77:259-282, 1972.

Alabiso, F. P.: Operant control of attention behavior: A treatment for hyperactivity. *Behavior Therapy,* 6:39-42, 1975.

Allport, F.: *Theories of Perception and the Concept of Structure.* New York, Wiley, 1955.

Bekhterev, V. K.: *Objective Psychology.* Leipzig, Teubner, 1913.

Berlyne, D. A.: Stimulus intensity in attention in relation to learning theory. *Quarterly Journal of Experimental Psychology,* 2:71-75, 1950.

Berlyne, D. A.: Attention, perception and behavior theory. *Psychological Review,* 58:137-146, 1951.

Bestor, M. L.: A study of attention in young children. *Child Development,* 5:368-380, 1934.

Bijou, S. L.: Rapid development of multiple schedule performances with mentally retarded children. *Journal of Experimental Analysis of Behavior,* 8:7-17, 1961.

Broadbent, D. E.: A mechanical model for human attention and immediate memory. *Psychological review,* 9:205-215, 1957.

Brooks, D. T., Morrow, J. W., and Gray, W. G.: Reduction of autistic gaze aversion by reinforcement of visual attention responses. *Journal of Special Education,* 2:307-309, 1968.

Brown, D. C.: *Operant conditioning of attending and verbal imitation of deaf children with deviant behaviors.* (Doctoral dissertation, University of Illinois) Ann Arbor, Michigan, University Microfilm, 1968, No. 68-8031.

Brown, M. P.: Continuous reaction as a measurement of attention. *Child Development, 1*:255-291, 1930.

Burnham, W. H.: Attention and interest. *American Journal of Psychology, 19*:14-18, 1908.

Cromwell, R. L., and Foshee, J. G.: Studies in activity level. IV. Effects of visual stimulation during task performance in mental defectives. *American Journal of Mental Deficiency, 65*:248-251, 1960.

Crosby, K. G., and Blatt, B. I.: Attention and mental retardation. *Journal of Education, 150*:67-81, 1968.

Dashiell, J. N.: *Fundamentals of Objective Psychology.* Boston, HM, 1928, p. 285.

Deutsch, J. D., and Deutsch, D. R.: Attention: Some theoretical considerations. *Psychological Review, 70*:80-90, 1963.

Egeth, E.: Selective attention. *Psychological Bulletin, 67*:41-57, 1967.

Ellis, N. R., and Pryer, M. S.: Primary vs. secondary discrimination learning in mental defectives. *Psychological Reports, 4*:67-70, 1958.

Ellis, N. R., Giardeau, F. L., and Prior, M. W.: Analysis of learning sets in normal and severely defective humans. *Journal of Comparative and Physiological Psychology, 55*:860-865, 1962.

Ellis, N. R., Hawkins, C. W., and Jones, R. P.: Distraction affects in oddity learning by normal and mentally defective humans. *American Journal of Mental Deficiency, 3*:576-583, 1963-1967.

Fechnerl, E. T.: Psycho-physidiza. In Geissler, L. R.: The measurement of attention. *American Journal of Psychology, 2*:473-529, 1854.

Fisher, L. R.: *A comparison of matched groups of brain-damaged children on externally validated attention measures.* (Doctoral dissertation, University of Cincinnati) Ann Arbor, Michigan, University Microfilm, 1969, No. 69-6338.

Foshee, J. G.: Studies in activity level: In simple and complex task performances in defectives. *American Journal of Mental Deficiency, 62*: 882-886, 1958.

Gardner, W. I., Cromwell, R. L., and Foshee, J. G.: Studies in activity level. II. Effects of distil visual stimulation in organics familials and hyperactives. *American Journal of Mental Deficiency, 63*:1028-1033, 1959.

Geissler, L. R.: The measurement of attention. *American Journal of Psychology, 20*:473-529, 1909.

Harlow, H. F.: Learning set and error factor theory. In Koch, S. (Ed.): *Psychology: A Strategy of Science,* Vol. 2, New York, McGraw, 492-537, 1959.

Harter, S., Brown, L., and Zigler, E.: The discrimination learning of normal and retarded children as a function of penalty condition and etiology of the retarded. *Child Development, 42*:517-536, 1971.

Hebb, D. O.: *The Organization of Behavior.* New York, Wiley, 1948, pp. 236-251.

Herring, A. T., and Koch, H. S.: A study of some factors influencing the interest span of preschool children. *Journal of Genetic Psychology, 38*:249-275, 1930.

Hermelin, D. C., and O'Connor, N. R.: The response of self-generated behavior of disturbed children in severely subnormal control. *British Journal of Social and Clinical Psychology, 2*:37-43, 1963.

James, W.: *Principals of Psychology.* New York, Hope, 1890.

Jensen, A. L.: Learning ability in retarded, average, and gifted children. *Merrill Palmer Quarterly, 9*:123-140, 1963.

Johnson, H. M.: Definition and measurement of attention. *American Journal of Psychology, 36*:601-614, 1925.

Kagan, J. W., and Huntsman, N. J.: Selective attention in mental retardates. *Developmental Psychology, 5*:151-160, 1971.

Kaspar, J. C.: *Research in distractibility and activity level: A review.* Paper presented at the proceedings of the 86th Annual Convention American Psychological Association, New Orleans, September, 1968.

Kaspar, J. C., Millichap, J. G., Backus, R., Child, D., and Schulman, J. L.: A study of the relationships between neurological evidence of brain damage in children and activity in distractibility. *Journal of Consulting and Clinical Psychology, 3*:329-337, 1971.

Kaspar, J. C., and Schulman, J. L.: Organic mental disorder: Brain damages. In Wolman, B. B. (Ed.): *Psychopathology of Childhood.* New York, McGraw, 1972, pp. 207-229.

Kaspar, J. C.: *The relationship between activity level and distractibility and performance on WISC in a sample of children with neurological dysfunctions.* Paper presented at the proceedings of the 81st Annual Convention of the American Psychological Association, Washington, D.C., September, 1973.

Kaspar, J. C., Personal communication, 1974.

Kaspar, J. C., and Koshaba, J. E.: *Distractibility.* Unpublished research, 1975.

Kassinove, H. O.: Developmental attention tests: A preliminary report on objective test of attention. *Journal of Clinical Psychology, 24*:76-78, 1968.

Kaufman, M. E., and Peterson, W. M.: Acquisition of a learning set by normal and mentally retarded children. *Journal of Comparative and Physiological Psychology, 51*:619-621, 1958.

Kennedy, D. A., and Thompson, I. J.: Use of Reinforcement techniques with a first-grade boy. *Personnel Guidance Journal, 46*:366-370, 1967.

Knowles, P. K., and Prutsman, T. D.: Behavior modification of simple hyperkinetic behavior and letter discrimination in a hyperactive child. *Journal of School Psychology,* 6:157-160, 1968.

Kulpe, O. A.: Outline of psychology. In Giessler, L. R.: The measurement of attention. *American Journal of Psychology,* 20:473-529, 1895.

Leontiev, A. N.: The development of voluntary attention in children. *Journal of Genetic Psychology,* 40:52-83, 1932.

Lipps, A. S.: Grudtatshere d seelenlebens. In Geissler, L. R.: The measurement of attention. *American Journal of Psychology,* 20:473-529, 1883.

Martin, G. L., and Powers, R. P.: Attention span: An operant conditioning analysis. *Exceptional Children,* 33:565-570, 1967.

Mentz, L. N.: Philosophical studies. In Geissler, L. R.: The measurement of attention. *American Journal of Psychology,* 2:473-529, 1893.

Meyer, W. J., and Offenbach, S. I.: Effectiveness of reward and punishment as a function of task complexity. *Journal of Comparative and Physiological Psychology,* 55:532-534, 1962.

Milner, B., and Penfield, W.: *The effects of Hippocampal lesions on recent memory.* Transactions of American Neurological Association, 80:42-48, 1955.

Moyer, K. G., and Gilmer, B. S.: The concept of attention spans of children. *Elementary School Journal,* 54:464-466, 1954.

Moyer, K. G., and Gilmer, B. S.: Attention spans of children for experimentally designed toys. *Journal of Genetic Psychology,* 87:187-201, 1955.

Nelson, T. O.: *The effects of training in attention deployment on observing behavior in reflective and impulsive children.* (Doctoral dissertation, University of Minnesota) Ann Arbor, Michigan, University Microfilms, 1969, No. 69-2659.

Obersteiner, H. B.: Experimental researches in attention. *Brain,* 1:439-453, 1879.

O'Donnell, J. P.: Observing hyphen response training and subsequent discrimination performance. *Child Development,* 40:191-199, 1969.

Packard, R. F.: The control of classroom attention: a group contingency for complex behavior. *Journal of Applied Behavior Analysis,* 3:13-28, 1970.

Pillsbury, W. C.: *Attention.* New York, Macmillan, 1896, p. 346.

Quay, H. F., Spague, R. D., Werry, J. S., and McQueen, M. W.: Conditioning visual orientation to conduct problem children in the classroom. *Journal of Exceptional Children,* 5:512-517, 1967.

Reeves, J. L.: *The effect of reinforcement and punishment on retardate attention and discrimination learning.* (Doctoral dissertation, Texas Technical University) Lubbock, Texas, 1973.

Ross, A. C.: The application of behavior principles in therapeutic education. *Journal of Special Education,* 1:276-286, 1967.
Schrater, H. A.: A method for measuring the sustained attention of preschool children. *Journal of Genetic Psychology,* 42:339-371, 1933.
Schulman, J. L., Kaspar, J. C., and Thorne, F. M.: *Brain Damage and Behavior.* Springfield, Thomas, 1965.
Sirvastava, R. K.: *The effectiveness of the type of reinforcement and the function of mental age.* (Doctoral dissertation, University of Kansas) Ann Arbor, Michigan, University Microfilms, 1968, No. 68-1796.
Skinner, B. F.: *Science and Human Behavior.* New York, Macmillan, 1965.
Strauss, A. A., and Lehtinen, L. E.: *Psychopathology and Education of the Brain-Injured Child.* New York, Grune, 1947.
Strauss, A., and Kephart, N. C.: *Psychopathology and Education of the Brain-Injured Child,* Vol. II. New York, Greun, 1955.
Stumpf, T.: *Tonpsychologie.* II. In Geissler, L. R.: The measurement of attention. *American Journal of Psychology,* 20:473-529, 1890.
Sullwold, F. R.: Contribution to an analysis of attention. *Zeitschritt Fuer Experimentelle und Angewandte,* 2:495-513, 1954.
Sully, P. N.: Outlines of psychology. In Geissler, L. R.: The measurement of attention. *American Journal of Psychology,* 20:473-529, 1885.
Titchner, E. B.: *Experimental Psychology.* New York, Macmillan, 1908, p. 189.
Tizard, B. E.: Observation of over-active imbecile children in controlled and uncontrolled environments. I. Classroom studies. *American Journal of Mental Deficiency,* 540-547, 1968-1972a.
Tizard, B. E.: Observation of over-active imbecile children in controlled and uncontrolled environments. II. Experimental studies. *American Journal of Mental Deficiencies,* 72:548-553, 1968b.
Turnure, A. E.: *Children's reactions to distraction: A developmental approach.* (Doctoral dissertation, Yale University) Ann Arbor, Michigan, University Microfilms, 1966, No. 66-4940.
Turnure, J. E., and Zigler, E. F.: Outer directedness in problem solving of normal and retarded children. *Journal of Abnormal and Social Psychology,* 4:427-436, 1964.
Wachtel, P. M.: Conceptions of broad and narrow attention. *Psychological Bulletin,* 68:417-429, 1967.
Walker, H. A., and Buckley, N. S.: The use of positive reinforcement in conditioning attention behavior. *Journal of Applied Behavior Analysis,* 1:245-250, 1968.
White, S. H., and Plum, G. E.: Eye movement photography during children's discrimination learning. *Journal of Experimental Psychology,* 1:327-338, 1964.

Woodrow, H. R.: The measurement of attention. *Psychological Monograph.* 17(No. 76):6-34, 1914.

Wright, A. C., and Dahler, M. S.: *Shaping children's observing behavior for an oddity problem learning set.* Paper presented at the meeting of the Psychonomics Society, St. Louis, October, 1966.

Wright, A. C., and Smothergill, D.: Observing behavior and children's discrimination learning under delayed reinforcement. *Journal of Experimental Child Psychology,* 5:430-440, 1967.

Wunt, W.: *Vorleswngen.* Berline, Kline, Vol. 1, 1892.

Zeaman, P. O., and House, B. A.: The role of attention in retardate discrimination learning. In Ellis, N. R. (Ed.): *Handbook of Mental Deficiency.* New York, McGraw, 1963.

CHAPTER 5

COGNITIVE DYSFUNCTION IN HYPERACTIVE CHILDREN

COGNITIVE DYSFUNCTIONS are viewed as specific learning disorders separate from those caused by mental retardation. This chapter will be concerned with the relationship between the specific cognitive dysfunctions exhibited by hyperactive children and their efficiency in learning. It will exclude those cognitive dysfunctions associated with infection, disease or trauma. In effect, the cognitive dysfunctions described will be those associated with lag in physiological development, focusing on a biosocial model which views the hyperactive child in terms of his efficiency of learning within the social environment. We will examine the interaction between the child's lag in physiological development and the learning environment in which he finds himself. Just as we have treated each of the characteristics associated with hyperactivity as separate and at times as unrelated processes, the cognitive dysfunctions will be treated in the same manner. It is very unlikely that all of the cognitive dysfunctions described in this chapter would be found in a single individual. The hyperactive child typically possesses only a few of them.

Since we are viewing the cognitive dysfunctions as variables which lower the child's efficiency in acquiring knowledge, it is important that at each step of the way we take into consideration the numerous social and environmental variables which also affect his efficiency in learning. The nature and content of instructional material, the interpersonal environment and the teacher's attitude are important variables in assessing efficiency of learning. These factors are so important that it is not possible to assess a child's efficiency in learning independently of them.

The importance of early identification of the child with cognitive dysfunction cannot be overstated. Indeed, early identification has proven itself repeatedly to be a crucial factor in determining the child's success in adjusting to special remedial programming. In stressing the importance of early identification of cognitive dysfunctions in hyperactive children, Schrager and Lindy (1970) referred to hyperactive children with cognitive dysfunction as the "population-at-risk." This concept suggested that, given certain negative variables, this population of youngsters was likely to react by developing an increased likelihood of school failure. In other words, given the child's hyperactivity, his specific cognitive dysfunction, a classroom situation not suited to his learning abilities at the primary level and late identification of his dysfunction, the likelihood of school failure and eventual school dropout was high. Using a student population of five hundred kindergarten children from six public schools, Schrager and Lindy used a forty-four-item check list to identify sixty behaviors associated with hyperactivity. The items from the list focused on indicators of minimal cerebral dysfunction, disturbed family dynamics, genetic composition and social pressure. Each of the children were rated by their teachers on the forty-four items on the check list. In addition, pediatricians, teachers, psychologists, psychiatrists and social workers were surveyed in order to obtain consensual validation of six behavioral attributes which they felt are most commonly associated with hyperactivity. These attributes were listed as: being fidgety and restless, inattentive, hard to manage, and the inability to sit still, pay attention and take frustration. Of the five hundred children sampled, those who scored highest on the forty-four-item checklist were targeted as the population-at-risk. Schrager and Lindy had hoped that, by making an in-depth analysis of the school performance and social adjustment of these youngsters, they could identify those factors which when combined would identify the child as a member of the population-at-risk.

The results of this study indicated the presence of four such factors. First, the high-risk children were found to be those children who, in the teacher's opinion, were observed to be fidgety, restless, easily frustrated, hard to manage and unable to sit quietly. These variables were viewed as the skills necessary for achievement of success in a child's early school experience. The second factor related to the interaction between the first factor and the school demands. In effect, the classroom expectations for conformity, adherence to instructions and behavioral control in interaction with the characteristics of the hyperactive child resulted in negative responses from teachers and peers. Schrager and Lindy predicted that this second factor was the basis for the child's negative feelings toward school and himself. The child was identified as having little probability of success in mastering the social demands of the school situation at the kindergarten level. Poor performance on readiness tests was identified as the third factor contributing to a child's likelihood of failure in school. Regardless of the child's level of intelligence, his ability to perform on academic tasks such as tests of readiness was found to be an important factor contributing to his perception of himself and to the perceptions that others maintained of him. Finally, high absenteeism was determined to be the fourth high-risk factor. In studying the population-at-risk, Schrager and Lindy found that hyperactive children had a significantly higher frequency of time absent from school than did non-hyperactive children. A careful study of the hyperactive group's absentee pattern demonstrated that these children are usually absent due to factors other than physical state of health. Indeed, the highest single category of absent hyperactive children were those whose absenteeism could be traced back to a lack of interest in school. In effect, what Schrager and Lindy had pointed out was that the greater the number of factors associated with a particular child, the higher the probability that his school experience would end in failure.

Using a biosocial model of treatment, two strategies aimed at reducing or eliminating the high-risk factors associated with hyperactivity were proposed. First, schools can set up a program for parents. The objective of this program is to sensitize parents to the special school problems of their children. Parent-teacher conferences can be established to share concerns over the child's school performance, and to anticipate the unique problems which were likely to be faced by both parents and teachers. A major job of the teacher and other school learning specialists is to help the parents as well as the child to develop competency in managing behavior. Second, the classroom teacher can receive consultation in helping to assess and cope with the child's behavior. In addition, this phase of the strategy includes helping the teacher to develop special techniques within the classroom that would accomodate the learning environment to the child's needs. In effect, the proposed strategies emphasize familiarization with the factors associated with hyperactivity in order to free the child of his membership in the "population-at-risk."

The remaining sections of this chapter focus on the identification of specific cognitive dysfunctions and classroom approaches to them. The child's ability to learn will be understood in terms of the efficiency of his learning systems. One such system, referred to in this text as the cognitive system, is controlled by the cerebral cortex. This system is controlled by the brain, and as such the cognitive dysfunctions associated with the inefficiency of this system relate to both verbal and nonverbal abilities. The second system, known as the receptor-effector system, relates deficiency in learning to the ability of the child's sense organs to receive, process and respond to environmental stimuli. The third system is one which involves the child's attitudes and learning habits. This threefold process of reception, organization and motor response represents an arc of learning much like an electrical arc. The learning arc requires the efficient interaction of all three processes.

COGNITIVE ABILITIES

Research in the nature of intelligence has shown us that there are at least ten basic cognitive abilities from which all other cognitive skills seem to stem (Wechsler, 1965). While the number of cognitive abilities is probably limited only by our ability to identify them, the ten major cognitive abilities seem to be generic. Presumably, the child's performance on measures of these ten abilities represents his level of intelligence.

Wechsler (1965) and others (Spearman, 1927, and Thurstone, 1947) defined intelligence as the "... measure of the mind's ability to do intellectual work" (p. 12). An understanding of the measurement intelligence is essential to our full comprehension of the hyperactive child. Indeed, it is on tests of intelligence that we are able to make the differentiation between mental retardation and cognitive dysfunction associated with hyperactivity. Typically, the mentally retarded child shows serious deficits on all measures of cognitive ability. The hyperactive child shows deficits in only some of the cognitive abilities, while others continue to function at a high level of efficiency.

Most of the cognitive abilities under the control of the cerebral cortex relate to the use of verbal skills. For instance the information cognitive ability refers to the child's ability to collect, store and retrieve information about the world around him. It requires that he use associative thinking along with a comprehension of facts which are acquired from his environment. While this ability is basically controlled by brain centers, the degree to which it is developed can also be affected by the child's level of interest, cultural background, degree of alertness and motivation for acquiring knowledge. Comprehension ability refers to the child's ability to use previous experiences in dealing with novel situations. This problem-solving ability measures the child's ability to integrate commonsense, judgment and reasoning. It serves as a measure of his adaptability in practical situations.

Arithmetic reasoning ability refers to the child's ability to apply basic arithmetic reasoning processes in personal and social situations. This ability is a complex one as it requires the child to manipulate complex thought patterns, follow verbal directions, concentrate on selected stimuli and utilize abstract concepts of number and numerical operation.

One of the cognitive abilities most central to the overall efficiency in learning is the abstract reasoning ability. This ability requires the child to use both abstract concepts and concrete materials in problem solving. It involves verbal concept formation, the capacity for associative thinking and remote memory. A well-developed abstract reasoning ability helps the child to understand and to formulate concepts for size, color and shape as well as a variety of other concepts. Eventually, developmental maturation helps him to understand the rules for classification of stimuli into conceptual categories. This ability calls for a high degree of abstraction as the child becomes older. The ability to conceptualize abstractly requires him to categorize symbols rather than tangible objects.

The vocabulary ability is one that determines the child's level of understanding of words. It also reflects his level of education and the amount and quality of verbal stimulation available to him in his environment. This area of cognitive functioning serves as a "reservoir" for accumulated verbal learning, range of ideas, fund of information and qualitative levels of reasoning ability.

One of the most important of the cognitive abilities for the child's adaptation to the environment is his ability to comprehend and understand social interactions. This comprehension ability is one which calls for an insight into a total social situation based on visual comprehension and organization of environmental experiences. It requires the child to perceive, evaluate and predict the responses of others based on the social situation in which he finds himself.

A number of other cognitive abilities also are considered in determining a child's level of cognitive dysfunction. These abilities are essentially nonverbal in nature, although they require the use of verbal concepts. One such ability helps the child in the reproduction of visual images. This ability helps the child to perceive, analyze, synthesize and reproduce abstract visual designs. It calls for the utilization of nonverbal concepts, a capacity for sustained effort, visual-motor coordination and abstract as well as concrete thinking. It represents an ability for overall planning and organization.

Another important nonverbal ability is the eye-hand coordination ability, which measures a child's flexibility in new learning situations. This ability requires the child to learn visual and motor skills from repetitive experiences. It brings into play his eye-hand coordination, as well as his ability to absorb new materials in an associative context. It is a general factor which relates to the child's overall psychomotor functioning. This ability is affected by visual-motor dexterity, speed and accuracy.

Finally, the last of the cognitive abilities is that of visual-motor coordination. This ability requires the child to master simple assembly skills while comprehending special relationships. It calls for the synthesization of concrete parts into meaningful wholes. In effect, it relates to his overall skill in generalizing from one learning situation to another.

A critical concept in understanding cognitive development is that of patterning. This concept refers to the relationship between various cognitive abilities. In a child of average intelligence not suffering from any form of cognitive dysfunction, the usual pattern is one in which all of the verbal and nonverbal cognitive abilities are relatively evenly matched. Figure 2 demonstrates graphically the patterning of cognitive abilities associated with normal intellectual development. In this particular example, all of the subtest scores representing the levels at which the various cognitive abilities have developed fall within the average range (scores 9-11).

Scores within the superior area of cognitive development (scores approximately between 11 and 20) are absent. While there is some minor deviation between scores on the various subtests, the overall picture is one in which all of the ten abilities are approximately equally developed. The child shows no exceptionally high scores nor are any significantly low scores represented. Assuming that motivational factors and emotional factors are also within normal limits, one could expect a child having a pattern of cognitive abilities similar to the one depicted in Figure 2 to do average classroom work in all subjects. The importance of patterning lies not in the degree of development of the cognitive abilities but rather in the relationship between various abilities. Of course, when scores are exceptionally high or exceptionally low, the patterns are then associated with superior intelligence or mental retardation respectively.

Figure 3 exemplifies the typical pattern associated with mental retardation. The overall pattern is one in which the majority of the cognitive abilities are poorly developed. While there can be much variability between various cognitive abilities

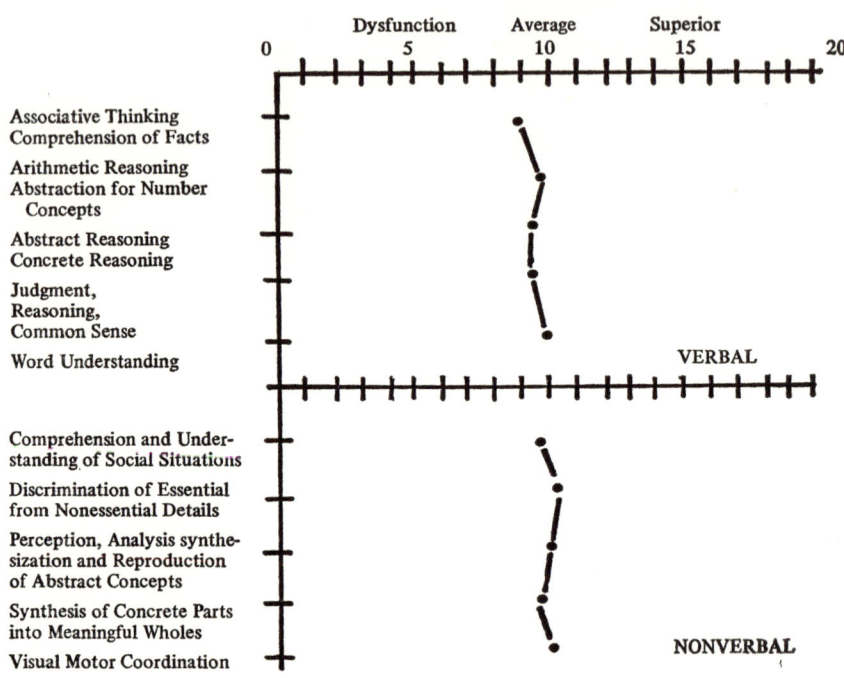

Figure 2. Pattern of cognitive abilities associated with average intellectual development.

in the mentally retarded child, the most common pattern is one in which nearly all of the abilities are fairly evenly matched while being significantly below average. Here again as was the case in Figure 2, the relationship between the various cognitive abilities is one in which they are developed approximately to the same degree.

As is the case with most children suffering from one of the various forms of learning disability, the pattern of cognitive abilities associated with hyperactivity is one that is typified by unevenness of the development of the various cognitive abilities. Even though the average of the verbal abilities may be close to the average of the nonverbal abilities, the pattern is character-

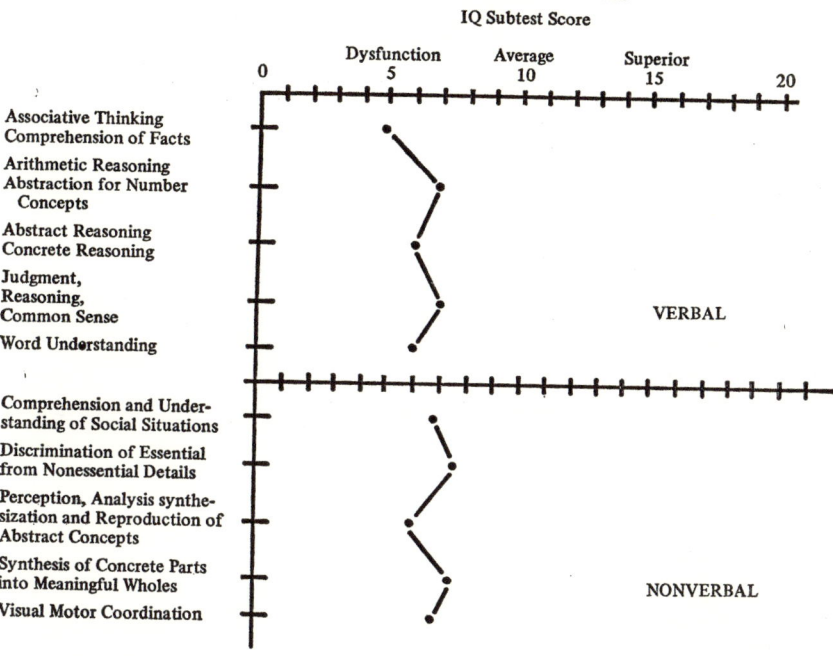

Figure 3. Pattern of cognitive abilities associated with mental retardation.

ized by a wide spread in the scores representing the level of development of the various cognitive abilities. Figure 4 exemplifies this pattern. The verbal and nonverbal abilities span all three of the ranges of cognitive functioning.

In the profile depicted, the child's ability to store and retrieve information is within average limits, while the ability to use previous experiences when dealing with novel situations is within the dysfunctional range. Other abilities such as the ability to synthesize and reproduce abstract concepts may be within a superior range. Even though the average of all of the abilities places the child within the range of average intelligence, he is faced with the fact that his intellectual functioning in certain areas is far below average while his intellectual functioning in other areas is superior. Generally, a five-point difference between various cognitive abilities is significant on tests of intelligence. However, it is quite frequently the case that hyperactive children

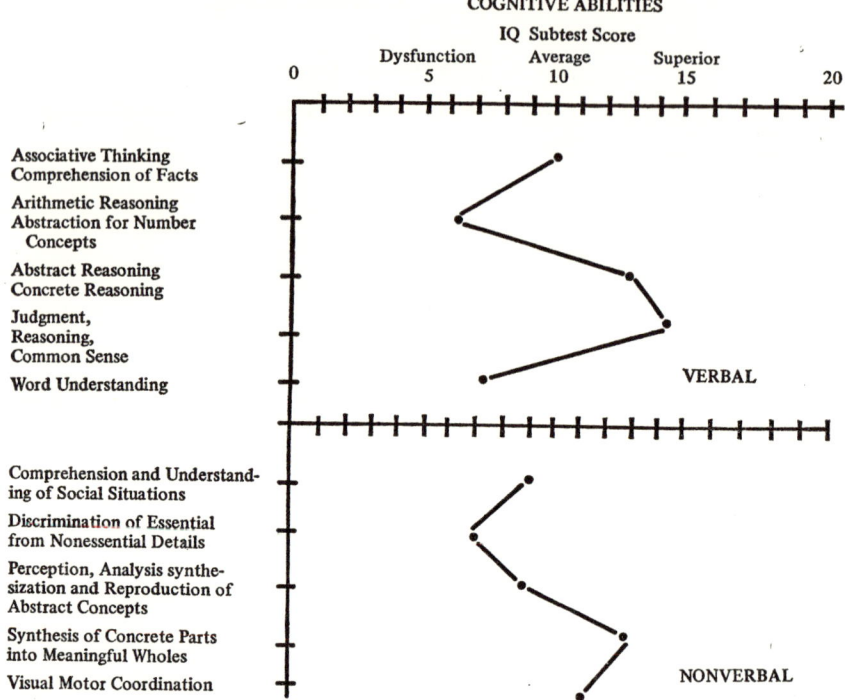

Figure 4. Pattern of cognitive abilities associated with learning dysfunction.

exhibit as much as a ten-point difference between various abilities.

A second pattern of cognitive abilities frequently associated with hyperactivity is one in which the verbal abilities are relatively well matched with one another and the nonverbal abilities are also relatively well matched with one another, but there is a significant discrepancy between the average of the verbal abilities and the average of the nonverbal abilities.

On tests of intelligence this form of cognitive dysfunction is usually represented by a fifteen-point disparity between the average of the verbal subtest scores and the average of the nonverbal subtest scores. Figure 5 represents a typical pattern of cognitive abilities associated with this form of cognitive dysfunction. Generally speaking, the child's overall intelligence is within the average range. The verbal abilities are relatively

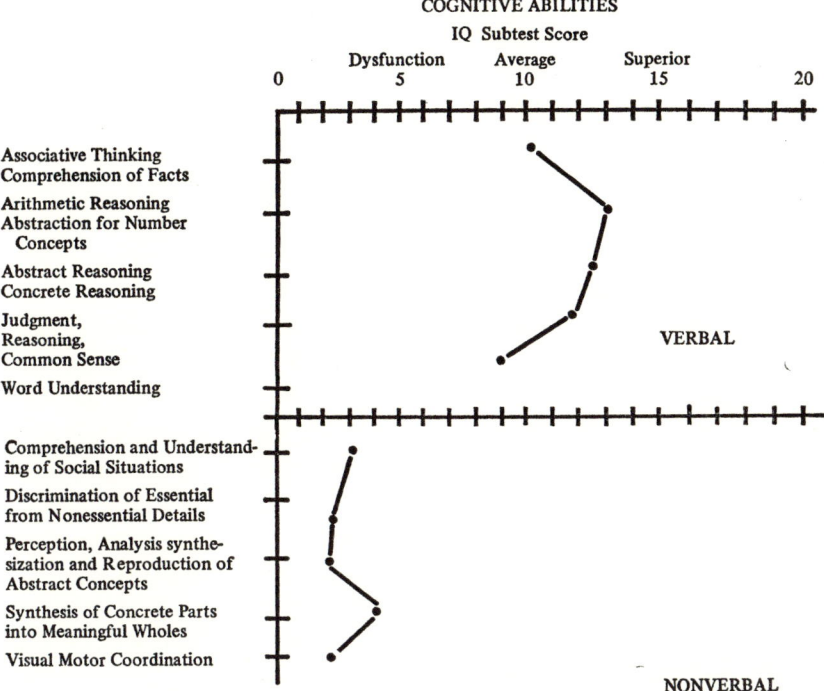

Figure 5. Pattern of cognitive abilities associated with learning disabilities.

well matched with an evenness of development demonstrated by the fact that the discrepancy between various subtests never exceeds five points. The nonverbal abilities, even though evenly matched, show an average score of fifteen points less than the verbal abilities. Quite typically, a hyperactive youngster who demonstrates this pattern may have a verbal IQ between 90 and 110 with a nonverbal IQ ranging between 70 and 90. This pattern is quite common in hyperactive children. It generally reflects a lag in the development of the nonverbal abilities. This lag in nonverbal abilities generally reflects the unevenness of physiological development associated with hyperactivity as discussed in Chapter 2. Unfortunately, the child's ability to do superior work in some areas while producing failing grades in other areas is often mistaken as a motivational problem. Frequently, these children are performing at capacity in both areas even though they are attaining an exceptionally high grade in some area while doing failing work in other subjects.

Frequently, these children develop a misconception of themselves as students. They are often told that they are lazy. The fact that they have achieved high grades in certain subjects is held up to them as "proof" that they can "do it if they want to." Such children are often chastised by both parents and teachers for their "low motivation and lack of self-discipline" when in fact their performance in school reflects the uneven development of their cognitive abilities. When a child operates under this misconception of his own abilities, it is not long before his self-image is one which fosters a rejection of success. Indeed, such children often refuse to perform to their capacity in the cognitive areas in which they have average or above average ability because their performance in these areas has often been held out as "proof" to them that they are not "living up to their potential."

Limited understanding of the developmental lag theory and of the concept of patterning of cognitive abilities leads to the recommendation that the child be retained in the same grade for the following school year. While this treatment approach can have positive results, it is very limited in that it proposes that a child's problems in learning may be ameliorated by repetition. While repetition in itself may be helpful for some children in overcoming cognitive dysfunctions, it is a very limited approach because it relies on only one treatment strategy. Such an approach often forces the child not to continue to progress as rapidly in the areas in which his cognitive abilities are well developed. At the same time it assumes that repetition alone will result in improvement in the abilities which are poorly developed. Actually, it is likely that a high percentage of children who seem to improve as a result of being retained actually improve due to the fact that they have had another year during which physical maturation takes place. Based on developmental lag theory, many of the poorly developed cognitive abilities may improve dramatically over the course of a school year due to rapid maturation in the physiological areas responsible for the development of these abilities. For some children suffering from cognitive dysfunctions who are also immature in their psychosocial development, retention may be of help. Here again, all other alternatives should be explored first. Many children come to look on the retention as both a punishment and as a sign of their failure. In spite of the best attempts of teachers and parents to undo these concepts, peer rejection is the rule rather than the exception. A far more effective approach is one which allows the child to progress with his age mates. The educational program should be one which offers the use of a resource room and special education techniques to facilitate learning in the areas where cognitive abilities could benefit from remediation, while allowing the child to progress at an average or above level in the areas of cognitive development in which his abilities show no deficits.

MEMORY ABILITIES

The cognitive abilities mentioned in the last section serve as a basis from which derive several other cognitive abilities all playing a key part in determining a child's academic performance level. These are the memory abilities. Although these abilities are controlled by the cerebral cortex and are of central importance to learning, they are not to be confused with intelligence or the ten generic cognitive abilities. In themselves, these abilities are necessary but not sufficient for learning. At the risk of making a very complex process appear simple, memory abilities may be considered to be either recent or remote, and as either visual or auditory. In other words, the memory abilities refer to the child's skill in recalling both visual and auditory stimuli from the recent as well as the distant past.

The process of memory involves the three stages of registration, retention, and recall or recognition. One of the most recent theories of recall has made a strong argument for the hypothalamus as the brain center which determines which sensory experiences will be stored for retrieval by the hippocampus fornix system (Smythe, 1966). As pointed out in other chapters of this text, it is a disturbance of synaptic transmission in the hypothalamus which plays a central role in the development of the most common forms of hyperactivity. In this section we will be concerned with recall and the effect that the recall abilities have on learning.

Recent memory involves the child's ability to recall and to recognize events, experiences and stimuli from the recent past. It is the measure of a child's ability to store and retrieve bits of information which are current. Remote memory, as the name suggests, involves the child's abilities to recall events, experiences and stimuli from the distant past. Many hyperactive children experience deficits in either or both of these areas. For instance, it is quite common for a hyperactive child to have fairly adequate recall for past events, but little ability to remember what he has just heard or seen. Frequently, such children are accused of not paying attention or of being disobedient, when in fact their ability to recall what has occurred earlier in the day is limited.

Another important form of memory involves the ability to store and manipulate bits of information in order to solve a problem. In other words, this form of memory is one in which the child is required to store and then retrieve bits of information in a different order than the one in which it was originally stored. More commonly, this memory ability is called mental control. Children suffering from dysfunctions in this area find it difficult to do such commonplace academic tasks as counting backwards and counting by threes. The memory ability of such children is affected in such a way as to prevent them from doing even the most simple cognitive manipulation of stored information. On a very practical level, for instance, such children may find it nearly impossible to go back and retrace the steps they went through in solving an academic problem.

Another variation of the mental control ability is that of sequential memory. This memory ability is responsible for the child's skill in recalling events in their proper sequential order. The hyperactive child with this cognitive dysfunction is unable to follow instructions in their order of presentation. Such children become confused or literally do not recall essential items in a series of instructions. For these children, presentation of instructions one at a time, with the next instruction being given upon the completion of the previous one, is necessary.

These inabilities make progressive learning extremely difficult as the child is confronted with the fact that he is unable to identify the stage in a problem-solving task at which he has made an error. Children with this problem are often accused of being unwilling to accept criticism or look at their mistakes. Here again, many assumptions are made about the hyperactive child which lead him to think negatively about himself.

In the area of immediate short-term memory, the child may experience deficits in logical memory, immediate short-term auditory recall and memory for visual reproductions. Each of these three memory abilities involves the recollection of stimulus materials presented shortly before the child is expected to recall them. However, each represents a different aspect of short-term memory ability.

Logical memory ability involves the child's skill in recalling events in their logical rather than sequential order. This particular memory ability is an important one in understanding the cause-and-effect relationship between past events. Many children who experienced a dysfunction in logical memory are unable to identify the logical relationship between two past events. Here again, children who suffer from this deficit are often criticized as not being willing to accept accountability for their responsibility in producing problematic behaviors. Such children are often unable to recall the relationship between the behaviors they have exhibited in the classroom and the outcome which resulted from them. On an academic level, they are frequently unable to recall the logical order of events leading up to the solution of a problem. This differs somewhat from sequential memory in which the child merely has to recall items in the order in which they were presented. Logical memory requires the child to recall the logical relationships between items which quite often do not occur in sequential order.

Immediate short-term auditory memory ability refers to the child's ability to recall auditory stimuli from the recent past. Here again, this ability can be affected by problems of sequencing. That is, the child may not be able to remember what he has heard in the order that he has heard it. More likely though, children with deficits in this area find it difficult to recall most of what they have just heard a short time before. Such children often find it difficult to recall new instructions or to remember what they have been told a short time previously.

Visual reproduction memory ability requires a child to reproduce symbols and designs which he had exposure to in the past. Children with a dysfunction in this area often experience difficulty completing simple tasks such as reproducing the alphabet or drawing a picture of something which they have recently seen.

Perhaps one of the most important memory abilities is associative memory ability. It is this ability which allows the child to make and recall associations between related and unrelated stimuli. This ability helps the child to use one symbol as a cue for recalling another less familiar symbol. This ability is very important in everyday functioning. For example, a child may learn to recall the name of the President of the United States by associating it with the name of the state in which that individual was born. The child, who has already memorized the names of the states, uses his memory for the states to serve as a cue for storing the name of the President, i.e. associative memory. The ability to associate one stimulus with the other for purposes of recall is a complex one as it requires the use of symbols rather than concrete stimulus objects. The greater the degree of abstraction called for by the task, the more important this memory ability becomes.

Dysfunctions in the areas of the memory abilities are a particular source of frustration to youngsters in their attempts to achieve academically. Each of us has had the experience of forgetting what we have done with something that we just set down a moment ago. It occurs so infrequently for most of us that we are able to laugh at how irritated we become over such a minor frustration. One can imagine how the degree of frustration multiplies for the child whose daily experience is one of repeated forgetfulness.

The Receptor-Effector Systems

A significant avenue of learning is that of the receptor-effector system. This three-part process involves integration and coordination of the various sense organs with the brain. It is primarily a physiological, perceptual-motor process involving the efficiency with which the various sense organs receive incoming stimuli, the efficiency with which the nervous system processes units of information about the stimuli received, and the accuracy and efficiency with which the nervous system produces a response. In this chapter we shall refer to this three-part process as the *learning arc*. Basically the process involves the reception of stimuli or units of information by the sense organ, the organization and transmission of these units of information by the nervous system and the production of a motor response. Cognitive dysfunctions may be the result of a deficit in the efficiency in any one of the components of the learning arc, as well as a deficit in the interaction between various components of the arc. The receptor-effector systems are particularly important in understanding learning disabilities because they call for the interaction between the cerebral cortex and the brain stem.

Technically speaking, physical traumas resulting in damage to one of the components of the learning arc do not qualify as a learning disability but rather are considered to be physical handicaps. However, for illustrative purposes it is convenient to use the example of sensory and motor aphasia to demonstrate how an interruption in the functioning of one of the components of the learning arc affects the whole process of learning itself. For example, in the case of auditory receptive aphasia, the external sense organ of the ear is able to efficiently receive and transmit sound to the brain. It is the task of the temporal lobe of the brain to recognize the information transmitted by the ear, that is, to develop a symbol or mental image of the object which the sound symbolizes. In cases of auditory receptive aphasia, the temporal lobe fails in its task of organizing the incoming stimuli and does not develop a mental image which the sound represents.

As a consequence, the individual suffering from this form of brain injury is unable to understand what the sound represents and thus is not able to produce the correct verbal response. While learning disabilities are not considered to be the result of direct physical injuries, a learning disabled youngster may experience a similar type of deficit such that he may not be able to develop a mental image of the object which a particular spoken word represents.

With respect to the learning arc, it is possible to conceptualize the acquisition of information about the environment in terms of the efficiency of each of the arc's components in receiving, processing and responding to stimuli. The threefold process of reception, organization and expression constitutes a major area of potential cognitive dysfunction in the hyperactive child.

Visual-Motor System

Actually, there are several receptor-effector systems. The visual-motor system is probably the best understood of these. This is probably due to the heavy emphasis in education, over the past several decades, on identification of visual dysfunctions in school age children. In simple terms, the visual-motor system processes incoming visual stimuli, i.e. it receives a visual image through the eyes. The next phase of the process involves the "conversion" of the visual image into nervous (electrochemical) impulses which are transmitted across nerve fibers to the brain. The brain receives the nervous impulses, organizes them in such a way as to produce a mental image, selects an appropriate response, and relays an impulse to the muscles of the body which results in the execution of a motor response. Eye-hand coordination tasks and reproduction of visual image tasks call the visual motor system into play. In the past, psychologists and other learning specialists have been able to identify the most frequent types of errors resulting from a malfunction in the visual-motor learning arc. These errors are frequently associated with hyperactivity as well as other forms of learning disabilities (Koppitz, 1962).

Visual motor dysfunctions show up primarily in the classroom when the child attempts to reproduce with a motor response what he receives visually, i.e. when a child attempts to copy or draw what he sees in a textbook or on the blackboard. Of course, the source of the dysfunction may be in any of the components of the learning arc, so that the child may experience difficulty in perceiving the stimulus which he sees in precisely the same manner as other children who are free of dysfunction. He may perceive the visual image quite accurately but may experience a dysfunction in his ability to execute a response. That is, he may perceive the visual stimuli accurately but may not be able to execute an accurate reproduction of that image. Usually, the child himself can identify whether the dysfunction is in the receptive component or the expressive component of the learning arc. He is usually able to tell his teacher that he is not able to draw it the way he sees it. In other instances he may not recognize that the image which he has reproduced does not accurately match the sample. Deficits in the ability of the brain to organize and produce mental images of incoming stimuli are more difficult for the child to identify.

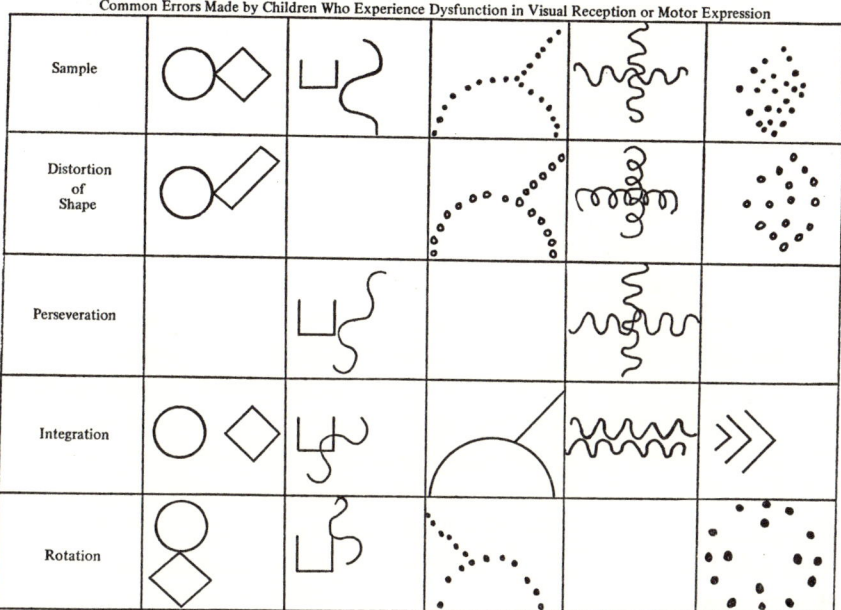

Figure 6. Errors in visual-motor reproduction associated with dysfunction of the visual-motor learning arc.

Regardless of the locus of the dysfunction, four basic categories of visual motor errors have been identified. Figure 6 gives examples of each of the different types of errors. It would be highly unlikely that any one youngster would produce all four of the errors in attempting to reproduce a single visual image. However, it is possible that each of the four errors may show up in his classroom work. Some of the primary types of errors are those associated with distortions of shape. These errors involve excessive flattening of figures so that what is perceived as a square may be reproduced as a rectangle. Distortions in shape also include reproductions of visual images which are characterized by missing angles or by one axis of a figure being twice as long as the other axis. Extra or missing angles are common errors along with the reproduction of figures in such a way as to show one figure to be disproportionate in size compared to another figure. This category also includes the substitution of angles for curves. The example shown in Figure 6 represents a common distortion of shape in which excessive flattening is exhibited.

Perseveration is also a common error. This form of visual-motor dysfunction involves the tendency to repeat a motor response excessively on successive attempts at reproducing a visual image. In the example given in Figure 6 the perseveration involves the production of numerous sinusoidal curves when the test stimulus in fact contains only three such curves.

Deficits in integration are also quite common. These deficits represent one of major areas of visual-motor dysfunction. Basically, these deficits show themselves in the form of an inability to perceive two objects as touching or as in close proximity to one another. This type of error is highly representative of visual-motor dysfunction and may be assumed to be present when the faliure at integration is as little as 1/8 of an inch. Children who experience this form of visual-motor dysfunction are unable to draw two images close together. Another form of dysfunction in the area of integration involves the inability of the child to see two images as separate or as touching one another without overlapping. In this case, the child is likely to draw one image as overlapping the other. Finally, the youngster may express difficulty in dealing with integration by blending the separate components of a complex design together in such a way as to lose the shape of the design. This type of error is seen quite frequently in elementary school children. An example of this is the familiar problem that some children exhibit in drawing the American Flag. Even though the child attempts to use different colors to designate different components of the Flag, the stars and stripes blend together to the extent that it is barely recognizable.

Rotation constitutes the fourth category of basic visual-motor dysfunction. Children who make errors in this category usually rotate their reproduction of a visual image by forty-five degrees or more. The rotation may be either in the actual figure which they produced or may be in the fact that they actually turn their paper by forty-five degrees or more. When the paper is replaced in the proper position, the figure does not appear to be rotated. It should be remembered that each of these dysfunctions in visual-motor ability occurs at various levels in the development of the visual motor system. It is not uncommon for preschool children to exhibit several, if not all of these errors. By the time a child reaches third grade the maturational process should have reduced the frequency of such errors significantly.

Visual-Verbal System

This system, like the visual-motor system, involves reception of visual sensory stimuli through the sense organ of the eyes. However, the output response is verbal rather than manual. This system calls for the reception of visual stimuli followed by an internal mediating process which involves the use of language. This process is highly complex, as it calls for the manipulation of complex, abstract concepts which are symbolized in the form of language. Dysfunctions in the abilities to think abstractly and utilize words as symbols for visualizations may result in learning dysfunctions.

The complex task of learning through the sense of vision involves the integration of several major systems of learning. In the past, defects in visual learning had been considered synonymous with defects in visual acuity. In other words, visual learning was considered to be a function of eyesight. In reality, eyesight is necessary but not in itself sufficient for visual learning. If visual learning were dependent on eyesight alone, the only requirement for visual learning tasks such as reading would be that the child be able to see the print. Both eyesight and vision are prerequisites for adequate visual learning.

The process of vision itself calls for the integration of four systems. The vestibular system is responsible for orienting the child's body and his posture to a central stimulus. This system facilitates visual learning by directing the child's body orientation, his posture and his position correctly in relationship to the stimulus. Deficits in this system are quite common but often go unnoticed since they involve posture which, to many individuals, seems remote from the learning process. Some children for example develop a posture which compensates for deficits in other visual learning systems by tilting their head to one side. Depending on the severity of the head tilt, this dysfunction may be hardly noticeable. By cocking the head slightly to one side the child attempts to compensate for failure of the depressor or elevator muscles of the eye to function properly. This compensation may create spasms of the neck muscles. In effect, the child compensates for the fact that one eye may be elevated or depressed slightly above or below the other eye. The resulting distortion of body posture may create backaches and headaches. When the child with reading problems complains of backaches or headaches while reading he may be accused of fabricating somatic complaints as excuses for his wish to avoid reading. Often the child's pains are not imagined.

Another system involves centering various sensory modalities on the stimulus to be observed. The function of this system is to converge all sensory modalities on a particular sensory stimulus. It is the task of the centering system to locate the stimulus object and to bring all sensory modalities in line with the visual object. In short, the centering system must line up all sensory modalities with the target. This task requires that both eyes work together as a team (teaming). Deficits in teaming can result in overlooking words on the written page. In addition to teaming, this system must simultaneously coordinate the movements of both hands and both feet in such a way that all the sensory modalities converge at the same time. In a sense, total body centering locates and holds stimulus objects.

Still another system is that of identification. In essence this system involves accomodating to another stimulus. This system calls for focusing on various visual stimuli located in different areas in the child's visual field. The ability to accommodate or focus rapidly is essential to visual learning. Children with deficits in this area for example may be well accomodated to the visual stimuli in the textbook located on their desk. However, when asked to shift focus from the textbook to the blackboard, the time lapse between shifts may be excessive. Many children with this dysfunction are forced to bear the frustration of having the example erased from the board before they have been able to focus on it. This process is a multi-sensory process involving both the ability to recognize familiar stimuli and the reaction time necessary to focus on them.

Finally, the completion of the visual process involves the communications system. This system is responsible for verbal expression. It brings into play the child's language skills which are necessary for labeling the visual object while making complex abstract manipulations of the visual symbols. The work of Skeffington (1968) provides us with a convenient model for understanding the interactions of these systems. Skeffington's model depicts each of the four systems overlapping with the remaining three systems. Figure 7 graphically represents the interaction of the four systems. According to Skeffington the most accurate level of visual learning occurs at the point at which all four systems intersect. The gray area in Figure 7 represents the integration of all four of the systems. While each of the various systems may overlap with one or two of the remaining systems it is only when all four systems integrate that visual learning is free of dysfunction.

Auditory Input-Output Systems

The ability to receive auditory stimuli and to produce either a verbal or manual response is controlled by the auditory input-

Skeffington's (1968) Model of Visual Processes

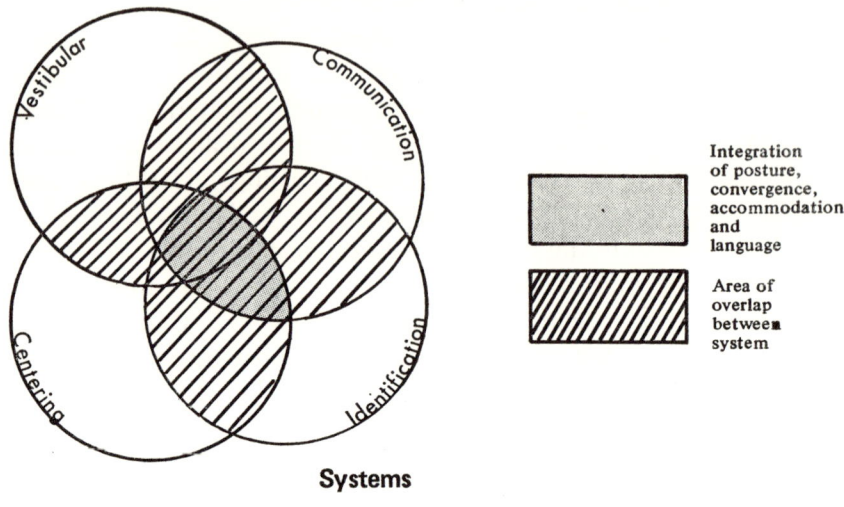

Systems

Vestibular
Responsible for Body Orienting Responses and Body Posture

Centering
Responsible for Converging all Sensory Modalities on a Central Stimulus

Identification
Responsible for Accommodating by Bringing the Stimulus Object into Focus

Communication
Responsible for Verbal Language Expression

Figure 7.

output system. The effectiveness of the system in learning depends on several factors. Similar to the case of the visual input-output system, hearing alone is not sufficient for auditory learning. The process of hearing itself depends largely on the structure of the inner ear. Auditory stimuli must be conducted to the cerebral cortex. This process involves the distortion-free conduction of air, the conduction of sound by the bones located in the inner ear (vibration) and sensorineural transmission. Dysfunctions in these areas are usually considered to be physical handicaps. Assuming that the auditory stimuli are transmitted accurately by the components of the inner ear, these stimuli must be received via sensorinueral transmission to centers in the brain. It then becomes the job of the cerebral cortex to match the sound with a mental image of that object which the sound represents. Some hyperactive children are well able to receive a sound but are unable to produce a mental image or a word to represent the stimulus object which the sound symbolizes. The auditory input-output system also calls for motor output following auditory reception. This process calls for the production of a motor response to auditory stimuli.

Using Osgood's (1957a, b) model, Kirk, McCarthy and Kirk (1968) developed an expanded model of the auditory input-output learning arc. According to Kirk et al., each input-output system (that is, each learning arc) represented a channel. Similar to our concept of learning arc, the components of these channels were reception, mediation and expression. While Kirk and McCarthy were primarily interested in auditory input and output channels, they also described visual input and output channels. They postulated that these two input-output systems were so closely linked that an adequate understanding of one system could only be achieved by a full understanding of its interaction with the other system. According to these authors, the receptive component of the channel involved the ability to recognize and to understand stimuli that are seen or heard. The expressive component of each channel involved the utilization of skills necessary for the expression of ideas both verbally and through gesture and movement. The mediating or organizing process required the internal manipulation of abstract concepts, precepts and linguistic symbols. This organizational process is the second of the three processes in the channel and is considered to act as a mediator between the activities of the receptive and the expressive components of each channel. According to Kirk and McCarthy, the mediating process was organized on two levels. The automatic level of the organizational process was one which called for the use of highly organized and highly integrated response chains. These response chains were thought to be of a less voluntary nature and involved such factors as speed of perception, ability to reproduce a sequence and the synthesization of sounds. The second and higher level of the organizational processes is the representational level. This level involved a complex mediation process calling for the utilization of symbols to represent the meaning of incoming stimuli. This process involved visualization, abstract thinking ability and complex manipulation of abstract symbols prior to the commission of a verbal or manual response.

The closeness with which visual learning arcs and auditory learning arcs are linked can be deduced from the fact that, with the exception of the fact that the incoming stimuli is received by different sense organs, the organizational process and the expressive process serve identical functions. In other words, regardless of which sense organ it is that receives the incoming stimuli, the cognitive activity at the organizational level and the verbal and manual activities at the expressive level are nearly identical. According to Kirk, McCarthy and Kirk the receptive process involves the child's ability to receive and comprehend visual and auditory stimuli. The auditory receptive process calls for the execution of several activities such as auditory reception. This activity is one which allows the child to derive meaning from verbally presented stimuli. Similarly, the activity of visual reception involves the child's ability to gather meaning from visually presented stimuli.

As mentioned above, the organizing process performs a mediating function which is carried out on two levels. On the representational level, this mediating process facilitates learning by allowing the child to make auditory-vocal associations. This activity calls for the association of concepts which are presented orally. It involves the manipulation of linguistic symbols. Concepts for size, texture, shape and other abstractions are called into play.

The second activity on this level involves the child's ability to relate concepts which are received visually. This ability to associate visual concepts with one another and to produce a motor response is one of the basic components necessary for visual-motor learning. This particular activity, for instance, performs the crucial learning task of allowing the child to associate visual stimuli. It is this level of association which permits the child to develop concepts for various objects in the visual stimulus field by permitting him to classify those objects according to the similarity of their visual characteristics. At its higher levels this activity involves categorizing visual stimuli which appear to be dissimilar into the same category based on other symbolic meaning. For example, the words "blue," "green" and "red" come to be classified in the category of colors even though the words visually are dissimilar.

Activity on the automatic level of the organizational process is more reflexive since it involves well-established automatic habits which have become integrated as a single unit of learning activity. Two of these basic units involve closure and sequential memory. Closure calls for the ability to generalize to the whole from its parts. That is, the ability to integrate discreet stimuli into meaningful wholes. It also allows for the child to utilize his abilities of habit and abstraction to fill in missing parts from an incomplete visual or verbal stimulus. On a verbal level, the grammatical redundancies in everyday language allow for the child to develop expectations for grammatical form. These redundancies, which are commonplace in everyday language, allow the child to more or less automatically predict or anticipate the next word. When these words are left out, his habit of expecting these words will allow him to close the gap by filling in the missing parts. Grammatical closure then involves the acquisition of habits necessary for the utilization of syntax in grammatical expressions.

A second form of closure on the auditory level allows the child to predict the sounds which have been left out of an auditory sequence. This ability to predict the missing sound allows the child to produce the completed word without all of the components of the word having actually been given. It is this ability which permits us to understand speech defects and other communications in which parts of the sound associated with a particular word are absent. Perhaps one of the most important forms of closure is that of sound blending. This activity, like the other forms of closure, is at the automatic level.

It represents a child's ability to blend various component sounds into a meaningful whole in order to produce a single word. Essentially, this activity involves the synthesization of the separate sounds associated with a particular word into an integrated whole. Many children who are able to successfully use various attack skills in dividing a word into its separate sounds are unable to say the word due to a dysfunction of their ability to blend sounds into an integrated whole.

Finally, visual closure comes into play on the automatic level of the organizational process. This activity is one in which a child is able to identify a familiar visual stimulus from an incomplete visual presentation. In essence it requires the child to fill in the missing visual component based on his repetitive experiences in encountering that visual stimulus and other similar visual stimuli in their intact forms. Many children who lack this ability are initially thought to be careless or lacking in their ability to attend to details.

Sequential memory also occupies an important place on the automatic level of the organizational process. This form of memory is similar to the one described in the section on the memory abilities. This ability allows the child to reproduce both visual and auditory stimuli in the sequence in which they were originally presented. Auditory sequential memory oftentimes depends on the length of time the item is present in the sequence. Some children, for instance, are unable to remember items in their sequential order when they are presented orally at intervals of more than two seconds apart. As in auditory sequential memory, visual sequential memory allows the child to reproduce visual stimuli in their proper order of sequence. Just as was the case with auditory sequential memory, the interval between visual presentations of items in the sequence is an important factor. For some children, an interval between presentations of as little as five seconds is enough to disrupt their ability to recall visual stimuli in the proper order.

The expressive process is the third component of each channel. This process is one involving the expression of an idea through the use of verbal or motor responses. Because it is the third of the three components, its activity is greatly affected by the processes of reception and organization. However, even when the receptive and organizational processes have functioned efficiently, cognitive dysfunctions can occur in the expressive process. For example, the neurological condition of apraxia, which is usually caused by infection or by trauma of the brain, results in an inability to carry out purposive, useful or skilled acts in the absence of paralysis. This neurological condition is limited to the expressive process, since individuals suffering from this condition are very able to receive and mediate incoming stimuli. From a learning disability point of view, deficits in the expressive process are considered to be the result of neither trauma nor infection but rather as a result of dysfunctions in neuronal structure. Verbal expression involves the child's ability to express concepts orally. From a qualitative point of view, oral concepts must be discreet, relevant and factual. Manual expressions, on the other hand, call for the child to express ideas through motor acts. The child must be able to manipulate objects as well as various body parts. He must also produce gestures in order to communicate a concept. Surprising as it may seem, some children express themselves very well verbally, but are unable to express the same concept through gestures or in pantomime.

Figure 8 outlines the three processes described by Kirk, McCarthy and Kirk (1968). Whether the input be visual or auditory, the activity of the cerebral cortex at the organizational level and the activity at the output level are similar for the two modalities of reception. A most important concept in understanding cognitive dysfunctions is the recognition that deficits in any of the abilities outlined in Figure 8 can occur independently of deficits in intelligence. Indeed, each of the ten cognitive abilities associated with intelligence can be operated at a high level of efficiency while dysfunctions may be operative within the learning arc.

Tactile Input-Output Systems

While references in the educational literature have been frequently made to tactile learning, little is actually known about this component of the learning arc. As with audition and percep-

PROCESS			
External Environment	Receptive (input)	Organizational: Automatic Level / Representational Level (Mediation)	Expressive (output)
→	→	→	→
Visual Stimuli	Visual Reception (eye)	Visual Closure; Visual Association; Visual Sequential Memory	Verbal Expression (vocal responses); Manual Expression (motor responses)
Auditory Stimuli	Auditory Reception (ear)	Auditory Closure; Auditory Association; Grammatical Closure; Sound Blending; Auditory Sequential Memory	Verbal Expression (vocal responses); Manual Expression (motor responses)

Components of the Learning Arc by Function

Figure 8.
Components of the learning arc by function.

tion, the tactile learning arc involves reception, organization, and expression. The primary receptor organ for the processing of tactile stimuli is through the sense organs of the skin. Through the sense of touch, information about external stimuli is conducted through the receptors of the skin to the brain where the organizational process via the associative and automatic levels produces visual imagery and abstract concepts to match the sensations received. Once organized and synthesized, these tactile concepts may be expressed either through gesture, motor responses or verbalizations. Frequently, errors occur in one or more of the components of this learning arc. For example, some children suffer from a disturbance in tactile reception which renders them unable to differentiate between texture and degree of softness of tactile stimuli. At the organizational level, some youngsters are unable to associate the feel and shape of an object, nor are they able to associate an object with the mental image of that object received via the sense of touch with other objects in the same category and class. In other words, at the organizational level they have difficulty in dealing with abstract concepts for tactile stimuli. On the expressive level they may be unable to make a gesturing response to represent the idea. For instance, some children may be able to recognize the shape of a square with their eyes closed by holding a cardboard cutout of a square in their hand while exploring it with their finger. However, when asked to draw that figure, they are unable to do so.

LEARNING SET

There is still another way in which cognitive dysfunction may occur even when intellectual ability, memory ability, perceptual motor ability and tactile ability are found to be intact. A learning dysfunction may appear in the area of learning set. This concept refers to the fact that the learning dysfunction may lie in the child's manner of approaching the acquisition of information. Learning sets represent learned habits which the child has acquired over a course of time. These habits represent his customary approach to acquiring knowledge.

Harlow (1959) identified four learning sets which he found to be highly dysfunctional. He referred to these learning sets as "error factors." He believed them to be relatively well-fixed approaches to learning that were repeated by the child regardless of whether they were reinforced or not. One set which commonly impairs the efficiency of learning is that of position preference. Children having this set exhibit a tendency to consistently respond to left or right positions in a discrimination task. In other words, these children tend to respond to location rather than other more relevant characteristics of the learning task. Such children consistently may identify an item in the lower left hand corner of the test sheet as a correct answer regardless of the nature of the problems to be solved.

Another learning set described by Harlow is associated with dysfunction in response shifts. The child utilizing this set would be characterized by a tendency to respond differently from trial to trial regardless of the correctness of his response. Such children have a tendency to shift from one response to another, though one of the two responses may be consistently reinforced while the other is consistently not reinforced. Another form of response shift has to do with the child's inability to change responses. In this case the child often exhibits a learning set in which, when given a different set of instructions, he continues to repeat a previously given set of instructions. Such children, for example, when given the task of identifying the differences between two objects, may proceed to give the similarities between the two objects if the previous task which they were working on was one which called for the identification of similarities.

Some youngsters exhibit a response characterized by repetition of incorrect responses on subsequent trials of the same problem. This learning set is a form of perseveration because it involves the nearly continuous repetition of the same response. Frequently, such a child will repeat the same incorrect response trial after trial, even when he is given feedback in the form of nonreinforcement for the incorrect response. Such children often give the impression of being fixated on repetition itself.

Finally, a child's cognitive set may be characterized by differential cue errors. This dysfunctional set refers to the relative frequency of errors on successive trials of a test in which the stimulus object to be learned changes position from the previous trial, compared with the frequency of errors made on successive trials in which the stimulus remains in the same position. Certain children who exhibit a learning set characterized by differential cue errors are likely to exhibit significantly more errors in learning when the correct stimulus is moved from one position to another in the perceptual field, as compared to their performance on successive trials in which the correct stimulus is held stationary. Such children often appear very rigid in their learning patterns. Indeed, even minimal changes of learning material within the perceptual field seem to result in a high incidence of errors. Everyday classroom occurrences, such as placing material to be learned in a different section of the blackboard, may prove to be confusing to these children. Differential cue errors seem to be the result of competing response tendencies. That is, the tendency to respond to a particular location appears to compete with the tendency to respond to the stimulus associated with reward. In effect, such children do not seem to understand whether a certain stimulus is the correct one to learn because of some characteristic of the stimulus itself, or because it occupies a certain position in their perceptual field.

COGNITIVE STYLES

Within the context of this chapter, learning sets have been used to refer to relatively simple cognitive responses which characterize a child's typical approach to acquiring information from the environment. When learning sets become interrelated they take on a quality which represents a child's general approach to problem-solving tasks. This general approach represents a more complex and widespread characteristic. This interrelation of sets, along with accompanying habits and associations, may develop into a general style of learning. These styles of learning involve a multiple of interrelated learning sets which characterize the child's orientation to learning in general.

One way of understanding the development of cognitive styles is to view them as strategies which the child has acquired through trial and error. These strategies represent an accumulation of reinforced responses from past experiences which have become associated with one another. Over a period of time, these problem-solving strategies cluster together to take on the quality of a style of cognition. In the hyperactive child such cognitive styles often represent the manner in which the child has adapted to the demands of the environment in conjunction with his own specific cognitive dysfunctions.

Campbell, Douglas and Morgenstern (1971) sought to identify learning dysfunctions in hyperactive children and to evaluate the effects of certain types of medication on these dysfunctions by comparing the cognitive styles of hyperactive children with those styles exhibited by nonhyperactive control subjects. Campbell and her associates identified four basic cognitive styles.

A Reflection-Impulsivity style referred to the child's cognitive tempo. As described in Chapter 6, this style relates to the speed with which a child makes the decision, especially in those situations in which he is not likely to know whether his response is correct. Kagan, Rosman, Day, Albert and Phillips (1964) found a negative correlation between correct responding and response speed. In other words, the more impulsive a child was in responding, the less likely he is to produce a correct response. Impulsive children tend to be characterized as those children who exhibit little latency between instructions for completing the task and making a response. The reflective child, on the other hand, is one who generally exhibits noticeably longer response latencies. These children tend to make few errors. Another characteristic of the child with an impulsive cognitive style is his tendency not to make a critical evaluation of all the response alternatives. Such children then are characterized by short response latencies, high frequency of errors and little critical evaluation of alternative responses. The child exhibiting a reflective cognitive style would tend to take more time in responding, exhibit fewer errors and make a more critical evaluation of his response alternatives. Hyperactive children are typically found to have an impulsive cognitive style. Indeed, there seems to be a high correlation between impulsive cognitive style, distractibility, short attention span and high activity level.

In earlier research on cognitive style, Witkin (1959, 1962) identified a cognitive style which he termed *field dependence-independence*. Witkin identified certain learning-disabled individuals as having difficulty in structuring and analyzing visual stimuli. The field-dependent style was one in which the child's typical strategy for dealing with the visual field is to treat his perceptions as if they were global and undifferentiated. That is, instead of separating the visual field into its various substructures or individual parts, these children tend to treat all visual learning materials as if they were diffuse. The field-independent child is one who isolates various characteristics of the figure from the background in visually presented material. Hyperactive children showing extremes in activity level along with diffuse motor output and poor impulse control tend to exhibit a field-dependent cognitive style. These children responded globally to even the most intense aspects of the stimulus field. Such children may respond more to a whole stimulus itself than to other, more essential characteristics of the test stimulus.

In learning concepts for shape and color, such children may respond to the fact that a visual presentation of a circle and a triangle are both colored red, rather than to the fact that they are different forms. The field dependent child gives the impression that his style of learning is controlled by the characteristics of the whole stimulus rather than by his own ability to analyze and structure his perception of the visual field.

Still another form of cognitive style was identified by Santostefano and Paley (1964). In his review of the research related to the various types of cognitive style, he emphasized the important role which the constricted-flexible control played in learning. This style refers to differences in the child's ability to ignore distracting and contradictory characteristics of learning materials. It also takes into consideration the child's ability to inhibit incorrect verbal responses. Santostefano's research on hyperactive and learning-disabled children demonstrated that such children tended to have a more constrictive cognitive style than nonhyperactive children. Supposedly, this was due to the fact that hyperactive children exhibit deficits in focusing on relevant stimulus characteristics. In their own study, Campbell et al. (1971) hypothesized that hyperactive children would have greater difficulty than nonhyperactive children in ignoring unessential and irrelevant stimulus characteristics. They also predicted that these children would have difficulty inhibiting incorrect verbalization. In other words, hyperactive children were predicted to demonstrate a constricted cognitive style of control.

Perhaps one of the more important cognitive styles is that of automatization. In his research on dimensions of cognitive styles, Broverman (1960, 1966) used the term automatization to refer to the ability to respond rapidly to simple repetitive tasks. This style involved the ability to resist fatigue and distracting stimuli while making rapid responses. Strong automatization is exhibited when a child is able to resist distractors in dealing with familiar stimulus materials. Individuals whose cognitive style is associated with a weakness in automatization tend to fatigue easily and are unable to maintain rapid response rates. Of course, a cognitive style associated with strong automatization calls for the accompanying skills of concentration and persistence. Here again the typical picture of the hyperactive child with poor concentration skills, poor tolerance for frustration and high distractibility suggest a cognitive style of low automatization. Indeed, Campbell et al. (1971) expected that on measures of automatization, hyperactive children would maintain less efficient response rates to repetitive tasks.

Deficiencies in cognitive styles represent a crucial factor in the ability of hyperactive children to learn. As pointed out by the research of Douglas, Weiss and Minde (1969), hyperactive children tended to be less attentive, more disruptive and on a lower academic achievement level than the control subjects. However, when the two groups were compared on a thorough diagnostic battery of tests of learning disabilities, the only difference which emerged between the two groups was in the area of perceptual motor disturbance. It is quite likely that the strong differences between the two groups with respect to academic achievement was related to the difference between the two groups in their cognitive styles. That is, the learning strategies of normal youngsters were probably much more efficient than those of the hyperactive counterparts. Douglas et al. (1969) concluded that the differences between the two groups contributed at least partially to overall differences in behavioral approaches to problem solving.

Campbell et al. (1971) compared the performance of a matched group of hyperactive subjects with nonhyperactive controls on various measures of cognitive styles. The Matching Familiar Figures Test (MFFT) (Kagan et al. 1964), the Children's Embedded Figures Test (Karp and Konstadt, 1963), the Naming Repeated Animals Test (Campbell, 1971), the Color Distraction Test (Santostefano and Paley, 1964) and an adapted form of the Color Distraction Test (Campbell et al., 1971) were used to measure reflection-impulsivity field dependence-independence, automatization and constricted-flexible control respectively.

The results of the study were in the expected direction. Hyperactive subjects were found to be significantly more impulsive while normals were found to be significantly more reflective on the measure of reflection-impulsivity. Data measuring the field dependent-independent cognitive style indicated that hyperactive subjects were significantly more field dependent than their normal counterparts. In other words, these children exhibited significantly greater difficulty in analyzing the components of their stimulus field. As a group they tended to respond to the whole field rather than to the separate parts of the stimulus. Performance on the two measures of automatization produced contradictory results. On the Naming Repeated Animals Test, no significant difference was found between the groups. However, on the Color Distraction Test hyperactive subjects were found to have significantly greater difficulty in learning to master simple repetitious tasks. On the constricted-flexible control dimensions of cognitive style, no significant differences were found between the two groups with respect to distractibility, interference or types of errors. A further analysis of the performance of hyperactive subjects on this measure of cognitive style did indicate that they committed significantly more errors of commission than did normal subjects. In other words, the hyperactive children had a significantly greater frequency of totally wrong responses. A scrutinization of their errors indicated that they tended to respond more to the stimulus presented to them than to the instructions about how to respond to the stimulus. For example, when the instruction was to observe a picture of a blue apple and to name the correct color, hyperactive subjects often responded with the answer "blue" or "apple" rather than "red."

It is evident that cognitive style plays an important role in learning efficiency. Cognitive style particularly seems to be affected by the presence of hyperactivity. Within the classroom, remedial programming will need to involve the identification of various response sets and cognitive styles along with the development of a program for correcting dysfunctions in these areas.

The Learning Arc

In retrospect we can see that the learning arc involves a complex system of interrelated processes involving physiological structure, external stimuli, response patterns and general approaches to learning. Figure 9 traces the complex interaction of various processes which interact to form the visual-vocal learning arc.

In this particular case, the visual-vocal learning arc for reading is described. Each of the boxes represent a different cognitive element which is critical to efficient reading. Visual input stimuli are received by the eyes, which are under control of the autonomic nervous system. The function of this receptive process is that of decoding. This task calls for the adequate functioning of the vestibular system, the centering process and the identification process. Dysfunctions in these areas may result in body disorientation, incorrect posture, deficits in convergence and failures in accommodation. Any one of these dysfunctions in reception is enough in itself to create a serious reading dysfunction. Superimposed on this component are the cognitive abilities which are under the control of the cerebral cortex. An adequate visual-motor coordination ability and an adequate ability to visualize essential details is essential to the receptive process.

Information received by the eyes is transmitted to the organizational process. This process, also under the control of the cerebral cortex, serves a mediational function. Certain aspects of this process, such as visual closure, are automatic. A dysfunction in this area may result in the failure to identify missing components. This function is critical to reading, as it allows the child to fill in grammatical structure and syntax which are not actually transmitted through the receptive process. On a more abstract complex level the organizational process involves representational activities. These activities, such as visual association and vocal association, involve the complex manipulation of visual linguistic symbols. This component of the system allows the child to make associations with the written words that he sees. This process is essentially that of visualization. That is, this system is needed to develop a visual image of the stimuli that are symbolized by the words on the written page. This component also allows him to store and retrieve concrete facts as well as abstract concepts. Both the automatic and the representational components' efficiency depends largely on the memory

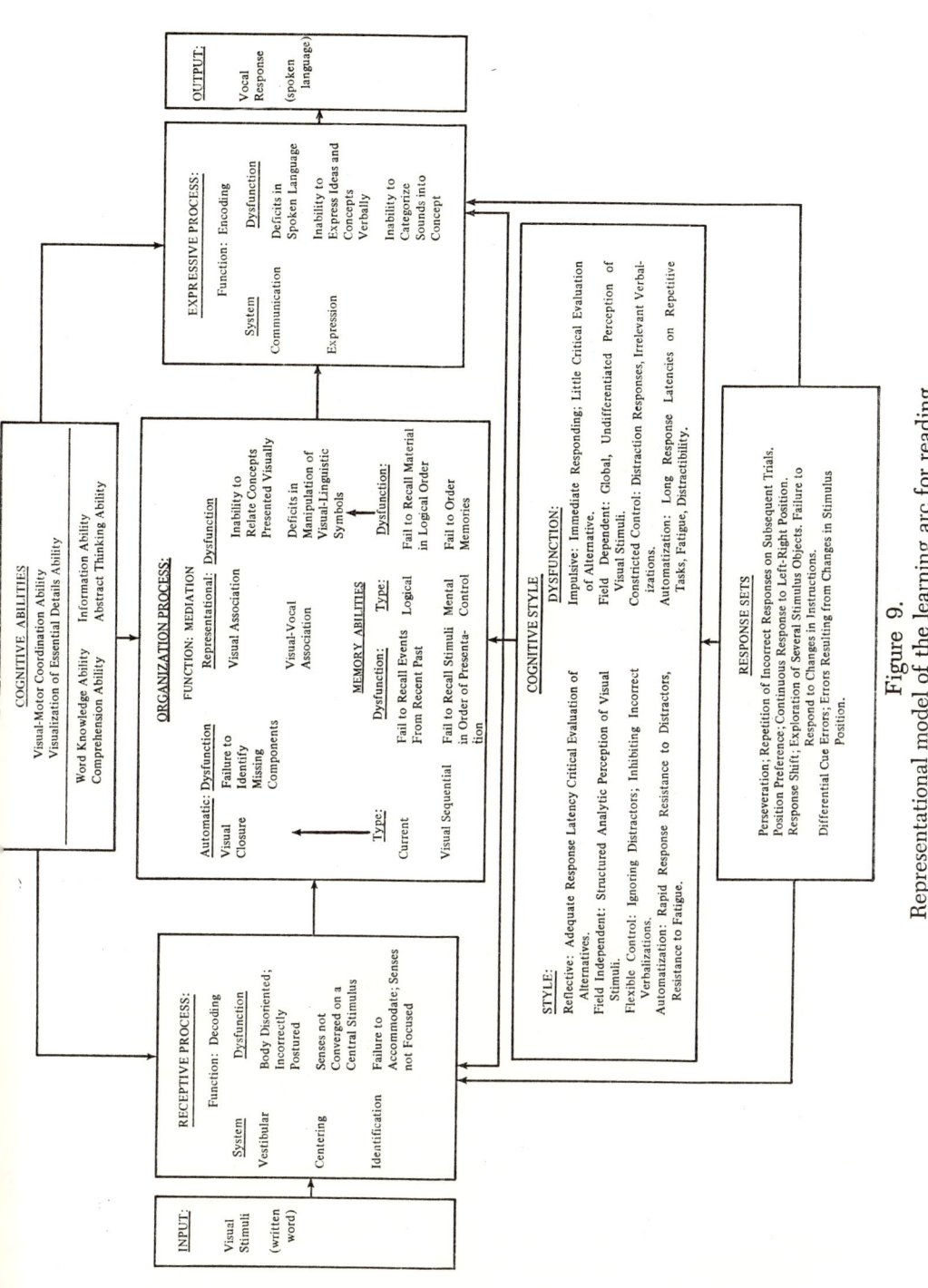

Figure 9.
Representational model of the learning arc for reading.

abilities. The ability to use current memory to recall recent events from the past, as well as visual sequential memory in order to recall visual stimuli in the order of presentation, are essential abilities for visual closure at the automatic level. The ability to systematically recall visual stimuli in an order other than the order in which it was presented (mental control), and the ability to recall visual stimuli based on their logical connections rather than on their actual physical position (logical memory), play a critical role in the mediation at the representational level. Cognitive dysfunctions of the organizational process may be the result of deficits in the interaction between the automatic and representational levels and the memory abilities. Even though each of the components in themselves may be intact, the interaction between the various levels in the organizational process and the memory abilities may be dysfunctional.

Superimposed on the organizational process are several other cognitive abilities under the control of the cerebral cortex. These abilities are associated with intelligence and play an important role in the efficient processing of stimuli at the organization level. The ability to understand words, use previous experiences in dealing with new situations, store and retrieve information and think abstractly are important cognitive components which directly affect the mediation functions of the organizational processes.

As information is transmitted through the organization process it is received by the expressive process. This process involves the physical structures associated with speech. Like the receptive process, it is under the control of the autonomic nervous system. The primary function of this process is that of encoding. The expressive process controls both the communication and the expression systems. These systems are primarily responsible for expression in the form of spoken language. Deficits in this area may take the form of an inability to use language in the spoken form, or they may involve an inability to express ideas and concepts verbally. These deficits may even take on the form of an inability to categorize sounds into concepts. Adequate functioning at this level results in the vocal response that we call reading.

The efficiency with which accurate vocal responses are produced may be impaired by the child's response set. These fixed response patterns can override the system of communication and expression. Inadequate response sets may present themselves in the form of a tendency to repeat incorrect responses in subsequent trials, as is the case with perseveration. Other children demonstrate position preferences which result in a continuous response based on positioning of the words on this page. Such children are often observed to verbalize more of the words physically situated on one side of the page than on the other. Other response sets, such as response shift pattern, may be observed in a child who gives the impression of exploring the entire written page without focusing on the words in any systematic order. At other times these children find it difficult to change their response patterns with changes in instructions. Finally, response set patterns, such as differential cue errors, may be exhibited. These errors are exhibited by the child who is unable to accommodate to reading written words when the words to be read shift their physical location on the written page.

Response sets can also affect functioning at the organization process level. Various combinations of response sets can become associated in such a way as to broadly affect a child's attitudinal approach to learning. The fixed network of several response sets may result in the development of a dysfunctional cognitive style. Like the cognitive abilities controlled by the cerebral cortex, the dysfunctions associated with a cognitive style have a broad impact on reading. These generalized approaches to learning affect all three of the main processes in the learning arc. Styles characterized by impulsive responding, global undifferentiated perception of visual stimuli, high distractibility with irrelevant verbalization, long response latencies on repetitive tasks and fatigue associated with distractibility can impair functioning at any point in the reading process.

Actually, what appears to be the simple task of reading involves a highly complex cognitive task which depends to a great extent on the interaction between various components. The development of a remedial program calls for the analysis of the various components of the learning arc as well as an evaluation of the efficiency with which these components interact. In many cases, deficits in this learning arc occur between components. That is, they occur at a sensorineural level. A prescriptive program will depend largely on the learning specialist's skill in identifying the component in which efficiency breaks down. The visual motor learning arc as well as the auditory vocal and auditory motor learning arcs are equally complex. While many hyperactive children experience deficits in the areas of those processes which are under control of the autonomic nervous system, it is quite common to find deficits in the other components.

Education Programming for Cognitive Dysfunction

Historical Perspective

Prior to Strauss and Lehtinen's (1947) identification of the hyperactivity, i.e. minimal brain dysfunction, as a diagnostic entity separate from that of mental retardation, special education programming for the hyperactive child was nonexistent. Indeed, the prescribed "treatment" was exclusion. In the years that have followed since Strauss first put forth his theories, educational programming for the hyperactive child has undergone a series of changes. Originally, it was thought that the most effective educational program for such children was one which completely adjusted the classroom environment to the child's dysfunction. Such "destimulated classrooms" were barren of all but the most essential visual and auditory stimuli. The academic program itself was one that focused on repetition as the main mode of learning. The program was designed to teach only the basic skills necessary for social and vocational adjustment.

As our knowledge of the hyperactive child's cognitive dysfunctions increased, educational programming underwent a series of evolutional changes. Eventually, the hyperactive child came to be viewed as being more capable than was originally thought. A shift in educational programming took place which emphasized strengthening the child's intact cognitive abilities. Fewer limitations were placed on the child's ability to learn. During this phase, educational programming was characterized by both environmental destimulation and specific remedial programming which encouraged the child to work to his fullest potential. Such programs typically produced noticeable changes in the classroom setting. However, the ability of such programs to bring about a generalization of the behaviors and levels of achievement attained in the classroom to other environmental situations was limited. At present, educational programs for the hyperactive child typically stress not only adaptation of the learning environment and the use of special remedial techniques in order to help the child attain his fullest potential, but also focus on teaching the generalization of these behaviors and levels of achievement to the world outside of the classroom.

As was the case with the entire educational system in America, the technology of teaching and the understanding of learning took major strides during the 1950's. During this era in American education, Bloom (1957) surveyed the types of academic approaches used in teaching learning-disabled children. His review of the literature described the developmental approach as the one most widely used. This approach involved limiting the child's education to exposure to various school experiences necessary for effective living. The educational program for the hyperactive child was based on repeated exposures of the child to these experiences only. The emphasis was on guaranteeing that the child would be able to be functional as an adult. This approach was revolutionary in its time in that it abandoned the regimentation of a fixed sequence of courses. In addition, it considered social adjustment to be an important factor in the child's academic program.

There was also a trend towards modification of the academic program for learning-disabled children. This approach involved modifying the quantity and the content of material contained in the child's academic curriculum. Information which was considered to be unessential was deleted in favor of providing adequate opportunity for extensive repetition of academic materials thought to be essential to adjustment in later life. Another characteristic of academic programming for the learning-disabled child was that of simplification of all academic materials. This approach involved reducing all academic material and terminology to its basic components.

All of these approaches were basically underwritten by the philosophy that it was the environment that must be changed because a child could not. Teaching the child only the basic materials essential for social and vocational adjustment was the goal of such programs. Mastery of basic academic tasks such as reading and counting were the main goals of these approaches. The child was expected to acquire these skills at his own level of understanding and capacity.

The concept of individualization of instruction had become increasingly accepted to the point that tailoring the program to the child's disability had become a byword in special education.

During the early stages of our changing educational attitudes toward the hyperactive child, educational researchers reflected a view which depicted the hyperactive child as unchangeable in his learning disabilities and as limited in his ability to become a fully functional adult. Indeed, such notable educators as Shainman (1951) urged that any educational training program for hyperactive children be focused on teaching them basic manual skills for vocational adjustment. The hyperactive child was viewed as a youngster whose learning disabilities primarily stemmed from "pent-up emotions." Classroom teachers were urged to permit such children to release their inhibitions while providing a school program which called for the child to spend half of his time in the classroom with the remaining half of his time to be spent in on-the-job training. While such approaches did emphasize the importance of practical learning experiences, they seemed to do so to the detriment of a child's potential for achieving academically.

At a point somewhat later in the development of educational programs for learning-disabled children, Kirk (1953) suggested that such programs call for the modification of both academic materials and the learning environment. It was urged that the complexity and quantity of materials in the academic curriculum be reduced. Kirk suggested that classroom instruction be adapted to the child's level of intellectual functioning. He urged that such children be educated in special classroom designed to work with a homogeneous group of learning-disabled children. Such classrooms were to be established in order to develop a special educational program for children with cognitive dysfunctions. These programs focused on the utilization of special, noncomplex academic materials. Instructional materials were to be concrete in nature. They emphasized the deletion of abstract material. Much emphasis was placed on teaching the child methods of transferring his learning from classroom to out-of-class situations. Instructional materials were to be more systematic and more repetitious than the materials utilized for average children. For the first time, much emphasis was placed on helping parents understand the concept of learning disabilities. Parent education programs were to be established by the school.

As the acceptance for these types of programs increased among members of the educational community, those interested in educational research began to focus on specific instructional techniques which could help the child to compensate for his learning deficits by strengthening his intact learning abilities. This was a minute but important change from the previously held attitude that special education solely involved simplification of the learning environment. While this approach still viewed certain learning deficits as fixed and unchangeable, it did represent a change in the educational viewpoint because it considered the child's intact learning abilities to be amenable to improvement.

Kaliski's (1955) position paper was timely as it presented a viewpoint that was representative of the general growing trend towards focusing on the child's abilities rather than his disabilities. In his paper, Kaliski emphasized that remedial educational programs should be focused on assisting the child to compensate for perceptual, auditory and kinesetic disturbances by emphasizing learning through intact learning modalities. Kaliski suggested that most learning-disabled children needed training in learning to focus their attention on a stimulus object, as well as special training in learning techniques for recall and differentiation. Indeed, his was one of the first articles to suggest that children with visual-reception deficits could learn the concepts of shape through tactile training. Kaliski recommended that the "total child" be taken into consideration. He stressed the importance of the classroom teacher having a full understanding of the child's medical history and family background.

This represented a changing attitude towards the role of the classroom teacher. Prior to this point in the development of these special education programs such information was considered to be out of the teacher's realm of expertise. Kaliski further advised that the classroom teacher must be knowledgeable about techniques for motivating students. He especially advised that special education teachers become well acquainted with the techniques for helping learning-disabled children to learn through association.

At about the same time, other researchers had begun to report on the effectiveness of special education programs. Jolles (1956) reported on one such study in which modifying the physical characteristics of the classroom, and making instructional materials simple and concrete, resulted in significant gains in academic achievement and social adjustment for hyperactive children. Jolles recommended that each learning-disabled child undergo a three-year remedial program before he enter regular classes. This program not only involved simplification and concretization of academic materials but also called for destimulization of the classroom.

Schrager, Lindy, Harrison, McDermott and Wilson (1966) summarized the emergent educational trends for hyperactive children. They urged that such programs take into account the "whole child." These authors outlined a special education program in which the child's entrance into the classroom was preceded by extensive consultation and preparation of both teacher and parent in order to make the child's school experiences "less eventful." The object was to help both parent and teacher to structure the child's interpersonal environment in order to take his special learning problems into consideration. The classroom program was one that called for limiting physcial stimuli within the classroom to allow for a stuctured program in which academic changes were gradually introduced. Repetition of instructional material was used as the major teaching strategy. This repetition was to be concrete in nature with as much deletion of abstract instructional materials as possible. It was urged that all instructional materials and learning tasks be segmented into the smallest possible units for learning. Each child was to be evaluated in order to determine which of the sensory modalities was the most efficient. Educational training through the use of these modalities was to be emphasized. Teachers and parents were urged to develop a high tolerance for troublesome behaviors. For the first time, strong emphasis was placed on the concept that treatment of such children largely fell within the domain of educational programs. Schrager and his colleagues urged that such children not be considered as psychiatric patients but rather as children with learning deficits. It was pointed out that the "treatment of choice" was to be within instructional classroom programs designed to identify and remediate specific learning deficits. A growing emphasis was placed on the teacher's ability to identify the child's specific learning dysfunctions and to identify an educational program designed to not only help compensate for those deficits but also help reduce them (Carter and Lockey, 1967).

Cruickshank's et al. (1966) now famous textbook specified the environmental characteristics which promoted learning in children with cognitive dysfunctions. More importantly, this text specified the specific cognitive dysfunctions of the hyperactive child. Cruickshank outlined a classroom program which called for reduction of environmental stimulation. He proposed that all extraneous and unessential stimuli be removed from the classroom in order to reduce distractibility. In addition, he recommended that the size of the classroom be reduced and the child's daily program be highly structured by the classroom teacher. He suggested that the daily routine be repetitive and unchanging and that the instructional materials be of high stimulus value in order to help the student to focus on them. Most importantly, Cruickshank identified five general characteristics of the hyperactive child. He described such children as being overly distractible in the sense that they were thought to be "hyperaware" of visual, auditory and tactile stimuli within their perceptual field. Such children were described as suffering from motor disinhibition. In other words, the child's inability to prevent himself from responding to extraneous stimuli was considered to be a learning dysfunction. Cruickshank also pointed out that such children frequently exhibited an inability to perceive the totality of the perceptual field. Such children were thought to be able to identify specific stimuli in their perceptual field without being able to visualize the perceptual gestalt. Cruickshank identified this dysfunction as dissociation. In addition, Cruickshank restressed the importance of cognitive dysfunction associated with figure ground disturbances.

Children suffering from this disturbance tend to confuse the figure with the background of their perceptual field. Occasionally hyperactive children are unable to see the difference between these two. Cruickshank also noted that such children give the same response repeatedly with little apparent ability to shift from one response set to another. Finally, Cruickshank noted that such children often exhibit catastrophic responses to frustration. These youngsters were described as overreacting to stress in the form of crying and tantrums. They were observed to be highly unstable in their performance in that they were frequently observed to regress. Gains made in academic achievement appeared to be lost without any apparent reason. The child was observed to progress well, then to return to his former level of functioning. Cruickshank's observations were especially important in the overall development of instructional programming for hyperactive children. These observations reflected a turning point in that they called for a close scrutinization of specific learning dysfunctions. The educational program not only became one of environmental control, but also one of diagnostic and prescriptive educational programs. Recently, Gofman (1970) summarized cognitive dysfunctions as stemming from disorders in language development, deficits in auditory discrimination and auditory sequencing, visual and auditory memory deficits, fine motor coordination deficits, genosis, praxis, left-right discrimination deficits, or auditory, visual and tactile kinesetic tracking deficits. Over the past several years, educators have become very sophisticated at identifying the specific areas of cognitive dysfunction.

As the ability to identify these specific dysfunctions has increased, the technology for remediating such dysfunctions has also increased. This technology has focused both on the use of special equipment in the classroom and on the engineering of the classroom's social environment. Martinson's (1967) description of the role of the classroom teacher was one that depicted her as a behavioral engineer. It was her task to identify the specific behavioral components associated with each of the child's cognitive dysfunctions. The teacher was charged with the responsibility of identifying specific behavioral objectives for each child. Targeting the specific behavioral components associated with each of the cognitive dysfunctions and identifying behavioral objectives was part of an overall classroom approach which called for the use of learning theory in treating the hyperactive child.

Modification of Cognitive Dysfunctions

Werry (1969) advocated the use of behavior modification techniques in the classroom in order to increase attention span, reduce distractibility and improve perceptual motor skills. Several other authors have strongly endorsed the use of behavior modification techniques as a means of treating learning dysfunctions within the classroom (Clarizio and Yelon, 1967; Ross, 1967; Wehlen and Haring, 1966). Alabiso (1972) strongly advocated the use of learning theory techniques in the treatment of cognitive dysfunctions associated with hyperactivity. Each of the dysfunctions cited in this chapter have been viewed as responses subject to modification through reinforcement procedures. Indeed, the cognitive dysfunctions are viewed as inefficient learning characteristics which are more or less subject to extinction procedures. At each point in this chapter, efficient learning has been considered to constitute a series of shapeable responses subject to the laws of reinforcement.

The teacher has also been cast in a new light. She is viewed as both a learning specialist and as a behavioral engineer who uses reinforcement principles to shape correct responses. It is her task as a behavioral engineer to structure the classroom environment in such a way as to increase the likelihood of the occurrence of specific correct cognitive responses. It is also her task to take into consideration the child's social environment, his relationship with peers, his concept of self, his attitudes towards authority, his fears of success and his struggles with counter-dependence and lack of trust.

Since we have viewed hyperactivity as primarily a developmental problem, this chapter advocates for an educational program which is prescriptive as well as diagnostic. It is the hope of the authors that this chapter will aid in the identification of specific cognitive dysfunctions which the teacher may come to identify and target for remediation. The concept of uneven development of the cognitive abilities is used as a rationale for an educational program which calls for keeping a child within the mainstream of education. Indeed, mainstreaming helps to undo a child's sense of failure, punishment and alienation. The so-called use of retention as a form of treatment is viewed as a last alternative. On the contrary, the emphasis should be placed on maintaining the child at his age and peer level while offering him special remediation in the resource room for those cognitive abilities which are at a lower developmental level than his chronological age. In essence, this treatment appoach is truly an ecclectic, multi-disciplinary one because adequate educational programming for the hyperactive child calls for the integration of the medical, psychological and educational resources. The ideal instructional program would be one that would integrate all of these resources into the child's education.

The classroom should be one which reflects the use of behavior modification techniques as a means of facilitating learning and maintaining high motivation. The interpersonal environment should be one that emphasizes the child's positive abilities. It should act to enhance, not destroy, his self-concept. The social milieu should be one that is rich in interactions with other children of average and above-average abilities. The instructional program should be aimed at assigning learning tasks in their smallest identifiable units so that at each step along the way correct cognitive responses can be reinforced. The classroom teacher should be an individual who is familiar both with the specific cognitive dysfunctions as well as with the personality characteristics of the hyperactive child. Emphasis should be placed on strengthening the intact cognitive abilities along with the development of specific programs designed to facilitate the generalization of in-classroom learned behaviors to the outside world. Parents should be made knowledgeable of the types of problems and frustrations they can expect to encounter in living with a hyperactive child. When appropriate, medical evaluation, with an eye towards chemotherapy, should be encouraged. Hyperactivity should be viewed as a deficit in the child's efficiency in learning rather than as a psychiatric entity.

Reinforcement Strategies

Developing reinforcement strategies as a treatment for cognitive dysfunction in hyperactive children is a complex process calling for integrating the principles of reinforcement with a social environment conducive to learning with a high degree of motivation. The teacher must also have a thorough understanding of the learning arc and its various components in order to plan for a remedial program which focuses on compensating and correcting for dysfunctions at various points in the learning arc. In short, the teacher must be able to combine her skills in reinforcement theory with her knowledge of cognitive dysfunctions within the learning arc in order to create a classroom environment which minimizes the damaging effects of cognitive dysfunction. The reinforcement strategies outlined in this section emphasize the integration of reinforcement into various elements in the learning environment. The studies presented emphasize structuring of the physical classroom, the introduction of appropriate instructional materials, the utilization of a variety of reinforcement strategies and the promotion of a social environment conducive to motivation.

STRATEGY I: THE TEACHER AS ENVIRONMENTAL ENGINEER. Often the classroom setting and social attitude play as important a role in facilitating learning as do the specific instructional materials and the utilization of positive reinforcement for working on classroom assignments. Glavin, Quay, Annesley and Werry (1971) demonstrated the impact that the proper classroom environment can have on learning in hyperactive children. These authors utilized the concept of a resource room as an alternative to special class placement for learning-disabled and hyperactive children. They had hoped to demonstrate that placing hyperactive children in a resource room for brief periods of time would allow them to progress academically to a point where they could be fully reintegrated into their regular classrooms. The success of the program was to be evaluated in terms of both improvements in academic performance as well as reductions in disruptive behaviors. Glavin and his colleagues integrated the concept of the highly motivating environment, i.e. the resource room, with reinforcement theory. Reinforcement was made contingent on increases in academic achievement.

Fifty-five second to sixth grade public school children who had been rated as either extremely disruptive or extremely withdrawn on the Quay, Peterson Behavior-Problem Checklist (1967), and who were found to be two or more grades behind academically, were included in the study. While all of the children studied were diagnosed as learning disabled, the majority of them were also determined to be hyperactive. The average child in the experimental group was ten years of age with a measured IQ of approximately eighty-five and a mean achievement level for reading and math at second grade fourth month and second grade first month respectively. Subjects in the experimental group were matched with a comparable control group.

All subjects were observed in their regular classroom settings. A baseline was kept of the periods of time during the day which they were observed to be most disruptive. The classroom conditions during these periods of time were closely scrutinized. The children in the experimental group were then assigned to the resource room for brief periods each day. These periods coincided with the times during the day during which the child was encouraged to maintain his identity as a regular classroom student. The time spent in the resource room was treated as would be any other special activity such as gym or art. While in the resource room each child received token reinforcement as well as praise for appropriate behavioral and academic improvement. Tokens were exchangeable at the end of the day for items available at a token store located within the school. For each child the resource room program was based on the concept of shaping positive behavioral responses. In other words, positive classroom behaviors as well as improvements in academic achievement were considered to be shapeable responses. By shaping each individual component and linking these components together through the use of intermittent reinforcement to form response chains, entire new patterns of appropriate classroom behaviors and academic performance were formed. In order to increase motivation at the onset of the child's initiation of the program, reinforcement was given liberally. When the child began to show progress, increases in motivation were stimulated by manipulating the learning environment. For example, as a child's time in the resource room increased, items in the token store went up in price for that individual child requiring a greater performance in order to earn the same amount of rewards. The principle of nonreinforcement was also incorporated into the learning environment. Disruptive behavior in the resource room was dealt with through the use of a time-out room. Reinforcement was unavailable to those children during periods of time in which they behaved in a disruptive manner. These children were allowed to participate in the reward-rich resource room program after they had demonstrated one or two minutes of appropriate silence and behavioral control.

Weekly meetings between the teachers and the teacher's aide focused on reviewing reinforcement strategies and increasing the response-reinforcement ratio for each child. The emphasis in this component of the program was on developing the most highly motivating reinforcement condition for each child. Much emphasis was placed on the importance of increasing academic achievement. Baselines were made of each child's performance within the resource room. Records were kept of the frequency of on-task behaviors, disruptive behaviors and pupil-teacher contacts. Baselines of these behaviors for the control group were made in the regular classroom. These baselines were repeated several times over the course of the entire academic year. In addition, pre- and posttesting for achievement in reading and math was completed for both groups. The duration between pre- and posttesting was six months, with all of the experimental subjects having been in a resource room for at least five months.

The results of the study showed that all of the children in

the experimental group showed significant improvement in grade achievement for reading and math over the control subjects. In addition, when their performance on the posttest measures of math and reading were compared with their performance on the pretest measures of math and reading, they showed significant improvement.

The children in both the experimental group and the control group were observed in the regular classroom following the completion of the study in order to determine any possible differences between the two groups for the three-target behaviors. No significant differences in the frequency of on-task behaviors, disruptive behaviors and frequency of pupil-teacher contacts were observed between the two groups. The authors' observations suggest that what was learned in the resource room was not transferred to the regular classroom. In other words the improvements and behaviors learned in the resource room did not generalize. This suggests that these behaviors had been maintained by the stimulus of the resource room and the response-reinforcement relationship. This observation has been repeated in many of the other reinforcement strategy studies presented in other chapters of this text. The fact that improvements in behavior did not generalize from the resource room to the regular classroom does not suggest that the program was ineffective, nor does it suggest that the children were not motivated. On the contrary, it points out an important weakness of many such programs, namely, that it is usually assumed that the behaviors learned in the highly motivating reinforcement-rich environment will be generalized to a stimulus environment characterized by fewer motivating influences. Generalization of behaviors learned in the resource room should not be assumed. On the contrary, an important component in any such program should be the reinforcement of generalizing these behaviors to the regular classroom.

A final observation in this study was that almost all of the gains made by the experimental group in classroom behaviors and in academic achievement occurred shortly after the student's entry into the resource room. This suggests that perhaps the gains observed could be accomplished in a time period as short as two months. This would have certainly allowed an adequate amount of time to develop a program for reinforcing generalization of behavioral and academic gains back to the regular classroom.

A valuable aspect of this particular study was that the greatest percentage of school time for each child in the experimental group was spent in his regular classroom. This approach fits with the concept of mainstreaming and permits the child to retain his identity as being like his classroom peers. The teachers in this study served as environmental behavioral engineers. They carefully assessed the social, academic and reinforcement components of the learning environment and developed each to its maximum level of efficiency in promoting student motivation.

STRATEGY II: REINFORCEMENT OF ACADEMIC ACHIEVEMENT THROUGH THE USE OF SCHOOL AND HOME REINFORCERS. The identification, management and dispensation of reinforcement within the classroom can present a problem itself. This aspect of the program calls for locating and stocking a variety of primary reinforcers to be used as purchasable items in the token store. Funding problems and managing a token program can demand much time for the teacher to spend in performing what amounts to an administrative function. Many classroom teachers prefer not to use their time in this way. In addition, the reinforcing value of tokens in the classroom can be quickly diminished by the fact that many of the reinforcers are available for the child at home. It often happens that a well-planned classroom reinforcement program is undermined by the fact that the student is able to obtain reinforcers outside of the classroom.

McKenzie, Clark, Wolf, Kothera and Benson (1968) addressed themselves to this problem by developing a token reinforcement, behavior modification classroom program which integrated the use of reinforcers in the classroom as well as in the child's home in order to decrease disruptive classroom behaviors while increasing the academic achievement. Recognizing that token reinforcement often involves expense and much administrative time in tallying, exchanging and managing tokens, and also recognizing that parents often feel excluded when the motivational program in the classroom is totally outside of their control, McKenzie and his colleagues sought to develop a token reinforcement program for improvement in academic achievement and in classroom behaviors without having to purchase or stock primary reinforcers. By enlisting the cooperation of their students' parents, McKenzie et al. established a program whereby tokens received in the classroom were applied towards the child's allowance at home. These authors were also interested in comparing the effectiveness of token reinforcement for home reinforcers as compared with token reinforcement for reinforcements usually available within the school, i.e. teacher attention, classroom privileges, etc. In order to reduce the administrative time involved in establishing the token program, McKenzie and his colleagues introduced the concept to the children by informing them that their grades would serve as tokens which they could exchange at home for an allowance.

Ten hyperactive, learning-disabled students in an elementary school learning abilities classroom were included in this study. All of the children were of average intelligence and ranged in age between ten and thirteen years. The classroom was a self-contained resource room with screened desks. The emphasis in bringing classroom behaviors under control was on the development of techniques for implementing reinforcement. With the exception of the screened desks, the classroom was like any other regular classroom. In keeping with the principle of structuring all of the components of the classroom, instructional materials were programmed for each child, depending upon his level of ability and degree of behavioral control. All of the instructional materials used required the child to make overt measurable responses which could then be reinforced.

During the first two days of the school program, all of the children in the experimental group were given achievement tests in reading, penmanship, arithmetic, spelling, English comprehension and grammar. Academic assignments were individualized to the extent that each child received the weekly assignment in each of the five areas based on his proficiency in each of these areas as measured by the pretest.

Each child's assignment sheet listed the materials he worked with each day, the total number of responses assigned for the day, and the starting and finishing time for each assignment by day. The teacher's assignment was to record the number of completed responses per assignment along with the number of correct responses per assignment, and to assign a grade accordingly. Weekly home allowance was made contingent on the grades received in each of the subject areas. "A" grades received the highest denomination, "B" grades received slightly less and "C" grades received still less. "I" grades resulted in a fine of the amount equal to that earned for an "A" grade. The monitary value of grades was determined by the parents according to their budgets, social values, attitudes and the age of their own child. This element of the program required a parent-teacher conference in which parents worked together with the teacher to develop an individualized reinforcement system for their child based on what they saw as an acceptable allowance. The importance of making reinforcements within the home environment contingent on improvements in the classroom, and of controlling the home environment so that access to reinforcers was dependent on performance within the classroom was stressed. Parents agreed with the classroom teacher that all incomplete work would result in a token fine. The child could work off the fine by doing certain predetermined home chores. Grades or tokens were redeemable at the end of each week at home. Parents not only distributed the child's allowance according to grades which he received, but they also insured high motivation by structuring rewards within the home in such a way that the child was not able to horde tokens. The children were required to use their allowances to pay for their own toys and special activities. An important factor in the success of this program was the parent's willingness to be sure that their children did not have access to money from any other source. Money received from relatives as gifts was placed in a savings account. This type of parental cooperation guaranteed the high reinforcing value of the allowance. Finally, in order to facilitate generalization, the parents of the children in the study were encouraged to continue their reinforcement program when the child returned to the regular classroom situation. Parental conferences were held once each month. Parents were in full agreement with the reinforcement program in the classroom. They agreed that academic behavior should be reinforced while inappropriate behaviors should result in nonreinforcement.

Within the classroom, access to certain reinforcers was available to those children who had completed their daily assignments. Recess was available to those children who had completed their assignments. In addition, the child was permitted to participate in free-time activities should he complete his assignment before the period was up. These activities included drawing, painting, reading and choice of a seat in the classroom. Special privileges such as going on school errands were also made available to children who showed recent improvement in the quality of their work. Those children who showed a consistent improvement in completing their assignment were also given the opportunity to join the rest of the school in the cafeteria for lunch. Children whose baseline was characterized by incompleted assignments were required to remain in the classroom while eating lunch at their desks. Of course, teacher attention was given liberally to those children who were working on their assignments.

The results of this study showed significant increases in reading achievement in only nineteen days. Over the course of the entire study, significant increases in arithmetic achievement were also observed. By the end of the school year, all of the subjects were working successfully at one to four grade levels above baselines. Sixty percent of the students in the study had returned to their regular classes. Half of the students who had returned to their regular classrooms earned grades of B or better, while the grades for the remaining half averaged C.

This study proved to be successful in several ways other than improving the child's academic achievement. For one thing, it brought parents and teachers closer together to facilitate an understanding of reinforcement and the role which it plays in increasing motivation. The study also demonstrated that an effective token reinforcement system could be established without the need for special funds and without a great deal of investment in administration time. Other than scoring the weekly assignment sheets, there was no need for teachers to keep long daily lists of tokens earned and tokens spent, and since grades became associated with token reinforcement, it is likely that the reinforcing power of grades themselves was increased.

SUMMARY

The relationship between hyperactivity, cognitive dysfunction and IQ has come to be more fully understood within the past few decades. Our present level of knowledge of these three processes allows us to view them as separate but related phenomena. Perhaps most important in terms of the history of cognitive dysfunctions is the understanding that the hyperactive child suffering from dysfunction constitutes a diagnostic entity separate from that of mental retardation. In viewing the hyperactive child as one who quite often suffers from cognitive dysfunctions, we have moved away from a medical model which classifies such children as "sick." On the contrary, the emphasis has been on the similarities between the average child and the hyperactive youngster. The child is best served by a philosophical approach which views him as an individual who is a member of a population-at-risk.

Our increased sophistication in understanding the nature of human intelligence and the variables which affect it has helped greatly in our understanding of the differential abilities found in hyperactive children. Generally speaking, the hyperactive child presents an IQ picture characterized by a pattern of unevenly matched cognitive abilities. While the ten basic cognitive abilities have been equated with intelligence, our review in this chapter has pointed out that many other cognitive variables affect child learning. The memory abilities play a particularly important role in the child's overall level of cognitive functioning. The memory process itself may be visual, auditory or tactile, and involves the stages of registration, retention and recall. The dysfunctions associated with deficits in recall are particularly important to the average classroom teacher. While most teachers have an understanding of the deficits in remote memory, little is generally known about dysfunctions of recent memory. Quite frequently, this particular form of memory dysfunction is found in the hyperactive child. Immediate short-term memory, mental control ability and sequential memory play important roles in the hyperactive child's cognitive profile. Of course, as the material to be recalled becomes more abstract, the memory deficits themselves become more difficult to understand. Dysfunctions of logical memory and associative memory have far-reaching effects on the hyperactive child's ability to learn.

Our understanding of cognitive dysfunctions has been helped greatly by the development of the receptor-effector system concept. This concept is one which views learning as a three-stage process involving reception through the sense organs, mediation by the cerebral cortex and either verbal or motor expression which is controlled by the autonomic nervous system. These receptor-effector systems involve visual or auditory input followed by the mediational process and verbal or motor output responses. One of the valuable secondary contributions of this conceptualization of the learning process is that it helps us to view the hyperactive child as a youngster who experiences inefficiency in learning. A full understanding of these systems and their functioning helps the teacher to dismiss many of the stereotype explanations which cast the hyperactive child in a "bad light."

The work of Skeffington (1968) has been particularly helpful in this area. His analysis of the vestibular system, the center process and the communication process has helped us recognize that many of the child's complaints in school are based on his faulty approach to learning tasks rather than on the wish to avoid learning itself.

The work of Kirk and McCarthy (1968) has also been very enlightening. By using Osgood's model (1957a, 1957b) these researchers were able to identify a number of important cognitive processes responsible for learning. Their explanation of cognitive activity at the organizational level has been particularly helpful for the classroom teacher. An explanation of such processes as visual closure and visual sequential memory, as well as visual association, have been invaluable. Their particular emphasis on the auditory processes has added much to the body of knowledge about cognitive dysfunctions.

Finally, the tactile receptor-effector system is one which has become increasingly important in understanding cognitive dysfunctions. While little has been written in the educational literature about this input-output system, its importance can be inferred from the fact that being able to form concepts through the sense of touch plays a critical role in helping the child who has been unable to learn through other senses.

The roles of attitudes and habits of responding also play an important part in cognitive efficiency. Response sets as well as cognitive styles may determine a child's learning efficiency even when no other form of cognitive dysfunction is operative. Response sets refer to specific habits in responding while cognitive styles represent approaches to learning on a molar level. These styles are particularly important because they represent the integration of attitudes and response sets into a general pattern which typifies the child's approach to learning.

One of the most important contributions of this chapter has been the introduction of the concept of the learning arc. The learning arc constitutes a representational model of the process of learning. It takes into account the receptive process, the organizational process and the expressive process as they are affected by cognitive abilities, response sets and cognitive styles. The learning arc represents the process of learning in its full complexity.

Recent changes in educational philosophy along with an understanding of the relationship between cognitive dysfunctions and developmental lag theory have brought about important changes in the academic curriculum for the hyperactive child. Our understanding of the fact that certain cognitive abilities may be poorly developed while others may be above average, and our understanding of the fact that retention is a form of treatment which relies mainly on developmental maturation to compensate for cognitive dysfunctions has laid the groundwork for the mainstreaming approach to the treatment of a hyperactive child with cognitive dysfunctions. This approach supports the child in the regular classroom while allowing him to attend special tutorial sessions in a resource room in order to work on improving those abilities which are least efficient.

The use of behavior modification techniques in the treatment of cognitive dysfunctions requires the teacher to utilize her expertise on several levels simultaneously. In effect she must become a learning specialist and an environmental engineer. Of all the reinforcement strategies used in treating the primary characteristics of hyperactivity, the strategies used in treating cognitive dysfunctions call for the greater integration of changes in the learning milieu, academic materials and implementation of learning theory to bring about a motivating environment.

REFERENCES

Alabiso, F. P.: Inhibitory functions of attention in reducing hyperactive behavior. *American Journal of Mental Deficiency*, 77:259-282, 1972.

Bloom, I., and Murray, W.: Some basic issues in teaching slow learners. *Understanding the Child*, 26:85-91, 1957.

Broverman, D. N.: Dimensions of cognitive style. *Journal of Personality*, 28:167-185, 1960.

Broverman, D. N., Broverman, I. K., and Klibern, L.: Ability to automatize an automation cognitive style: A validation study. *Perceptual Motor Skills*, 23:419-437, 1966.

Campbell, S. B., Douglas, V. I., and Morgenstern, T.: Cognitive styles and hyperactive children and the effect of methylphenidate. *Journal of Child Psychology and Psychiatry*, 12:55-67, 1971.

Carter, P., and Lockey, A.: Teaching the hyperactive child. *Provo Papers*, Summer, 124-131, 1967.

Clarizio, H. F., and Yelon, S. N.: Learning theory approaches to classroom management: Rationale and intervention techniques. *Journal of Special Education*, 1:267-274, 1967.

Cruickshank, W. T., Bentzen, F. P., Ratzenburg, F. L., and Tannhauser, M. N.: *A Teaching Method for Hyperactive and Brain-Injured Children*. Syracuse, Syracuse UP, 1966.

Douglas, V. I., Weiss, G., ad Minde, K.: Learning disabilities in hyperactive children and the effects of methylthenidate. *Canadian Psychologist*, 10:201, 1969.

Glavin, J. P., Quay, H. C., Annesley, F. R., and Werry, J. S.: An experimental resource room for behavior problem children. *Exceptional Children*, 10:131-137, 1971.

Gofman, H.: The physician's role in early diagnosis and management of learning disability. In Tarnobol, L. (Ed.): *Learning Disabilities*. Springfield, Thomas, 1970.

Harlow, H. F.: Learning set in error factor theory. In Koch, S. (Ed.): *Psychology: A Study of a Science*. New York, McGraw, 1959, 492-453.

Jolles, I. L.: A public school demonstration class for children with brain damage. *American Journal of Mental Deficiency, 60*:582-588, 1956.

Kagan, J., Rosman, B., Day, D., Albert, J., and Phillips, W.: Information processing in the child: Significance of analytic reflective attitudes. *Psychological Monograph, 78*:N. 578, 1964.

Kaliski, L.: Educational therapy for brain-injured retarded children. *American Journal of Mental Deficiency, 60*:71-76, 1955.

Karp, S. A., and Konstadt, N.: *Manual for Children's Embedded Figure Test.* Cognitive Test, New York, 1963.

Kirk, S. A., McCarthy, J. J., and Kirk, W. D.: *Illinois Test of Psycholinguistics Abilities.* Urbana, University of Illinois Press, 1968.

Kirk, S. A.: What is special about special education?: The child who is mentally retarded. *Exceptional Children, 19*:138-142, 1953.

Koppitz, E. M.: Diagnostic brain damage in children with the Bender Gestalt Test. *Journal of Consulting Psychology, 26*:541-546, 1962.

Martinson, M. E.: Education of a trainable child: an opportunity. *Exceptional Children, 34*:293-297, 1967.

McKenzie, H. S., Clark, M., Wolf, M. M., Kothera, R., and Benson, C.: Behavior modification of children with learning disabilities using grades as tokens and allowances as back-up reinforcers. *Exceptional Children,* Summer, 745-752, 1968.

Osgood, C. E.: *Contemporary Approaches to Cognition.* Cambridge, Harvard UP, 1957a.

Osgood, C. E.: *Motivation dynamics of language behavior.* Paper presented at the Nebraska Symposium on Motivation. Lincoln, University of Nebraska Press, 1957b.

Quay, H. C., and Peterson, D. R.: *Manual for the Behavior Problem Checklist.* (Mimeograph) Champaign, Children's Research Center, University of Illinois, 1967.

Ross, A. C.: The application of behavior principles in therapeutic education. *Journal of Special Education, 1*:276-286, 1967.

Santostefano, S., and Paley, E.: Development of cognitive control in children. *Child Development, 35*:939-949, 1964.

Schrager, J., and Lindy, J.: Hyperkinetic children: early indicators of potential school failure. *Community Mental Health Journal, 6*:447-454, 1970.

Schrager, J., Lindy, J., Harrison, S., McDermott, J., and Wilson, P.: The hyperactive child: an overview of the issues. *Journal of the American Academy of Child Psychiatry, 5*:526-533, 1966.

Shainman, L.: Vocational training for the mentally retarded in the schools. *American Journal of Mental Deficiency, 56*:113-119, 1951.

Skeffington, A. M.: Optometric case analysis. *Optometric Extension Program, 10*:1-39, 1968.

Smythe, J. R.: *The Neurological Foundations of Psychiatry.* Baltimore, Blackwell, 1966.

Spearman, C.: *The Abilities of Man.* New York, Macmillan, 1927.
Strauss, A., and Lehtinen, L. B.: *Psychopathology and Education of the Brain-Injured Child.* New York, Grune, 1947.
Ullman, L. R.: A sample of operant studies. *Journal of Special Education,* 2:319-321, 1968.
Wechsler, D.: *The Measurement and Appraisal of Adult Intelligence.* Baltimore, Williams and Wilkins, 1965.
Wehlen, R. I., and Haring, N. E.: Modification and maintenance of behavior through systematic application of consequences. *Exceptional Children,* 32:281-289, 1966.
Werry, J. S.: Developmental hyperactivity. In Chess, S. E., and Thomas, A. B.: (Eds.): *Annual Progress in Child Development.* New York, Brunner-Mazel, 1969.
Witkin, H. A., Duik, R. B., Faterson, H. S., Goodenough, G. R., and Karp, S. A.: *Psychological Differentiation.* New York, Wiley, 1962.
Witkin, H. A.: The perception of the upright. *Scientific America,* 200:50-56, 1959.

CHAPTER **6**

IMPULSIVITY IN HYPERACTIVE CHILDREN

Perspective

IMPULSIVE BEHAVIOR HAS been a source of concern for the classroom teacher for many years. Prior to the last decade there had been little research upon which the classroom teacher could draw to help in planning an educational program for the impulsive, hyperactive child. An early review of the literature brought Murray (1938) to the conclusion that impulsivity involved the tendency to respond rapidly without reflection. According to Murray, this tendency was subject to such variables as social pressure, intuitive behavior, emotional "drivenness," deficits in forethought and a willingness to work without a strategy for problem-solving. While Murray's work provided us with an overview of the research, it left many unanswered questions, particularly in view of the fact that hyperactivity had not yet been established as a separate diagnostic entity. The relationship between impulsivity and the syndrome of hyperactivity had yet to be explored.

Relatively little research appeared in the interim between Murray's review of the literature and the concepts presented by Diamond, Bolvin and Diamond (1963). Diamond and his colleagues focused on the physiological aspects of impulsivity. They attempted to link impulsivity to a deficit of the inhibitory process of the cerebral cortex. While their findings raised many interesting questions about the possible organic correlates of impulsivity, the results were limited to studies on brain-injured children. Actually, little of the research on the physiological causes of impulsivity in human beings has been applicable to the classroom situation. As we shall see in other parts of this chapter, a variety of other social factors and learning variables have a profound effect on the development of an impulsive cognitive style.

Within the past decade, research on impulsivity has increased. Hirschfield (1965) viewed impulsivity as a constellation of personality traits and behaviors. His definition of impulsivity included quick response time, deficits in the ability to reflect on response alternatives, restlessness, weaknesses in control over feelings and a tendency to react against authority. The core of this constellation was viewed as an inability to control motor and feeling responses. This deficit he equated with hyperactivity.

Schwebel (1966) focused more on the concept of impulsivity than on the relationship between impulsivity and hyperactivity. In his research in this area, he examined both the characteristics of impulsivity and the characteristics of reflectiveness. Most definitions of impulsivity have viewed these two traits as reciprocal inhibitors of one another. Schwebel viewed impulsivity as a deficit in the ability to reflect on a task. Indeed, he believed that impulsivity represented a dysfunction in the ability to critically evaluate response alternatives. That is, he viewed impulsivity as a weakness in the ability to be reflective. This view of the hyperactive-impulsive child depicted him as an individual who was unable to make a critical evaluation of his response choices. The quickness with which the impulsive child was described as responding was attributed to the fact that he spent little time in reviewing his choices. Actually, this concept of impulsivity and reflectiveness as being reciprocal inhibitors of one another leaves many unanswered questions about the nature of impulsivity. For instance, this theory would seem to suggest that as reaction time decreases, the ability to critically evaluate response alternatives increases. In other words the ability to make a critical evaluation of response alternatives was related to the speed with which the child responds. While this theory may have face validity, subsequent research shows reflection and impulsivity to be separate components of cognitive style.

Mercurio (1975) addressed herself to this issue. In her review of the literature she noted that the definition of impulsivity tended to be confusing. This confusion surfaced in her study in which she attempted to develop a teacher rating scale of impulsivity. Interestingly enough, the scale which she developed was based on teacher observation which did not correlate significantly with the other major measures of impulsivity currently in use. Apparently, there has been a lack of teacher consensus as to what constitutes impulsivity.

Kagan, with his colleagues (1964, 1965a, b, c; 1966; 1966a, b, c; 1971), has been a pioneer in this area of research. Indeed, his early studies on impulsivity have served as a standard by which other studies have been evaluated. Bypassing the confusing issue of physiological correlations of impulsivity, Kagan viewed impulsivity as a cognitive style. As mentioned in Chapter 5, cognitive style represents the child's overall attitude in approaching a learning task. It involves an integrated constellation of response sets, previous learning experiences and attitudes towards learning. He defined impulsivity as a cognitive style with two components. These components consisted of cognitive tempo, that is, the speed with which a child responds to a problem solving task and the ability to critically evaluate response alternatives when the correct response was not immediately obvious (Kagan, Rosman, Day, Albert and Phillips, 1964). In short, he defined reflection-impulsivity as the relationship between the child's decision time and the quality of his performance when he is faced with solving a problem that is characterized by a variety of solution alternatives. Kagan developed an instrument for measuring these two dimensions in elementary school children. The MFFT requires the child to examine a picture (the standard) and six highly similar stimuli (response alternatives). Only one of the response alternatives is identical to the standard. The test requires the subject to select the one response alternative which is identical to the standard. The child's score on the test reflects both latency in response time and the number of errors committed.

During the past several years, a second body of research has developed around the cognitive style associated with impulsivity-reflection. Interestingly enough, this body of research was generated by studies in the development of language. Kohlberg et al. (1968) identified four types of speech which form a developmental hierarchy. The lowest form of speech was that of self-stimulating private speech. As the child matured, this pattern yielded to outer-directed private speech which was followed by inner-directed private speech. Finally the child was observed to make indistinguishable self-mutterings. Essentially, the developmental process was one in which the child made the transformation from viewing words as concrete objects to utilizing them as internal symbols for the self-regulation of behavior. Level 1 in this developmental process depicted the child as engaging in such verbalizations as word play, animal noises, word repetitions and singing. At the second level, the child addressed remarks to inhuman objects while also, verbalizing descriptions of his own activities. When functioning at the third level the child was characterized by inner-directed self-guiding private speech. This speech was characterized by self-instruction which the child used to control and direct his own behaviors. The presence of indistinguishable self-mutterings indicated that Level 3 had become routinized to the point that word fragments had become symbols for entire sets of self-instructions.

Based on Kohlberg's research and the research of others (Bem, 1967, 1970; Vygotsky, 1962; Klein, 1963; Lovaas, 1964; Luria, 1959, 1961), Meichenbaum and Goodman (1969a) proposed that language serves a mediating function between the requirement of the task and the child's actual response. They viewed the impulsive children as experiencing a deficit in the hierarchy of language development. According to Meichenbaum, these youngsters had not learned to use inner speech to guide problem-solving behaviors. The reflective child on the other hand was one who functioned at the highest level in the hierarchy of speech development. These children were described as individuals who could use private speech to direct their responses. The short response latencies observed in impulsive children were thought to result from the absence of the use of private speech. Private speech was thought to serve a dual role. First, the child's private speech served to delay his response time. Second, private speech was thought to guide the child through a series of problem-solving strategies. Meichenbaum's findings in this area of cognitive development indicated that there is much merit to this theory.

THE NATURE OF IMPULSIVITY

Kagan's Concepts

The Kagan et al. (1964) monograph on impulsivity stands as the most authoritative publication on impulsivity. In this monograph, Kagan and his colleagues undertook eight studies to evaluate the nature of impulsive cognitive style.

In the first study the relationship between the ability to respond analytically to cognitive tasks and impulsivity-reflectivity was evaluated. The Conceptual Style Test (CST) was utilized in order to measure both ability to perform on an analytic level and impulsivity-reflectivity. This instrument is one which requires the child to select two pictures from an array of several pictures. The child's task is to select the two visual stimuli which are most alike. Correct responses reflected an ability to identify concept classifications and relational concepts. A large group of elementary school age children were evaluated to test the hypothesis that as analytic style increased, impulsivity would decrease. Among other findings, this study revealed that analytic attitude is associated with the tendency to inhibit impulsive, inaccurate responses. In other words, Kagan and his associates found an inverse relationship between analytic cognitive style and impulsive responding.

In the second study, the Design Recall Test (DRT) was utilized in order to test the hypothesis that a learning set for reflection would increase analytic concepts while a set for brief response latencies would interfere with analytic cognitive responses. The DRT requires the child to remember a geometric design which was presented to him fifteen seconds prior to observing an array of other designs in which the standard is present. Children were given different sets of instructions which either encouraged long response latencies or brief response latencies in favor of a longer time to reflect on response choices. The results of this study indicated that the response set significantly affected the ability to perform on analytic tasks. Long response delays were associated with high analytic performance. Under instructions to respond quickly, analytic performance decreased significantly.

The third study was established to test the hypothesis that

children with a highly analytic cognitive style would tend to be more reflective in their cognitive styles. That is, these children would be more critical in evaluating their response alternatives. The findings of this study supported the hypothesis. It led Kagan and his colleagues to confirm that reflection was a demonstrable aspect of cognitive style.

Based on the results of the first three studies, they concluded that when a child is faced with a task in which several response alternatives are simultaneously available, he may show a divergent cognitive response style characterized either by impulsivity or a tendency to be reflective. The first three studies focused on the aspect of response latency. In other words, these studies investigated the relationship between impulsivity and cognitive tempo.

The fourth through the sixth studies evaluated the dimension of reflectivity. This dimension addressed itself to the child's ability to make a critical evaluation of several response alternatives. It differed from cognitive tempo in that it refers to the correctness of a child's response rather than the speed in which he makes it.

In the fourth study the relationship between the ability to make a critical evaluation of response alternatives and analytic cognitive style was investigated. The results of this study indicated a positive significant correlation between the production of analytic responses and the ability to critically evaluate response choices. These findings confirm the theory that analytic cognitive style is related to the tendency to analyze the test stimulus into its essential components and the tendency to inhibit impulsive answers. The findings of this study were somewhat obscured by the fact that the instruments used to assess reflectivity required the child to use his visual memory abiltiy. It was thought that deficits in visual memory ability could have acted to confound the results of the study.

In the fifth study, to delete this variable, Kagan and his colleagues developed the now-famous MFFT. This test was one that removed the variable of visual memory by presenting the child with a standard test stimulus and its variants simultaneously. The subject's task was to select the variant that was identical to the standard. The standard consisted of a figure with which the average child would be familiar. Five of the six variants were similar but not identical to the standard with only one of the six variants identical. The child's task was to identify the variant which was identical to the standard. The MFFT provides measures of both visual analysis and reflection. The results of this study indicated that correct recognition of the essential stimulus characteristics as presented in the MFFT was positively related to analytic conceptual style as measured by the CST and the DRT. This study established reflectivity as a dimension of cognitive style. The findings of Study Five remained constant even when testing conditions changed from a friendly, encouraging test atmosphere to one in which the examiner withheld encouragement and was more technical in his dealings with the child. These findings indicated that regardless of testing conditions the relationship between impulsivity and analytic cognitive style remained stable. The sixth study replicated the findings of the fifth study.

The seventh study was critical in that it evaluated the relationship between the ability to make a critical evaluation of response alternatives, i.e. reflection, and rapid cognitive tempo. The results of this study for both male and female subjects demonstrated conclusively that an inverse relationship existed between the ability to respond reflectively and the tempo of response. The shorter the latency time between the presentation of the task and the first response, the greater the number of errors in the child's ability to make a critical evaluation of response alternatives.

The eighth study concerned itself with the broader relationship of impulsive-reflective cognitive style to two of the other primary characteristics associated with hyperactivity. This study focused on the interactions between impulsive-reflective cognitive style and distractibility, and between impulsive-reflective cognitive style and motor activity. A large group of male and female elementary school children was assigned to either the reflective or impulsive group based on their MFFT performances. With respect to attention-distractibility the results indicated that impulsive subjects were most likely to exhibit momentary lapses of attention while working on academic tasks. Reflective children on the other hand exhibited a greater degree of concentration, and less distractibility during academic performance. Observation of spontaneous displays of gross motor activity indicated that reflective children tended to show less spontaneous gross motor activity. They were observed to be more oriented towards individual tasks. No association was observed to exist between the degree of aggression and impulsivity-reflectivity. An inverse relationship was found between restlessness and reflective cognitive style.

In subsequent years, Kagan has completed other studies in order to assess the effects of cognitive style on academic achievement (Kagan, 1965) and the effects of cognitive styles across learning tasks (Kagan, 1966b). In his study on the relationship between impulsive-reflective cognitive style and reading ability, Kagan (1965) emphasized that the impulsive-reflective cognitive style was composed of two separate dimensions. The first dimension was that of response time or cognitive tempo. The second was that of critical evaluation of response alternatives. In this study Kagan sought to determine whether measures of impulsive-reflective cognitive style in first grade children would predict success in reading during the second and third grades. Kagan hypothesized that reflective children would commit fewer word recognition errors. Sixty-five male and sixty-five female first grade middle class public school children were selected for the study. Each subject was tested on two separate occasions, once at the beginning of the study and then one week following the completion of the study. During the first test session each subject completed the Design Recall Test, the Haptic Visual Matching Test, the Wechsler Intelligence Scale for Children and the MFFT. They also completed a visual analysis examination in order to determine if they were able to distinguish figures from background. Finally, each subject completed a reading ability test which consisted of measures of the child's skill in letter and word recognition. The results of this study indicated that word recognition errors were inversely related to response time. As response latencies increased, word recognition errors decreased. Kagan also observed that subjects who exhibited high verbal ability scores on the Wechsler Intelligence Scale for Children did well on the word recognition test. This was not attributed to native intelligence but rather the fact that these children appeared to have developed a conceptual strategy for problem solving. No sex differences were observed with respect to the findings. In addition, no significant relationship was found between performance on the pretest of visual ability and the incidence of word recognition errors. This finding was particularly important in view of the fact that reading disorders are thought to result solely from visual problems. Kagan's findings, to the contrary, indicated that for the subjects in his study, reading errors were mainly related to the nature of the child's cognitive style.

One hundred and thirteen of the one hundred and thirty subjects tested during the first grade were retested at the end of second grade. These children were given a word recognition test in which the experimenter read a word and the subject was required to identify it from a list of three printed words. This task was repeated thirty-nine times. Six months later, the MFFT was given and the scores on the two tests were correlated. The results of this part of the study indicated that scores on the MFFT and the word recognition test in the first grade were predictive of performance on the word recognition test in the second grade.

The same group of children was again tested six months later. During this testing each of the subjects took the MFFT and another test of reading ability. This test was more complex than the original word recognition test. It evaluated the child's tendency to make ten different types of reading errors. The results of this study tended to support the previous findings. Children classified as impulsive responders in the first grade had the highest reading errors on this more complex measure of reading ability which was administered over one year later. Kagan concluded that the study indicated that impulsive cognitive style was a major cause of reading disabilities in elementary school children. He cautioned, however, that his study assumed that subjects with long response latencies were utilizing the response time to make a careful consideration of response alternatives. He noted that this assumption may not always hold true, as in the case of the distractible child who utilized response latency time to attend to extraneous stimuli. The nonimpulsive hyperactive child, for example, may display a long response latency. It is not safe to assume, however, that such a child manifests a reflective cognitive style.

Kagan (1966b) sought to evaluate the generality of cognitive style across learning tasks. He investigated the relationship between impulsive-reflective and accuracy of performance on serial learning tasks. Serial learning tasks are ones in which a list of words are read to the child. Errors are scored when, in the process of recalling the word list, the child introduces a word which was not in the original presentation. These errors, known as errors of commission, are particularly important in a variety of classroom learning situations. Kagan also evaluated the motives, expectations and level of anxiety which characterize the reflective child. He further sought to evaluate the effects of "desire for success" and fear of failure on cognitive style.

This study involved the same group of first and second grade children who participated in Kagan's 1965 study. These children were evaluated upon entering the third grade. The MFFT and the Wechsler Intelligence Scale for Children were administered and the children were subsequently assigned to either the impulsive group or the reflective group. Three-and-a-half months later all subjects were given a serial learning task. After several warm-up trials, subjects listened to familiar words read to them from a tape recorder. They were then asked to repeat the word list. In order to study the variables of subject expectations and anxiety over failure, a new condition was introduced during the third testing trial. On this trial, described as the "threat" trial, suggestions were made that the next trial would be more difficult and that many children were expected to do poorly. The purpose of this instruction was to arouse anxiety over failure. For a second group of children, the third trial introduced the variable of anxiety. This trial known as "the rejection trial" was one in which children were told that their performances on the first two trials were poor. They were informed that they were expected to do better on the third trial. The purpose of this instruction was to arouse anxiety over disapproval. Finally, another subgroup of children were tested under control group conditions. For them, the third trial was administered under standard instructions.

Test results indicated that on the first two trials the reflective subjects exhibited significantly fewer errors of commission than did the impulsive subjects. In addition, the higher the recall score, the lower the number of errors of commission. No relationship was found between verbal intelligence, reflection-impulsivity or errors of commission for either males or females. Reflective subjects showed significantly better recall on the first two lists than did impulsive subjects.

All subjects, including the control subjects, did poorer on the third and fourth trials. This finding initially suggested that the experimental conditions of expectation for failure and disapproval had the same effect regardless of a subjects' cognitive style. However closer evaluation of the data did reveal important group differences. Reflective and impulsive subjects did not differ on latency of the first response during their trials. However, reflective subjects persisted longer in attempting to recall the list. This suggested a higher level of motivation. Threat statements seemed to discourage reflective subjects while rejection statements seemed to increase motivation. Reflective subjects showed a significant increase in errors of commission under the threat condition while showing no difference in the number of errors as a result of expectations of examiner disapproval. Changes in response scores between the first two trials and the third and fourth trials were greater for reflective than for impulsive subjects. Evidently, reflectives were more effected by threat than were impulsive subjects. However, this difference did not reach statistical significance. Kagan concluded that cognitive style affects both recall and the frequency of errors of commission. Reflective children seem to be more negatively affected by anxiety than do impulsive children. Evidently, one of the characteristics of the impulsive responder is that, within certain limits, anxiety level seems to have no negligible affect on his ability to perform.

In an overview of his research on impulsivity, Kagan (1966a) addressed himself to the implications that his research findings had for education. He encouraged teachers to become more sensitive to the pervasiveness and far-reaching effects of cognitive tempo. His findings challenged the long-held stereotype that the slow responder is a dull child and that fast response times are an indication of intellectual brightness. He further encouraged teachers to recognize that cognitive style can become a major source of reading disability. Finally, he encouraged teachers to develop programs for the teaching of a reflective cognitive style.

Meichenbaum's Concepts

Within the past several years, a second body of research has been developed around the dimension of reflective-impulsive cognitive style. Meichenbaum drew on the literature of the development of psycholinguistic ability in order to formulize his theory of impulsivity as a lag in development in verbal mediation ability (Meichenbaum and Goodman, 1969a, b; Meichenbaum and Goodman, 1971a; Meichenbaum, 1974; Meichenbaum, 1975a, b, c). In Meichenbaum's review of the literature on the development of verbal mediating ability he reported that Bem (1970) theorized that verbal mediation as psycholinguistic ability undergoes a series of refinements associated with increases in development level. According to Bem (1970), problem solving requires that the child be able to comprehend, produce and mediate overt behaviors with the use of verbal responses. The young child is viewed as not maintaining any ability to mediate or regulate his behaviors verbally. For such a child, words do not act to control his external behaviors. Like the young child, the impulsive child tends not to spontaneously produce verbal mediating responses, nor does he comprehend the aspects of problem solving that call for the use of verbal mediation. Vygotsky (1962) emphasized the importance of internalizing verbal commands in the child's development of voluntary control over his behaviors. Drawing on the findings of several authors, Meichenbaum (1971b) concluded that the development of the self-guiding private speech was a critical factor in impulse control. He further noted that the process of development self-guiding private speech appears to be integrally related to the child's developmental level. Essentially, the process of developing self-guiding private speech was described as one in which the child's behavior progresses from a level at which it is controlled externally to a level at which it is internally controlled. Meichenbaum viewed the process whereby the control that speech has over behavior becomes internalized as critical in development of a reflective cognitive style. ". . . early in development, the speech of others, usually adults, mainly controls and directs the child's behavior; somewhat later, the child's own overt speech becomes an effective regulator of his behavior, and still later the child's covert or inner speech can assume a regulatory role" (p. 116).

Perhaps the best description of the developmental process through which a child must go before covert, verbal mediation becomes effective is presented in the work of Kohlberg et al. (1968). This researcher identified four different types of speech, forming a hierarchy which ultimately results in the efficient utilization of self-regulating prviate speech. According to Kohlberg, children at the lowest developmental level in the hierarchy are characterized by speech patterns which contain self-stimulating private speech. These individuals are observed to make such verbalizations as animal noises, repeating words, singing songs and word play. At the next level of development, the child's verbal behavior is characterized by outer-directed, private speech. Children at this level direct remarks to inhuman objects and make descriptions of their own activity. At the third developmental level, inner-directed or self-regulatory private speech appears. Children at this level use their own inner speech as a guide for controlling their external behavior. In effect, they use their inner speech as a form of self-instruction. Finally, at the highest developmental level the child's speech is characterized by inaudible mutterings. These mutterings reflect external manifestations of internal speech. In effect these mutterings become shortened forms of symbols for groups of self-instruction.

Meichenbaum (1971a) used the verbal mediation model described by Kohlberg (1968) as a basis for his hypothesis that training in self-guided private speech would significantly improve the performances of impulsive children. He conducted a series of four experiments to evaluate the relationship between impulsivity and verbal mediation abiilty. Two of these studies were particularly instrumental in the development of his theory of impulsivity.

In the first study he sought to identify differences between impulsive and reflective children by analyzing the content and quality of their self-verbalization. Eight impulsive and eight reflective four and one-half-year-old nursery school children were selected from a larger group of nursery school children based on their performances on the MFFT. The reflective and impulsive groups were matched on age and IQ. The play behaviors of all the subjects were observed over a two-and-a-half-week observation period. Frequency and quality of play behaviors were recorded and modified according to Parton and Newhall's (1943) rating scale. Frequency of verbalizations and the content of private speech were also recorded. Reflective children gave significantly more verbalizations during the two-week observation period. Impulsive subjects exhibited a significantly higher frequency of egocentric speech patterns. Their speech patterns were characterized by speech which was not addressed to a listener. Reflective subjects used speech to give instructions or to ask questions. In addition they gave three times as many inaudible mutterings during solitary play. These mutterings represented external manifestations of internal speech. There was no difference between the groups in the amount of general communication observed. Meichenbaum concluded that both groups spent their playtime in the same manner, but that the quality of their verbalizations differed significantly. Reflective children were observed to use private speech in a more mature, more instrumental manner. Their pattern of private speech was one that was characterized by self-guidance as opposed to the impulsive preschoolers who did not seem to use speech as a means of controlling and guiding their behaviors.

In the second study reported (Meichenbaum and Goodman, 1969), Meichenbaum sought to evaluate the effects of self-instruction on the performances of reflective and impulsive children on a Luria-type task. This task was one in which the subject was instructed to depress a foot pedal when a certain visual cue was given. The pedal was to remain depressed until the visual cue was removed. When a second visual cue came into the child's focus, his instruction was to not depress the foot pedal. The performances of reflective and impulsive children on the task were evaluated under two conditions. In the first condition, the child was simply to complete the instructions as given by the examiner. That is, any self-instruction that the child might have practiced was on a covert level. According to the second condition the child was to overtly verbalize the instruction while completing the task. In other words, when the correct stimulus cue appeared the child was to say the word "push" aloud while depressing the foot pedal. When the other visual stimulus came into the perceptual field the child was to say aloud "don't push." The function of these instructions was to provide a testing condition in which an analysis could be made of the relationship between the subjects' frequency of correct responses and his overt verbalizations. The results of this study proved rather interesting. Only 40 percent of the impulsive subjects passed the Luria-type test to the criterion of 90 percent correct responses. On the other hand, 85 percent of the reflective subjects met this test criteria. Impulsive subjects exhibited less verbal control over their motor behavior. They were observed to use private speech in a less instrumental fashion than reflective subjects. Meichenbaum concluded that training impulsive children to talk to themselves in a self-regulatory manner could facilitate behavioral change and self-control.

In an overview on the cumulative research on impulsivity, Meichenbaum (1975, c) observed that reflective children differed from impulsive children in a number of ways. He noted that reflective children seem to use their eyes differently in scanning the visual field. Reflective children tend to make more eye fixations and examine more stimulus alternatives. On the MFFT they tend to look more at the standard stimulus. Impulsive children seem to be less systematic in their search of the visual field. They are generally less analytic than reflective children in evaluating stimuli in their perceptual field. He further described impulsive children as frequently interrupting themselves, thereby shortening the length of time they spent at any given activity. Their strategies for searching the perceptual field tended to be less thorough and less systematic. They seem less capable of keeping track of more than one focus of attention task at a time. Reflective children, on the other hand, seem to process visual information more efficiently. They were observed to use more systematic and more mature problem-solving strategies. They seem to be able to make better use of feedback about their performances and they asked more constraint-seeking questions which helped them by eliminating several of the response alternatives.

Meichenbaum suggested that no one theory of compulsive-reflective cognitive style was able to account for all of the observed differences. He suggested that present theories of impulsivity could be integrated in order to develop a broader conceptual base for a comprehensive theory of impulsivity.

In an attempt to integrate the cognitive tempo theory of impulsivity with verbal mediation theories of impulsivity, Meichenbaum developed an instrument which he called the cognitive-assessment approach (Meichenbaum, 1975c). This approach was one which involved an assessment of the child's cognitive strategies. He recommended that the interaction between the child's performance and the testing conditions be closely examined in order to analyze the interactions between deficits in attention, private speech and cognitive tempo. Meichenbaum further suggested that remediation involved analyzing the child's problem-solving strategies by dividing them into subunits. It was the job of the teacher to identify a hierarchy of the child's skills and to help the child translate those skills into self-statements that could be rehearsed. Self-instruction training would first involve having the child observe an external model who demonstrated and verbalized the response strategy. This phase was to be followed by the child's own performance of the response strategy under the direction of the model. Then the child was to continue to practice this response strategy while whispering the directions to himself. Finally he was to complete the task using only private speech to self-guide his response strategy. Teaching the child private speech involved learning a response strategy method in which the child is taught to define the problem. Second, he is trained to focus his attention by using self-instruction. Third, the child is encouraged to use self-verbalization to reinforce his own performance. He is encouraged to tell himself that he has done well and that he is improving. Finally, the child is taught to use self-guiding private speech to make an evaluation of his performance. He is to praise himself for correct responses and to identify errors in his own response strategy.

Conclusion

From a theoretical point of view, impulsivity seems to be affected by a variety of cognitive processes. The brief response latency which is usually thought of as characterizing the impulsive child refers to only one dimension of this cognitive style. The child's ability to critically evaluate his response alternatives constitutes an important variable in determining the degree of impulsivity. In addition, his ability to use inner speech to mediate his behavior and to control his responses plays a critical role in his problem-solving abilities. Impulsivity is a relatively stable trait which seems to resist change over time. Within limits, developmental level does not seem to assume the same position of importance with respect to impulsivity as it does with the other primary characteristics of hyperactivity. The subject's gender and level of intelligence seem to play only minor roles in this cognitive disposition. The instructions of others including those given by parents have little effect on cognitive style. Furthermore, impulsivity seems to affect the child in a variety of learning situations. The old axiom that the child with the quick response has the higher IQ does not stand up under the test of research on impulsivity. The generality of this cognitive style and its far-reaching effects across a variety of academic tasks presents substantial challenge for amelioration. A more in-depth understanding of the population characteristics and the relationship of impulsive cognitive style to the other primary characteristics associated with hyperactivity would facilitate a fuller comprehension of treatment approaches.

RELATIONSHIP TO OTHER CHARACTERISTICS OF HYPERACTIVITY

Impulsivity and Attention

Meichenbaum (1975, c) linked impulsivity to attention. In his review of the literature on the impulsive cognitive style, he reported that there was a strong relationship between impulsivity and the child's ability to attend to a given task. In view of our understanding of attention presented in Chapter 4, it seems likely that the length of time that a child spends at a given task (span) and his cognitive tempo influence one another. Meichenbaum reported that the research findings of Segel, Babich and Kirasic (1974) and Weiner and Berzonsky (1975) demonstrated a positive relationship between selective attention and reflective-impulsive cognitive style. While Meichenbaum makes no direct mention of the relationship between focus of attention and impulsivity, the relationship between these two phenomena seems apparent as evidenced by the fact that the primary measure of impulsivity (MFFT) is essentially a focus of attention task. As noted above, this task is a single-stage stimulus discrimination task of the type described in the section on focus of attention in Chapter 4.

Meichenbaum was not the first to comment on the relationship between impulsivity and attention-distractibility. Douglas (1972) noted the common property of these two characteristics. Both characteristics were described as responding positively to treatment with psychostimulant drugs. Douglas concluded that the impulsive children in her study lacked the ability to complete tasks that required concentrated attention and organized planning. She considered attention to be so closely linked to impulsivity that she viewed the ability to be attentive, and to control and organize response strategies as a single dimension. In a more recent article, Douglas (1974) studied the relationship between sustained attention and impulsive control. According to Douglas, attention required impulse control as the task of attending demanded that the child continue to focus on stimuli long after having lost interest in them. In addition, impulse control was thought to be necessary if the child was to use his attention skills in inhibiting tendencies to respond to incorrect stimuli. Finally, impulsivity was thought to interfere with attention span since deficits in impulsivity resulted in brief response latencies which prevented the child from making a careful search of response alternatives. Douglas saw these two characteristics as so closely linked that her description of them gave the impression that they could be considered reciprocal inhibitors of one another.

Harrison and Nadleman (1972) investigated the relationship between attention, distractability and impulsivity. He was particularly interested in the effects of distractability. He hypothesized that response tempo was related to the ability to inhibit responses. The results of his study demonstrated a significant positive correlation between performance on two measures of ability to inhibit motor movements and the MFFT. In other words, Harrison substantiated the presence of a positive correlation between the ability to inhibit responses and cognitive style. Generally, those children having the highest scores on the measures of ability to inhibit motor movement were found to be characterized by a reflective cognitive style. Those youngsters having low scores on the measure of ability to inhibit motor movement were found to be impulsive on the MFFT. In addition, a significant inverse relationship was found between the number of errors on a MFFT and the ability to inhibit motor responses. Harrison concluded that impulsivity correlates significantly with distractability.

Impulsivity and Activity

The relationship between impulsivity and activity level has not gone unnoticed. Douglas (1972, 1974) noted that activity level seems to vary independently of impulsivity. She supported this contention with the fact that activity level tends to decrease with age while an impulsive cognitive style is relatively permanent. Her studies generally suggest that there is no causal relationship between activity level and impulsivity. However, there does tend to be a qualitative relationship between these two characteristics. Impulsivity is one of the characteristics of activity level often found in hyperactive children.

Welch (1973) observed reflective and impulsive children in the free play setting. She observed the differences in behaviors of preschool, reflective and impulsive children who were matched on activity level. She found no differences between the groups on the number of activities in which they engaged. However, the reflectives were observed to remain at a given activity for a significantly longer period of time. The impulsive children in the study exhibited significantly greater transition behaviors. That is, they were observed to be either between tasks or to be engaged in idle time activities in which they seemed to be exhibiting no purposive behaviors. The impulsive youngsters did not demonstrate more activity than did reflective youngsters but the nature of the activity was observably different. The impulsive children, for instance, were observed to exhibit a higher frequency of dependency behaviors such as attention seeking. A most important finding of this study was the fact that reflective children exhibited twice as many simultaneous behaviors as did the impulsive children. In other words, the reflective children were observed to, at a higher frequency, engage in more than one task at the same time. The impulsive children, on the other hand, seemed unable to do this. Attending to one task was interrupted by any attempt to simultaneously complete another task.

As a part of an overall attempt to study the relationship between impulsivity and gender, Gardner, Percy and Lawson (1971) hypothesized that behavioral impulsivity and intellectual impulsivity were separate processes. Based on this hypothesis, they predicted that as activity level increased, errors on measures of impulsivity would also increase. Behavioral impulsivity was defined as the rapid shifting from one activity to another. A frequency count of various classroom behaviors was made by the researchers. They concluded that increases in behavioral impulsivity were accompanied by increases in activity level.

Impulsivity and Cognitive Dysfuncton

Several studies have demonstrated a clear-cut relationship between impulsivity and cognitive dysfunction. Kagan, with his colleagues (1965, 1966), conducted several studies to evaluate the relationship between impulsivity and cognitive dysfunction. In one such study, he found that impulsivity alone was enough to cause significant reading deficits in elementary school children. Impulsive readers were observed to have a high incidence of word recognition errors. In addition, they made numerous errors of commission as well as intrusion. Impulsive children were found to have significantly greater errors on measures of letter and word recognition. On tests of reading, these children were found to make a high number of substitutions. These substitutions usually had graphemic similarity to the correct word. For example, the impulsive children would substitute the word "nose" for "noise," "truck" for "trunk" and "eight" for "eat." The relationship between these errors and verbal ability was negative. In other words, the high frequency of errors was not related to the child's ability to use verbal concepts.

Kagan et al. (1966) also studied the relationship between impulsivity and errors of commission in serial learning tasks. A high correlation between errors of commission and errors on the MFFT was found. Those subjects in the study who were in the reflective group exhibited significantly fewer errors on the serial learning task. It would appear that impulsivity affects the child's ability to perform academically in the classroom even when his other cognitive abilities are functioning efficiently.

Campbell, Douglas and Morgenstern (1971) studied the relationship between hyperactivity and cognitive style. A group of hyperactive youngsters of normal intelligence was compared with the control group on four measures of cognitive style. The subjects in each group completed tests measuring their response latency and number of errors, i.e. reflection-impulsivity; their ability to analytically view visual stimuli, i.e. field dependence-independence; their ability to respond rapidly to routine tasks, i.e. automatization; and their ability to inhibit responses to distracting stimuli and contradictory cues, i.e. constricted-flexible control. No differences were found between the two groups on automatization and constricted-flexible control. However, the differences in performance between the hyperactive and control subjects on the measure of reflection-impulsivity and the measure of field dependence-independence were significant. The hyperactive subjects were found to be more impulsive and less analytic than normal subjects in their approach to visual stimuli. The investigators observed that hyperactive children tended to apporach cognitive tasks differently than nonhyperactive children. The hyperactive subjects in this study were observed to be more impulsive. They responded more quickly and made more errors than the normal subjects. They were less able to inhibit verbalizations and were less able to prevent responses to distracting stimuli. They were noticably less analytic and more global in their perception of the stimulus field. In addition, they were slower to respond automatically to routine tasks.

Although not all hyperactive children are impulsive, the relationship between impulsivity, activity level, attention-distractability and cognitive dysfunction give impulsivity a place of central importance in understanding hyperactivity. A further description of the characteristics of the impulsive child would help our understanding of the theoretical causes of this dysfunction.

POPULATION CHARACTERISTICS

A number of investigators have studied the relationship between impulsivity and a variety of psychosocial variables. Such variables as age, sex, IQ, style of parenting, stability of cognitive style and personality factors have been researched.

Intelligence

One of the most researched variables has been the relationship of impulsivity to intelligence. As part of Kagan's study (1965, b) on the relationship between impulsivity and reading ability, he investigated the effects of impulsivity on intellectual functioning. Sixty-five male and sixty-five female middle-class first graders attending a public school were tested on three measures of impulsivity, Wechsler Intelligence Scale for Children and a test of reading ability. One of the findings of this study indicated that high verbal ability tended to be associated with reflective cognitive style. However, there was no significant difference between reflective and impulsive children on the measure of IQ. In addition, there tended to be no significant relationship between intelligence and impulsivity. A highly impulsive child was found to be as likely to be of high as low intelligence.

Douglas (1972) made a longitudinal study of a large group of hyperactive middle-class children of normal intelligence. As a part of this comprehensive study she listed several important population characteristics associated with hyperactivity. The subjects in her study were all of average or above intelligence. Ninety percent of the subjects were made with no deficits in language abilities, comprehension, conceptual thinking or short-term memory. A full battery of psychological tests was administered to matched control group normal subjects in order to evaluate the possible relationship between attention, impulsivity and IQ. No significant correlation was found between impulsivity and level of intelligence in either group. They concluded that the ability to be attentive, the ability to control responses, and intelligence were not causally related.

Cohen (1969) administered the MFFT and two other measures of impulsivity to a population of lower income, low-achieving boys were found to be more impulsive. The low achievers were also more consistent in their cognitive styles than the high achievers. There was no significant correlation between performace on test of intelligence and measures of impulsivity.

In her review of the literature on impulsivity, Mercurio (1975) reported that impulsive children tend to have lower IQ scores and a lower self-confidence than do reflective children. However, she attributed this to the effects of impulsivity on test-taking ability rather than to any native difference in intelligence between impulsive and reflective children. Douglas' (1972) findings supported this observation.

The general consensus among researchers seems to be that there is no measurable relationship between impulsivity and lower intelligence. It appears that this dimension of cognitive style varies independently of the subjects' level of intelligence. Quite frequently, the impulsive child is taken for an intellectually dull youngster. To date there has been no research data to substantiate this assumption. The only relation between performance on tests of intelligence and impulsivity seems to be one which is generalized across performance tasks for impulsive children. That is, impulsive children tend to do poorly on measures of performance whether the measure is one of intelligence or academic achievement It would seem that the impulsive child's cognitive style obscures his ability to perform on tests of intelligence.

Sex

The relationship of gender to impulsivity is particularly interesting in view of the significantly greater incidences of the primary characteristics associated with hyperactivity in boys. Several researchers have found that the effects of impulsivity are differentially affected by the sex of the subject (Sutton-Smith, 1961, 1967; Seigel et al., 1967; Kagan, 1964). Generally, these studies have shown that attentiveness in planning, which is characteristic of reflective cognitive style, has a positive effect on academic performance in male subjects. However, this same variable seems to have a negative effect on the performance of female subjects. Ostensibly, these studies suggested that females perform better on standardized tasks when they become somewhat more impulsive while the performances of males on the same task improves if they become somewhat more reflective. Maccoby (1967) hypothesized that there would be a significant positive correlation between impulsivity and a high level of task performance in females, and a significant positive correlation between reflective cognitive style (or as Maccoby termed it "inhibited passive factor" p. 261) and a high level of task performance in male subjects. The results of his study confirmed these hypotheses.

In a rather extensive follow-up study, Gardner, Percy and Lawson (1971) examined the relationship between impulsive-reflective cognitive style, gender and intelligence. Using the term *passivity* to describe reflective cognitive style, and the term *activity* to describe impulsive cognitive style, Gardner and his colleagues hypothesized that females would tend to be more passive, i.e. reflective, while males would be more active (impulsive). They proposed a theoretical continuum with passivity at one end and activity at the other end and hypothesized a curvilinear relationship between gender and position on the activity-passivity continuum. They also predicted a negative correlation between impulsivity in boys and reflective cognitive style in girls. In other words, they hypothesized that as boys who tended to be impulsive became more reflective, IQ scores would increase. Girls who tended to more reflective were predicted to show increases in IQ performance as they became more impulsive. It was predicted that this relationship held true for points in the middle ranges of the continuum, however, as either gender approached the extremes of the continuum, IQ performance was predicted to decrease. Based on these hypotheses, Gardner and his colleages predicted that boys would be more active than girls. They also predicted that, regardless of the subject's gender, whenever he moved to either extreme on the passivity-activity continuum IQ performance would decrease. Based on this prediction, they also hypothesized that subjects in the middle ranges on the passivity-activity continuum would do best on measures of intelligence. In order to add power to their study, Gardner and his colleagues identified two types of impulsivity. Intellectual impulsivity was defined as a rapid responding to any problem situation. Behavioral impulsivity was said to occur when the subject rapidly shifted from one activity to another.

Fifty-five boys and and fifty girls from a public elementary school were selected from the study. Subjects were matched on age and intelligence. Both groups were tested for intellectual impulsivity and behavioral impulsivity. The tests for intellectual impulsivity was one that was similar to the MFFT. The test used by Gardner was one in which the subject was presented with a picture of a familiar object and then was required to identify a slightly different figure of an array of six pictures in which five were identical to the standard. Impulsivity was measured in terms of response latency and the number of errors. Behavioral impulsivity was recorded by using a rating scale to tally the frequency of certain behaviors which occurred during random, two-minute intervals in the classroom.

The results of the study were in the predicted direction. That is, male subjects scored significantly higher on measures of behavioral impulsivity. A low level of behavioral impulsivity in boys was found to correlate highly with heightened intelligence. A high level of behavioral impulsivity in males correlated negatively with heightened intelligence. As predicted, a high level of behavioral impulsivity in females correlated positively with intelligence, while a low level of behavioral impulsivity in females correlated negatively with intelligence. Interestingly enough, no differences between sexes were found for the measure of intellectual impulsivity. Males were not found to be significantly more intellectually impulsive than females. Another interesting finding was that both males and females who attained intermediate scores on the measure of passivity-activity did not do significantly better on measures of IQ than did individuals at either extreme of the scale. Evidently, the differential effects of gender on impulsivity hold true with respect to behavioral impulsivity only. None of the hypotheses were confirmed with respect to intellectual impulsivity. With respect to behavioral impulsivity, findings did confirm that active girls and inactive boys tend to be more reflective. Gardner et al. attributed this relationship between impulsivity and gender to the differential effects of the socialization process. Boys on the other hand were described as receiving early socialization which encouraged behavioral impulsivity. According to Gardner et al., both groups tend to perform the higher levels when they are encouraged to move towards the center of the passivity-activity continuum.

Harrison and Nadelman (1972) made a similar observation. While the main focus of his study was on the relationship of attention-distractibility to impulsivity, he did make several important observations about the relationship between gender and impulsivity. Male and female preschool children were studied. When the study data was analyzed according to gender, girls were found to be better able to inhibit motor responses. Males tended to have more difficulty in voluntarily controlling their tendency to respond quickly and in controlling their tendency to give only cursory evaluation to response alternatives. Harrison, however, contributed this difference in ability to inhibit motor response to developmental factors rather than to factors associated with socialization. He suggested that girls of the same age as boys tend to be more advanced developmentally.

Based on the literature reviewed, it would seem that a relationship between impulsivity and gender exists. It appears as if females tend to be more reflective while males are apt to be more impulsive. Whether this relationship is associated with socialization or the differences in developmental level between males and females when age is held constant is unclear.

Age

The question of the effects of age on impulsivity has been evaluated by several researchers. To date the findings have been contradictory. In her longitudinal study of hyperactive impulsive non-brain-damaged elementary school children, Douglas (1972) reported that impulsivity changed little with age. Indeed, the subjects who were identified as being impulsive during the first year of the study were found to be generally more impulsive several years later. Kagan (1965, b) followed a group of children from kindergarten to the completion of third grade. Students were tested each year for impulsivity as a part of a study on the relationship between reading failures and impulsive cognitive style. Generally, the child's status changed little over the three-and-a-half-year period of the study. Children who were determined to be impulsive at the kindergarten level were usually found to be impulsive at the third grade level.

Shelley and Riester (1972) studied a population of young adults who had a school history of hyperactivity, impulsivity and aggressiveness. He traced the school history of these subjects and found that academic achievement in high school was superior to that of elementary school. The adults were described as having learned to avoid tasks which required the use of perceptual motor skills. Other than this handicap, no residual effects of impulsivity were observed. Shelley concluded that impulsivity decreased with age to a point where it was no longer a liability during adulthood.

The research findings of Mosher and Hornsby (1966) seem to offer the most insight with respect to the relationship between age and impulsivity. These authors studied a large population of elementary school children at various chronological and developmental levels. Their findings indicated that impulsivity is a relatively stable trait between infancy and age six. Between the sixth and the tenth year, the child is involved in the process of developing more sophisticated response strategies. These strategies involve the use of symbols and abstract concepts. Mosher and Hornsby concluded that children who fail to develop symbolic and abstract response strategies tend to remain impulsive. Those children who develop these strategies tend to become reflective. In his studies on the relationship between impulsivity and response strategies, Ault (1972, 1973) concluded that the child's ability to develop a response strategy which inhibits impulsivity increases with age. He observed that impulsive children at the fifth grade level seem to be those children who do not develop sophisticated response strategies.

The combined findings of Mosher and Hornsby (1966) and Ault (1973) suggest that any changes in impulsive cognitive style that occur with increase in age are related to a general developmental factor associated with the ability to use symbols and to think abstractly. At this point more studies are needed in order to substantiate a developmental theory which would link decreases in impulsivity to physiological maturation.

Studies on the stability of impulsive-reflective cognitive style tend to substantiate the theory that physiological maturation alone is not sufficient to bring about a change in cognitive style. Kagan (1966) studied the stability of impulsive cognitive style in two independent samples of children. He used the MFFT response time score as a measure of impulsivity. In the first study, male and female third graders were administered the MFFT. One year later a different form of the same test was administered. The correlation between response time on the first test and on the second test was significantly high for both males and females. Kagan replicated this study with first graders. The test was administered at the onset of first grade and readministered one year later. No significant difference in response latencies was found between the two test administrations.

Kagan concluded that response latency was a relatively permanent dimension of cognitive style. Based on these two studies and several others, Kagan concluded that though response latency tends to increase somewhat with age, the child's cognitive style is a relatively permanent characteristic of his performance on learning tasks.

Messer (1970) devoted an entire study to the relationship between impulsivity and stability of cognitive style. He was particularly interested in the relationship between impulsivity, stability and school failure. Messer administered the MFFT to sixty-five elementary school children at the first grade level. The same group of youngsters was retested two-and-a-half years later on a more difficult form of the MFFT. During the initial testing, Messer identified three distinct cognitive styles. A subgroup of children presented a clearly reflective style. Another subgroup was determined to be impulsive. The third group was found to have long response latencies and a high frequency of errors, i.e. a slow inaccurate cognitive style. Finally, the fourth group exhibited a pattern characterized by brief response latencies with few errors, i.e. a fast accurate cognitive style. When tested two-and-a-half years later the subjects retained their subgroup membership. Those children who were determined to be impulsive-reflective, fast-accurate, or slow-inaccurate responders on the first grade administration of the test remained unchanged on the third grade administration of the test. Seven of the subjects in this study failed at least one grade during the two-and-a-half-year period. Five of those seven subjects had the highest impulsivity scores on the grade one testing. Two-and-one-half yaers later they were still among the most impulsive subjects in the study. Academic retention did not help to change their cognitive style. Their IQ's did not differ significantly from the other children in the study. Evidently, cognitive style is a relatively well-fixed response pattern which is established at an early age.

Mother-Child Variables

Several researchers have investigated psychosocial variables associated with cognitive style. Campbell (1973a, b, c) has investigated the relationship between maternal style of parenting and cognitive style in children. In the first study, Campbell compared reflective, hyperactive and impulsive subjects on a measure of field independence-dependence cognitive style. She also administered a measure of cognitive style to the mothers of the children in each group in order to examine any possible relationship between the cognitive styles of mothers and their children. Thirty reflective, impulsive and hyperactive boys from a suburban elementary school were selected for this study. These subjects were obtained from a larger group of second and third grade students. Each of the children was assigned to one of the experimental groups based on his performance on the MFFT. The groups were matched on age and intelligence. The mothers of the children in the experimental groups were tested on the MFFT. All of the children were given the Embeded Figures Test (Witkin, 1950), a test of field dependence-independence. The findings of this study indicated that significant performance differences were found between reflective children and impulsive and hyperactive children. As would be expected, the reflective children showed fewer errors and longer response latencies than either the hyperactive or the impulsive children on both the MFFT and the Embeded Figures Test. No performance differences were found between impulsive and hyperactive subjects. Most importantly, no differences were found in cognitive style between the mothers of the children and each of the three experimental groups. The performances of the mothers did not correlate significantly with the performances of their children. Campbell concluded that mothers and their children did not have similar cognitive styles.

In a series of further studies, Campbell (1973b; 1975a, b) continued to investigate the relationship between maternal cognitive style and the style of their children. In one study the mothers of hyperactive, impulsive and reflective children were observed while they watched their children who were attempting to complete standardized tasks. The mothers' cognitive styles and the nature of their interactions with their children were evaluated. The mothers of the hyperactive children did not engage in significantly more interactions with their children than did the mothers of reflective children or the mothers of impulsive children. In other words, the mothers of hyperactive, impulsive and reflective children all seemed to interact with their children to about the same extent. The mothers of the hyperactive children did, however, differ from the mothers of the reflective and impulsive children in their pattern of interaction with their children. Contrary to what one might have expected, the mothers of the hyperactive children gave a significantly greater amount of direct physical help. They offered significantly more encouragement and a greater number of impulse control suggestions. This finding is particularly interesting in that the interaction patterns of mothers of hyperactive children seem to be ones that would facilitate a reflective cognitive style. Further evaluation of these mothers indicated that they were not any more punitive or disapproving than the mothers of the other two groups of children. An analysis of the interaction pattern of the reflective mothers with their children indicated that they also tended to make specific suggestions regarding impulse control. They gave more direct physical help to their children than did the mothers of the impulsive children. The overall implication of this finding is that maternal intervention in the form of task structuring, suggestions regarding impulse control and direct physical help have little effect upon a child's cognitive style.

In a follow-up study, Campbell (1975b) studied the interaction pattern between various groups of mothers and their children. The study included a group of normal control subjects, a group of hyperactive subjects and a group of nonhyperactive, learning-disabled subjects. The primary characteristic differentiating between the subjects in the hyperactive groups and the ones in the learning disability group was that the hyperactive youngsters were characterized by a higher degree of distractability and a greater activity level. The learning-disabled youngsters were primarily characterized by academic failure. This group did not evidence a behavior problem. Each group contained thirteen elementary school boys matched for age, IQ and socioeconomic class. As in the previous study, the mothers of the children were observed and rated on the frequency and nature of their interactions with their children while their children were required to complete several tasks. Each mother's interactions were rated according to the frequency of their suggestions regarding impulse control, the frequency of encouraging statements, the number of nonspecific suggestions and the frequency of disapproving statements. No differences were found on these four variables between the mothers of the learning-disabled children and the mothers of the normal, control group children. The mothers of the hyperactive children did show a definite qualitative difference in their interactions with their children. These mothers tried to optimize their child's performance by attempting to provide direction in order to keep the child focused on the task. They seemed to view their child's approach to problem solving as impulsive and disorganized. The hyperactive children's pattern of interacting with their mothers was also observed to be qualitatively different from the patterns established by the normal and learning-disabled children. Hyperactive children were observed to make more requests for assistance. They more frequently asked for feedback and made a higher frequency of comments regarding their own performance and the nature of the task. The overall conclusion of this study was that impulsive cognitive style is not significantly affected by mother-child interaction, due to the fact that the comments of the mothers of hyperactive children regarding timing and critical evaluation did not improve the children's performances.

There has been no study which has been able to substantiate a causal relationship between the mother's cognitive style and that of her child. In addition, it appears that cognitive style is not significantly affected by the quality of the mother-child interaction. This is particularly surprising in the case of hyperactive, impulsive children whose mothers were observed to give numerous suggestions regarding the importance of the critical evaluation of response alternatives and allowing adequate time for the evaluation.

Personality Factors

The relationship between impulsivity and personality factors has been investigated by several researchers. Sutton-Smith and Rosenberg (1959) investigated the relationship between impulsivity and self-concept. These authors theorized that masculine and feminine self-image was linked to impulsive cognitive style. They predicted that there would be an inverse relationship between impulsive cognitive style in boys and masculine self-image. The findings suggested that boys who tended to be impulsive often preferred quiet, orderly and highly structured games of the type most usually preferred by females. Such youngsters were observed to avoid the more aggressive and open-ended games usually stereotyped as "boys games." Highly impulsive girls were observed to show a preference for games usually thought of as masculine. These authors felt that the relationship between gender, appropriate self-concept and impulsivity was so important that all measures of impulsivity should also include measures of gender and self-concept. While much work needs to be done in order to establish this theory, the findings do point to a general psychosocial theory which would suggest that early childhood socialization experiences of impulsive boys tend to be ones that discourage their impulsivity. This process of discouragement make take on the form of reinforcement for engaging in games typically participated in by young girls.

Schwebel and Bernstein (1970) viewed impulsivity as an adaptive response to the environment. They theorized that the impulsive child's history of social, academic and home failure resulted in the child's taking on a cognitive style which allowed him the most rapid degree of escape from a noxious situation, while still meeting the basic requirements of the task. Kagan (1971) also commented on the adaptive nature of impulsivity in some children. He described impulsivity as an adaptive response for children whose school history was characterized by failure. The impulsive cognitive style was seen as a means whereby the child invests less of his emotional energy on a task on which he anticipates failure. Kagan saw these children as being highly anxious over failure. The reflective child was described as having a high standard of performance with much overt anxiety over errors. The impulsive child, on the other hand, was described as having learned to adapt to his high anxiety over failure by developing a cognitive style characterized by low standards of performance, a counterphobic attitude about failure and a low level of investment in tasks on which failure was anticipated.

Kagan (1966, c) viewed impulsivity as the child's adaptive response to a learning situation which required him to produce mutually exclusive behaviors. The impulsive child was described as one who was trying to meet the demand characteristics of the typical classroom. The child was described as being caught between one set of values which called for him to produce an answer as quickly as possible and a second set of values which required him not to error. Essentially the child was pictured as being expected to give quick answers with few errors. Kagan described this as an approach-avoidance conflict in which the child sought to approach short response latencies while avoiding high frequency of errors. The reflective child was seen as adapting to this dilemma by becoming more sensitized to the anxiety associated with high errors than to the anxiety associated with not producing an immediate response. The impulsive child, on the other hand, was thought to be an individual who placed a higher value on quick response time.

Kagan made a longitudinal study on the personality characteristics of reflective and impulsive children. Of the 75 children who were studied from first grade to preadolescence, Kagan selected those male and female subjects who appeared to be most impulsive and most reflective. This subgroup consisted of eight impulsive males and eight impulsive females and eleven reflective males and eight reflective females. These children's behaviors were observed in the classroom and in a free-play situation. Their behaviors were rated on a seven-point rating scale. The reflective and impulsive children showed opposing personality traits. The reflective subjects maintained a higher standard of mastery for intellectual tasks. They exhibited a significantly greater degree of persistence. They were also observed to choose more difficult tasks and to remain more vigilant during those tasks. In social situations, reflective children tended to avoid peer group interaction. They tended to be fearful in strange situations and generally avoided any risk of physical harm. The impulsive children, on the other hand, were observed to quickly embark on new tasks in an unfamiliar social situation. They did not avoid physically dangerous activities to the same extent that reflective children did. They were also observed to be less persistent on difficult tasks.

From the standpoint of personality development it would appear that impulsive cognitive style may be modified or maintained by the child's level of anxiety and history of experiences with failure in social situations. It is quite possible that cognitive style may reflect an adaptive response to the demand characteristics of the social situation. Whatever the cause, it seems that impulsive cognitive style is a relatively stable trait which is not related to either parental cognitive styles or level of intelligence. Age does seem to play an important factor in the reduction of cognitive impulsivity, but only in as much as the child's age may be related to his level of sophistication in developing abstract and symbolic response strategies.

TREATMENT APPROACHES

A variety of approaches have emerged in the treatment of impulsivity. A number of studies have shown impulsivity to be responsive to chemotherapy. These studies present a convincing argument for the use of medication in the treatment of impulsive cognitive style. However, chemotherapy by no means exhausts the treatment possibilities. Indeed, chemotherapy alone does not seem to be sufficient for altering any of the aspects associated with impulsivity other than cognitive tempo. Learning theory has provided us with a variety of treatment approaches which facilitate the critical evaluation of response alternatives and the utilization of self-guiding speech along with increasing response latencies. Depending on the aspect of impulsivity, which has been targeted, the reinforcement program may consist of social modeling, reinforcement scheduling, i.e. delay training, or positive reinforcement. Training in reflective style may also include the instruction in the development of problem-solving strategies. In this section a variety of treatment approaches will be reviewed.

Chemotherapy

Studies by Freidberg, Douglas and Wiess (1968); Werry, Weiss, Douglas and Martin (1966) have shown that tranquilizing drugs have a demonstrable effect on cognitive style. As was the case with the other primary characteristics associated with hyperactivity, it appears that the psychostimulant drugs have the greatest effects on cognitive style. In an important report on this aspect of treatment, Douglas (1972) reported that psychostimulant drugs acted to reduce deficits in attention while improving the child's ability to perform on measures of sustained performance. Most importantly for this section was Douglas's observation that methylphenidate (Ritalin) facilitated an increase in the frequency of correct responses on measures of reflection-impulsivity. Impulsive children treated with this class of psychostimulant drugs tended to be less impulsive on the MFFT. Not only was there an increase in the number of correct responses, but there was also an improvement in cognitive tempo. These findings have been replicated by other investigators (Conners, Rothschild, 1968; Knights and Hinton, 1969; Sprague, Barnes and Werry, 1970).

In a more recent study, Douglas (1974) reported on the data accumulated from a series of studies on the relationship between impulsivity and chemotherapy. The overall conclusion based on these studies was that stimulant drugs mainly affect attention and impulse control. In one group of double-blind studies, the amount of methylphenidate was gradually increased from a minimal original dosage to a rather extensive dosage over a fourteen-day period. While receiving the medication, hyperactive youngsters made a greater number of correct responses, their reaction times improved and they exhibited more control over response tempo. They also exhibited longer response latencies and fewer errors on the MFFT than the control subjects who had not received medication.

The one study which seems to present the most clear-cut support for the theory that psychostimulant medication facilitates a reflective cognitive style was conducted by Campbell, Douglas and Morgenstern (1971). As described in Chapter 5, in the first part of this study, nineteen hyperactive and a matched control group of nineteen normal children were tested on four measures of cognitive style (reflection-impulsivity, field dependency-independency, constricted-flexible control, automatization). The impulsive hyperactive subjects differed significantly from the normal control subjects only on the measures of impulsivity and field dependence-independence. In the second half of this study the effects of medication on the four types of cognitive style were evaluated. Twenty-two hyperactive children ranging in age from five years nine months to thirteen years four months, with a mean IQ of ninety-nine, were given four measures of cognitive style. In this study each subject served as his own control using a double-blind drug placebo design. In other words, each subject was evaluated before and after drug administration. Eleven of the subjects in the study received a placebo while the remaining eleven actually received medication. This process was repeated so that the children who originally received the placebo during the first half of the study received medication during the second half of the study. The dosage was gradually increased over a two-week period of time. The results had strong implications for the value of using drugs as one form of treatment for impulsive cognitive style. The results indicated a significant difference in performance on the MFFT between groups which received the drug and the groups which received a placebo during the first part of the study. Those subjects who actually received the drug showed an improvement in reaction time and a decrease in errors. Campbell concluded that hyperactive children became significantly less impulsive while being treated with methylphenidate. The drug did not significantly affect the children's performances on measures of field dependence-independence nor did it significantly affect the child's skills of automatization or constricted-flexible control.

While drug studies show conclusively that chemotherapy tends to improve the deficits associated with impulsive cognitive style, studies in this area have not yet differentiated between possible effects on response speed as opposed to possible effects on the ability to critically evaluate response alternatives. It is not only possible but likely that the improvement in impulsivity resulting from chemotherapy actually reflects the effects of the drug on response latency time. The increased latencies resulting from the ingestion of the drug may then allow the child the time necessary to make critical evaluation of his response alternatives. The ability to make this evaluation is probably in itself not affected by the drug. As was the case with the other characteristics of hyperactivity, chemotherapy alone does not stand by itself as the only treatment for impulsivity. On the contrary, there are numerous drawbacks to this approach, the least of which is the fact that controlling response tempo through medication does little to actually help the child to internalize more efficient problem-solving behaviors.

Delay Training

Teaching the child to increase his response latency represents an important area of treatment for impulsive cognitive style. A number of researchers have reported that increases in response latencies are highly correlated with a decrease in the frequency of errors.

Kagan, Pearson and Welch (1966) evaluated the modifiability of impulse tempo. Impulsive first grade children were trained to delay their response by ten to fifteen seconds. After only three hours of response training the subjects demonstrated a significant increase in the ability to delay response time. While there was no decrease in the frequency of errors, the training program did suggest that response tempo was a modifiable behavior.

Lowery and Ross (1975) studied the effects of training in response delay on the performances of impulsive mentally retarded children. Fifteen impulsive retardates with a mean age of fourteen years two months were studied. Those subjects who demonstrated the shortest response latencies and the highest frequency of errors on the MFFT and on another similar test were selected for inclusion in the study. To control for any possible effects which the subjects' mental retardation may have had on their performance on the MFFT, a new form of the test was introduced in which six geometric drawings were introduced. Each drawing contained a standard in five response alternatives plus an identical match to the standard. The test was simplified by the use of color and geometric design. Performances of all subjects were recorded on this test. All subjects were involved in three phases of the study, which were carried out over a twenty-four session period. In Phase I, one-half of the subjects received no delay training; during Phase II, these individuals were trained to delay their responses; no delay training was offered during Phase III. The remaining subjects in the study received delay training followed by no delay training and the reintroduction of delay training. During each of the phases of the study, verebal praise and candy reinforcement were received for correct responses. That is, the primary reinforcement was made contingent on production of a correct response regardless of the subject's response latency. The results of the study indicated that subjects in all groups performed at a chance level during the no delay phases and the baseline phase of the study. When a delay of as little as five seconds was maintained by the subjects, correct responses rose steadily to a high level and were maintained. As soon as the reinforcement was withdrawn, all subjects quickly returned to their former level of responding. The overall importance of this study was that it demonstrated that learning theory techniques could have a significant effect on response tempo.

Schwebel and Bernstein (1970) sought to increase the latency of response time for impulsive children in order to better understand the relationship between cognitive tempo and the ability to make a critical evaluation of response alternatives. Eighteen lower class impulsive boys ranging in age from nine to fourteen years were included in the study. The children were divided into two matched groups. One group received response latency training while the other group received no training. Four subtests of the Wechsler Intelligence Scale for Children were administered to both groups. The delay training group took the test in the standard manner prescribed by Wechsler (1949). The delay training group completed the same four subjects under an imposed latency condition. The children in this group were instructed not to respond to the examiner's question until he gave the signal. During this interim period, the subjects were cautioned to carefully evaluate their response alternatives. The latency between asking the questions and the time the child was permitted to respond varied from six to twenty seconds depending on the complexity of the task. The results of this study demonstrated that the children who received delayed response training did significantly better on two of the verbal subtests and one of the nonverbal subtests. Subjects who did not receive delay training generally gave the first response that came to mind. The subjects who received delay training were reported to use response latency time to evaluate potential responses. They were observed to make fewer trial-and-error responses.

Based on the studies presented in this section, it would seem that delay training can make a significant difference in the child's performance, yet it only requires a minimum of training time. Perhaps more encouraging is the applicability of learning theory to delay training. In effect, delay training involves teaching the child to pause before responding. Pausing is a response characteristic which is quite predictable. Response pauses have been shown to characterize subjects' performances on various schedules of reinforcement. In effect, pausing can be created by simply designating the intervals during which reinforcement would be available as in a fixed interval schedule of reinforcement. In other words, by making reinforcement available only at certain fixed intervals following the presentation of the test stimulus, the child is likely to delay his responses until the time at which the reinforcement would become immediately available.

Such a treatment approach would be simple enough to translate into a practical classroom procedure. It simply would involve informing the child that he would not be reinforced for his response until the teacher gave the cue.

Another schedule of reinforcement which accomplishes the same results is the limited hold schedule of reinforcement. Initially, this schedule was devised to decrease pausing in reinforcement. In effect, it made reinforcement available during the fixed interval only if the fixed interval was preceded by a response which occurs in the interim between the presentation of the test stimulus and the onset of the fixed interval. The subject was required to make at least one response before the onset of the period during which reinforcement was available. A modification of the limited hold schedule of reinforcement schedule could be applied in encouraging response pausing. The modified schedule would be one during which the child was required not to make a response during the interim between the onset of the test stimulus and the time at which fixed interval reinforcement was available. The emission of a response during the limited hold period would result in the extinguishing of the test stimulus such that the entire procedure was started over again before the subject could go on and earn a reinforcement. Simply put, if the child responded in the interval between the time he observed the test stimulus and the time the cue was given for making a response, his response would go unreinforced and he would have to go back and start from the beginning. The reliability of fixed interval and limited hold schedules of reinforcement has been well established. Utilizing these schedules of reinforcement as a means of treating rapid cognitive tempo would undoubtedly result in the child's success.

Strategy Training

Whatever changes may occur in response tempo as a result of chemotherapy should not be allowed to minimize the importance of training the child to use effective response strategies in the critical evaluation of response alternatives. Strategy training has become a separate area of research. Early research in the area of cognitive response strategies suggested that the basic response strategy is one in which the child applies his skills in discriminating between the characteristics of a variety of similar but different stimuli (Gibson and Gibson, 1955). A more refined version of this theory was put forth by Solley and Murphy (1960). These investigators suggested that the basic response strategy involved the matching of visual input with a prototype which was stored in the child's memory. Improvements in problem-solving strategies were thought to be the result of a more highly developed memory storage for the prototype for the specific stimulus which the child was monitoring at any given time. Following this line of research, Odom, McIntyre and Neale (1971) studied the problem-solving strategies of impulsive and reflective children. Their findings indicated that reflective children tended to use a problem-solving strategy in which they identified the distinctive features of the standard stimulus. They then utilized these distinctive features as a standard of comparison from which response alternatives were evaluated. Impulsive children gave no indication of having mastered this response strategy.

Zelniker, Jeffery, Ault and Parsons (1972) theorized that the impulsive child's deficits in attention prevent him from making an effective evaluation of response alternatives on measures of impulsivity, which require the child to compare the standard stimulus with similar but different variants. Zelniker and his colleagues attempted to correct for the effects of deficits in attention on the performances of impulsive children by helping impulsive responders to develop a response strategy. Instead of using the procedure outlined in the MFFT, these authors required their impulsive subjects to canvas an array of response alternatives in which all of the alternatives were identical to the standard except one. This was different from the MFFT, in which all of the response alternatives except one differed from the standard. The nature of this task alone served to significantly increase response latencies because the child was required to search for the different stimulus. Searching for the differences between stimuli in itself taught the child an effective response strategy. This was particularly true for the impulsive responder who had been shown to have little skill in identifying the difference between stimuli. The results of this study indicated that training impulsive responders to find the differences between stimuli improved their ability to perform on the MFFT. Though their overall response latencies remained short, the number of errors decreased significantly. This finding suggested that training in critical evaluation of response alternatives did not affect a child's cognitive tempo. In other words, this study not only demonstrated that the training in response strategies could improve a child's ability to reflect on these response alternatives, but it also confirmed the hypothesis that cognitive tempo and critical evaluation of response alternatives represent different dimensions of impulsive cognitive style.

In a follow-up study, Zelniker and Openheimer (1973) sought to evaluate the effectiveness of several different response strategy training methods on perceptual learning in impulsive children. They hypothesized that impulsive children who were trained to differentiate between stimuli would make fewer errors, i.e. be more reflective, than those impulsive children who were trained in finding the similarities between visual stimuli. This hypothesis was based on their rejection of the prototype theory proposed by Solley and Murphy (1960). Zelniker's et al. (1972) earlier study lent support to the theory that an effective response strategy is one which teaches the child to find the differences rather than the similarities between response alternatives (Gibson and Gibson, 1955). Sixty impulsive and sixty reflective kindergarten students matched for age and sex were divided into their respective groups according to their cognitive style. The sixty reflective subjects constituted the control group. Thirty of the impulsive subjects were given training in the differentiation between stimuli. The thirty remaining impulsive subjects were given training on the MFFT. Their training was one in which they were required to identify the similarities between the standard stimulus and its variants. In each subgroup of impulsive responders, each subject received verbal feedback on the accuracy of his responses. If he was correct he received positive verbal reinforcement. Incorrect responses resulted in negative verbal reinforcement. The results of the study indicated that those children who received training in identifying the differences between stimuli performed the best on the generalization measure of the ability to critically evaluate response alternatives. This group made fewer errors than the control group subjects and fewer errors than the subjects who had received training in identifying the similarities between stimulus characteristics. No significant differences in number of correct responses were found between the impulsive subjects trained in identifying similarities and the control group of reflective subjects. The overall findings in this study confirmed the hypothesis that effective response strategy training involved teaching impulsive children to identify the differences rather than the similarities between response alternatives.

By making a more refined evaluation of children's performances on the MFFT, Ault (1973) identified two additional subgroups of problem-solving strategies. In addition to the impulsive cognitive style characterized by brief response latencies and high errors, and the reflective cognitive style characterized by longer response latencies and fewer errors, Ault identified what he termed fast-accurate problem-solving strategies and slow-inaccurate problem-solving strategies. In effect, individuals who belonged to these groups demonstrated an ability to maintain rapid cognitive tempo while making few errors in critical evaluation of response choices, or they exhibited a slow response tempo with a high frequency of errors in the ability to critically evaluate response choices. Ault hypothesized that performance deficits associated with impulsivity may be the result of ineffective response strategies rather than rapid cognitive tempo. In his study, he sought to compare the performances of impulsive children on the MFFT with the performances of fast-accurate and slow-inaccurate responders on the same test. One hundred-and-eighty-two male and female elementary school children at the first, third and fifth grade levels were evaluated for inclusion in this study. All subjects completed a modified form of the MFFT plus The Twenty Questions Test. Ault reported that as response time increased, the frequency of errors decreased.

He discovered a high, positive correlation between learning strategies as measured by the Twenty Questions Test and errors on the MFFT. The relationship between response time errors and learning strategies remained stable at all ages sampled. Response strategies improved somewhat with age. Impulsive responders were found to do poorer than reflective responders and fast, accurate responders at all ages. Young reflective subjects achieved scores equal to those of older impulsive subjects. This suggested that poor cognitive style in older children may be related to developmental lag. Reflective and fast accurate subjects were determined to have cognitive response strategies that were more abstract and at a higher developmental level than the impulsive and slow, inaccurate responders.

Modification of response strategies constitutes a major area of treatment for impulsive-reflective cognitive style. It is evident that training in cognitive tempo alone does not significantly alter the child's ability to make critical evaluation of response alternatives. From the literature reviewed it appears that the most effective approach to modifying response strategy is one that teaches the child to identify the differences rather than similarities between response alternatives.

Positive Reinforcement

Douglas (1974) reported on a series of studies on the effects of positive reinforcement on the performances of hyperactive impulsive children. She compared the results for hyperactive impulsive children with those of normal children. Douglas reported that reinforcement increased alertness in both groups of children. Only the normal subjects, however, seemed to become more critical in evaluating response alternatives. Douglas concluded that positive reinforcement alone was not sufficient for increasing critical evaluation of response alternatives in hyperactive, impulsive children. She recommended that general reinforcement of positive responses be supplemented by specific reinforcement for those behavioral responses which led to critical evaluation of response alternatives. Based on the research on distractability, Douglas theorized that the improvement in impulsivity as a result of introduction of positive reinforcement was minimized by the fact that the reinforcement itself served as a distracting stimulus for the impulsive child. She described the impulsive child as one who became fixated on the reinforcement itself. Indeed, in another study (Douglas, 1972), she suggested that when positive reinforcement was made contingent on activity level, impulsivity tended to increase. Here again she attributed this to the fact that impulsive children often become distracted by the presence of the reinforcer. Actually, not all authors have reported the same results. At this point, however, the effectiveness of positive reinforcement in decreasing impulsivity needs further investigation.

Douglas's findings do not necessarily verify that positive reinforcement has a negative effect on the decrease of impulsive behavior. What her findings do suggest is that there is an interaction between reinforcement and distractability. A carefully controlled study which regulated the distracting effects of the introduction of the reinforcer would be necessary before any conclusive statement about the effects of positive reinforcement on impulsive cognitive style could be given with certainty. It seems likely, however, that should such a study be undertaken, the outcome would be in favor of positive reinforcement. This hypothesis is based on the overwhelming body of literature showing that positive reinforcement favorably influences other primary characteristics associated with hyperactivity.

Social Modeling

As outlined in Chapter 3's section on reinforcement strategy, social modeling described the effects that observing another individual who is operating under a response-reinforcement contingency has on the observer's behavior. In effect, the observation of reinforcement of a social model's behavior tends to increase the frequency of those behaviors in the observer.

Yando and Kagan (1968) studied the effects of teacher cognitive tempo on the cognitive style of classroom children. In effect, these investigators sought to determine whether the teacher served as a social learning model for her students. Twenty-eight first grade teachers from a rural school district were interviewed and given an adult form of the MFFT. The final sample contained ten reflective teachers and ten impulsive teachers ranging in age from twenty-two to sixty-three years. The students consisted of twelve children (six males and six females) from each of the classes of the twenty teachers involved in the study. The children were selected at random and tested on the MFFT. Prior to the beginning of the study all children took the MFFT and the Metropolitan Reading Readiness Test, and were evaluated by their teachers. The MFFT was not scored until the end of the study so that the teachers had no way of knowing which of the children were classified as impulsive and which were reflective. The children were tested during both the fall and spring semesters.

The results of the study indicated that the children exhibited dramatic changes in response latency time between the fall and spring testings. Boys in the classroom of experienced, reflective teachers showed significant increases in the length of response time over the course of the academic year. Female subjects of reflective teachers also showed a considerable increase in response time. These effects were most dramatic when teacher experience was combined with reflective style. Boys and girls with impulsive but experienced teachers made no significant gains. Yando and Kagan concluded that the significant improvements in response latency time for the boys and girls who observed an experienced, reflective model were related to both positive reinforcement by the teacher and social modeling effects. Yando and Kagan recommended that impulsive boys be assigned to experienced reflective teachers as a standard classroom procedure. As we shall see in the section in this chapter concerning strategies, social modeling has become one of the primary methods of reinforcing reflective behaviors.

Combined Dimensions

A very effective approach to the treatment of impulsivity is one which combines various aspects of learning theories to produce combined effects. The verbal mediation theories espoused by Meichenbaum (1971a, b) lends itself to such an approach. The subject's words have been found to be powerul stimulus cues and effective reinforcers in the control of self-behavior. Indeed, one particular form of learning theory called a *covert sensitization* utilizes the subject's visual imagery ability plus his inner speech to bring about a conditioned change in the frequency of certain behaviors. This approach basically relies on the negative reinforcing value of certain visual images made more powerful by the use of words which carry a negative connotation. This approach is an adversive form of conditioning used to decrease the frequency of maladaptive approach behaviors. For example, the child who shows no fear of water is trained to visualize himself becoming violently ill and requiring hospitalization as soon as he steps into water over his waist. At the same time he would be required to visualize an angry lifeguard yelling "Stop! Go back! If you go any deeper you will become ill!" Basically, this form of therapy relies on the child's use of inner speech in order to pair a noxious stimulus with a maladaptive approach behavior. When applied to the child's covert thinking process this form of behavior therapy is known as *thought stopping*. Covert sensitization and thought stopping are particularly applicable to verbal mediation therapy because they deal almost exclusively with the use of words in controlling overt behaviors.

Social modeling also lends itself to the treatment of deficits in verbal mediation ability because the observation of what is said by both the model and the reinforcing agent is so important in helping the child to understand the response reinforcement relationship.

Meichenbaum (1971b) utilized both these approaches in the treatment of impulsivity. He viewed the impulsive child as one who was fixated at an immature level in the development of verbal mediation abilities. According to Michenbaum, as the child's age increased, his ability to use private speech to guide his responses improved. That is, the control of overt behavior shifted from external control to internal control. Early in the development of verbal mediation ability, the speech of others controls and directs the child's behavior. It is the parents admonition "Don't Touch!" that stops the eighteen-month-old child from putting his fingers in the light socket. As the child matures, his own overt speech comes to control his external behaviors. At age two, he can be overheard to say "Me not touch." Finally the child's own overt speech regulates his behavior. In other words, at age three he says to himself, "I should not touch it!"

Meichenbaum sought to train impulsive children to use their own internal mediating responses to control their overt behaviors. He had hoped that this approach would help them to overcome problems in comprehension, problem analysis and response production. In other words, he had hoped that training in verbal mediation would help the child to evaluate the demands of the task, to cognitively rehearse a solution and then to guide his own performance by means of self-instruction. This process was completed with the child's own self-reinforcement. Fifteen second grade male and female impulsive students having the mean age of eight years two months and an IQ of 85 or above were included in the study. The subjects were divided into three groups. The cognitive self-guidance group received four half-hour training sessions over a two-week period. During the sessions, the experimenter acted as a model to the child by performing the task while following the experimenter's spoken instructions. Next the subject was asked to complete the task while instructing himself aloud. This was followed by a period during which the subjects performed the task while whispering the response strategy to himself. Finally, the subject was asked to complete the task while covertly instructing himself. This phase of the study combined several approaches. First, it gave the child specific training at each level of development in the verbal mediation hierarchy. Second, it exposed the child to a social model. Third, it utilized a thought-stopping type of approach. By the time the child reached the last stage of training, he was to say to himself, "Okay, what is it I have to do? You want me to copy the picture with the different line. I have to go slow and be careful. Okay, draw the line down. Good; then to the right, that's it; now down some more and to the left. Good, I'm doing fine so far. Remember go slow. Now, back up again. No, I was supposed to go down. That's okay. Just erase the line carefully, then four dots. Good. Even if I make an error, I can go on slowly and carefully. Okay, I have to go down now. Finished. I did it" (p. 117).

This form of cognitive self instruction involved elements of the thought-stopping technique and self-reinforcement. A variety of tasks were used to train the subject in self-instruction and in controlling nonverbal behavior. The difficulties of the task increased over the four training sessions. The second, or attention, group was composed of youngsters who were seen for the same amount of time as the subjects in the cognitive self-training group. The same test materials were used but no instruction was received. The third group, known as the assessment control group, received only pretreatment, posttreatment, and follow-up evaluations. The children were required to complete three measures of impulsive-reflective cognitive style. Selected subtests of the Wechsler Intelligence Scale for Children measuring comprehension ability, abstract thinking ability and motor speed ability were also administered. Measures of generalization of treatment effects to the classroom were also made. The children were observed in the classroom using a rating scale and a time-sampling technique along with the teacher questionnaire. The follow-up was completed at two week intervals: one week before the end of the study and three weeks after the end of the study.

The results of the study showed that the cognitive self-guidance group did significantly better on all three measures of impulsivity as well as on the performance IQ subtest. During the follow-up study the cognitive self-guidance group showed itself to have significantly better scores over the other two groups. This study exemplified the powerful effects which verbal reinforcement and social modeling have over impulsive cognitive style.

This approach is particularly valuable to the classroom teacher. It is straightforward, uncomplicated and easily enacted in the classroom situation. It simply involves teaching the child to "internalize" the set of instructions before responding. The instructions should include direct self-reinforcement along with utilization of certain words as negative reinforcers for maladaptive approach responses.

STRATEGIES FOR CHANGE

Reinforcement strategies have centered mainly around the use of modeling techniques. A variety of methods of introducing social modeling to children have been utilized. The common element in all of the approaches is that the child learns by observing a social model who is reinforced while exhibiting a reflective cognitive style. Modeling techniques have been employed in the targeting of the various components of impulsive cognitive style. For example, in several studies, children have been given the opportunity to observe social models who received reinforcement for delaying their responses. Other studies have focused on the child observing a social model demonstrating a reinforced problem-solving strategy characterized by critical evaluation of response alternatives. Still other modeling procedures have focused both on response time and critical evaluation of response alternatives by using covert sensitization and self-reinforcement to bring about verbal mediation of overt behaviors. Evidently, the type of model plays an important role in influencing the child's learning.

In the strategy section of this chapter, various modeling techniques will be described. While none of these studies were actually carried out by classroom teachers, the methods employed readily lend themselves to classroom application. In view of the important role that the teacher herself plays in modeling reflective cognitive style for her students, and in view of the fact that reflective children may serve as models for their impulsive classmates, the research studies presented in this section should prove most helpful.

STRATEGY I: REINFORCEMENT OF REFLECTIVE CONCEPTUAL TEMPO THROUGH THE OBSERVATION OF CLASSMATES AS SOCIAL MODELS. Debus (1968) sought to evaluate the modifiability of impulsive tempo by having impulsive elementary school children observe several patterns of social modeling behavior. He had hoped that impulsive children would learn to change their cognitive response style by observing both impulsive and reflective social models performing a standard task in which positive reinforcement was contingent on a reflective cognitive style.

One hundred impulsive third grade elementary school children (fifty males and fifty females) were selected from a population of three hundred and twenty children. These children were found to be the most impulsive of the third grade school population based on their performances of the MFFT. Subjects matched on age were randomly assigned to each of four experimental groups. All subjects observed a model of their same sex. The models in this study were sixth grade elementary school children who were given special training to perform as models.

The experimental subjects in the various groups were exposed to a variety of modeling conditions. Debus hoped to determine which style of social modeling would be most effective with the impulsive responder. One group of experimental subjects observed a reflective model who received positive reinforcement for his responses. The second group observed an impulsive model. In other words, the impulsive experimental subjects observed an impulsive child who received less positive reinforcement. A third group observed what Debus called a change model. This model was one whose cognitive style from impulsive to reflective changed midway through the test session. Of course, as the cognitive style changed from impulsive to reflective a noticeable change could be observed in the frequency with which reinforcement was received. The fourth group underwent the dual modeling condition. In this condition, the impulsive child was given the opportunity to observe two models, one impulsive and one reflective responder. Of course, the experimental subjects also observed the contrasting frequency with which reinforcement was available. Finally, a control group of impulsive subjects received no training in social modeling.

During the training each experimental subject was brought into the test room in order to complete a standardized task. Just before the child was to begin the task, the social model entered the room explaining that the teacher had requested that he be tested immediately in order to return to the classroom as soon as possible. The experimenter asked the subject to observe the model as he completed the test. Following this observation of model behavior, the child was tested. The reflective models exhibited a twenty-five-second response latency. During that period of time they could be observed to look closely at the standard and the various response alternatives. The task was set up in such a way that the model exhibited a variety of behavioral cues associated with reflective cognitive style. Each correct response received positive verbal feedback and each incorrect response received negative verbal feedback from the experimenter. The model himself verbalized the strategy which he used in completing the MFFT items. During the impulsive modeling condition the initial response latencies were held to eight seconds. The models correctly answered only two of the ten test items. On four of the ten items they were trained to make one mistake. On the remaining four test items they were trained to make two errors on trials seven through nine and three errors on item ten. The models also exhibited typical behavioral cues observed in impulsive children. For instance, they were trained to hold their finger poised over the response alternatives before the experimenter had completed the instructions. The experimenter gave both positive and negative verbal feedback for the child's responses. The model actually verbalized that he was trying to respond as quickly as possible. The changed model condition was one which provided the subject an opportunity to observe an impulsive social model who changed his response style to become more reflective. On the first five items of the test, the social model responded in a manner identical to that of the social model described in the impulsive modeling condition. For the remainder of the test the social model exhibited a reflective cognitive style as outlined in the reflective modeling condition. Both models verbalized their strategies and received verbal reinforcement according to the correctness of their responses. Of course, the difference in frequency of response between the two models was obvious. When the model changed from impulsive cognitive style to a more reflective one, he verbalized this change as an insight, claiming that he could now see that there was a better way to solve the problem. Finally, the dual modeling condition was one in which two social models were introduced into the testing situation. One model acted in an impulsive fashion, giving the same behavioral cues and verbalization of response strategies, and the same low frequency of reinforcement as was described for the impulsive modeling condition. The other model demonstrated a reflective cognitive style in which a greater frequency of verbal reinforcement was received.

Several interesting findings were reported. Latency scores for females who observed reflective change in dual model were significantly longer than for either controls or male subjects. The latency scores for male subjects were significantly higher than for control subjects. In other words, females tended to be more responsive to cross modeling conditions for the social modeling form of behavior modification.

Another interesting finding was that, though the models in each of the conditions exhibited specific identifiable behavioral cues and verbalized their response strategies, only response latencies were affected. There seemed to be no significant change in the frequency of correct responses as a result of the modeling training. This was particularly important in view of the fact that training in the development of effective response strategies has been shown to be an important component of building a reflective cognitive style. The greatest degree of improvement was seen in the group who observed the reflective model. This group's response latency was twice that of subjects in any of the other remaining groups.

The change modeling condition seemed to be most effective in helping impulsive responders to identify the verbal cues which accompanied reflective style. Evidently, the contrast between impulsive and reflective style was sufficient for helping children to identify the specific verbal cues associated with reflective thinking. This effect lasted longer than any of the others in the study. This finding has particularly important implications for the classroom teacher, as it suggests that an effective social modeling program for the impulsive hyperactive child would be one which gave the child an opportunity to observe changes in cognitive style.

The author emphasized that the critical factors in reducing errors seem to be that of learning a more effective response alternative scanning strategy. Apparently, children in this study are capable of learning to alter their response tempo but require further specific training in altering their response strategies.

STRATEGY II: THE USE OF SOCIAL MODELING TO INCREASE THE FREQUENCY OF REFLECTIVE PROBLEM-SOLVING STRATEGIES. Ridberg, Parke and Hetherington (1971) addressed themselves to the problem of altering the impulsive child's problem-solving strategies. This study, unlike the one by Debus (1968), focused on using social modeling as a technique for teaching the child to alter his specific response strategies. Little emphasis in this study was placed on altering cognitive tempo. Ridberg and his colleagues sought to evaluate the effectiveness of different social modeling techniques on impulsive responders.

One experimental condition was designed to model the verbal behavior which accompanies the child's response strategy. The other condition was one which focused on having the subject observe a social model go through the actual motor movements associated with visual scanning, while making an evaluation of the response alternatives. This model traced his scanning strategy with his finger during the response latency period while taking the MFFT.

Ridberg selected one hundred fourth grade boys based on their MFFT scores and their level of intelligence. The subjects were randomly assigned to one of five matched groups. He further subdivided each of these into groups of subjects with high and low IQ's.

In order to assure that the social model observed was identical for subjects in each of the groups, Ridberg filmed the performances of the models as they completed the MFFT. The performance of an impulsive model on the MFFT was filmed. This model responded to test items within ten seconds. The correctness of the model's responses was indicated. The reflective model on the other hand delayed his response for up to thirty-one seconds. Correct responses were also indicated. Five different modeling conditions were depicted. The nonverbalizing nonscanning impulsive model delayed his response for less than ten seconds. No verbalizations were given, nor was his scanning technique demonstrated. The reflective model delayed his response for approximately thirty-one seconds. He also gave no verbalizations and did not demonstrate the scanning procedure.

The verbalizing-nonscanning models were those individuals who verbalized their response strategies (impulsive and reflective respectively) between the onset of the task and making the first response. The reflective model verbalized instructions to himself which included statements to respond slowly to avoid choosing the first stimulus that appeared to be correct. He also described his response strategy. The impulsive verbalizing-nonscanning model said that he should respond quickly and select the first response alternative that appeared to be correct. Similar to his reflective model counterpart, he described his response strategy. The scanning-nonverbalizing models did not describe their response strategies. They did, however, demonstrate their scanning techniques by pointing to the standard and then moving their fingers from the standard to each of the response alternatives in the manner that indicated that they were making comparisons between the two. The reflective model pointed to the standard and then to each of the other stimuli in order to compare them before arriving at a decision. The impulsive model, on the other hand, pointed to the response alternatives and then back to the standards. This was followed by pointing to the second response alternative and then back to the standard until he came upon the one which appeared to be correct. In most cases, this left several alternatives unevaluated. The verbalizing-scanning models, as the name suggests, not only verbalized their response strategies but also demonstrated them by pointing. A control group was also included in the study. These subjects had no exposure to the filmed modeling techniques described above.

All the subjects in the study except those who were assigned to a control group were told that they would have the opportunity to observe a film of a boy who did well on the same test that they were about to complete. The film was shown to all of the subjects except the control subjects. Following the film, Form 2 of the MFFT was administered. One week later, Form 3 of the MFFT was administered.

The results indicated that impulsive subjects who were exposed to the activities of a reflective model showed a significant increase in response time. Most importantly, however, was the finding that the subjects exhibited significantly fewer errors in their critical evaluation of response alternatives. The observed changes remained stable over a one-week period of time. The reflective subjects who were exposed to the impulsive model showed a paradoxical effect. Quite unexpectedly, the response time for these subjects was observed to have increased along with the frequency of errors.

Ridberg further observed a high correlation between high IQ and superior performance on the MFFT. The results suggested that low IQ subjects seemed to do best when the models both verbalized and demonstrated their scanning strategy. This modeling condition seemed to decrease the effects of intelligence on performance. This may have resulted in the fact that giving complex response cues to highly intelligent subjects interfered with their problem-solving strategies while lower IQ subjects did not have these established and therefore were able to more effectively utilize them.

The primary value of this study was that it demonstrated that both verbalization and behavioral demonstration of response strategies could be combined in order to effectively decrease the high frequency of response errors demonstrated by impulsive subjects. Classroom programs using this technique would be ones in which the teacher assigned a reflective child in her class to work with an impulsive child. The reflective child would need to be instructed to both tell his coworker how he went about problem solving and to demonstrate the strategy.

STRATEGY III: THE USE OF SOCIAL MODELING AND VERBAL MEDIATION TRAINING COGNITIVE TEMPO AND CRITICAL EVALUATION OF RESPONSE ALTERNATIVES. Meichenbaum (1971a) combined the techniques of social modeling and training in verbal mediation in order to study the effects of these two variables on the response latencies and frequency of error of impulsive responders. Fifteen kindergarten and first grade students who showed themselves to be most impulsive on an alternate form of the MFFT and who showed no significant increase in response latency when tested on an alternate form of the MFFT when instructed to "Take your time" were included in the study.

All subjects were matched for age and degree of impulsivity, and randomly assigned to either a modeling group, modeling plus self-instruction group, or an attention group. The subjects in the cognitive modeling group observed the experimenter as he modeled his performance. The experimenter then modeled the response strategy while verbalizing the strategy aloud. The subject was then given the opportunity to perform the task. Social reinforcement was received for correct responses but no explicit training was offered in self-instruction. The subjects in the cognitive modeling self-instruction group underwent the same modeling procedure as the subjects in the group performing cognitive modeling alone. However, these subjects differed in that they received explicit training and self-verbalization. This training took place over eight practice trial sessions in which the child was instructed to fade his verbalizations from an overt description of his strategy to a level of covert self-instruction. Finally, the attention group was composed of subjects that spent an equal amount of time as the subjects of the other two groups working with the same test materials. These subjects did not have an opportunity to observe a social model nor did they receive any training in self-instruction. All groups did receive social reinforcement for correct response. A reflective control group was also included in this study. Subjects in this group consisted of kindergarten and first grade students who were found to be reflective responders on the original prestudy screening test. These individuals went through the standard test procedure but received no modeling and no training.

The results indicated that during the initial screening procedure the reflective subjects improved with the simple instructions from the experimenter to "Go slower." In other words, these children demonstrated a significant increase in their response latencies as a result of a simple instruction to delay their response. No change, however, was observed in the number of correct responses. As might be expected, no significant change was demonstrated by the impulsive subjects as a result of the simple instruction to delay their responses. The modeling only group and the cognitive modeling self-instruction group showed a significant decrease in decision time as a result of treatment. As might be expected, the cognitive modeling self-instruction group did significantly better than the remaining groups. This group not only demonstrated a significant increase in response latency but they also demonstrated a significant reduction in errors. The modeling alone group did demonstrate a significant increase in response latency time. However, no comparable decrease was observed with respect to the frequency of errors. Apparently, the modeling of increased response latency time is an adequate treatment for cognitive tempo. However, it would appear that training to cover self-instruction is necessary if the child's ability to critically evaluate his response alternatives is to be changed.

SUMMARY

Our understanding of impulsivity has improved greatly since the early work of Murray (1938). The combined findings of many researchers have attributed to a growing body of knowledge which came to view impulsivity as a dimension of cognitive style. Kagan and his colleagues' (1964; 1965a, b, c; 1966, 1966a, b, c; 1971) research on impulsivity was a turning point in our understanding of this dimension of cognitive style. Kagan theorized that impulsivity was located at one end of a theoretical continuum which consisted of a child's length of response latency and his ability to critically evaluate response alternatives. For many years, Kagan's theories have stood as the authority on impulsive-reflective cognitive style. Within the past several years a second body of theory has developed around the research findings of Meichenbaum (1969a, b; 1971a, b; 1974. 1975a, b, c, d). Using findings from current research on the development of psycholinguistic ability in children, Meichenbaum hypothesized that impulsive children suffer from a lag in development of the verbal mediating responses used in private speech to control overt behaviors.

Impulsivity occupies a central location with respect to its

relationship to the other primary characteristic associated with hyperactivity. Several authors have commented on the interrelationship between attention-distractibility and impulsivity. The similarities between subject's performance on focus of attention tasks and the child's performance on measures of impulsivity are quite convincing. Numerous studies have reported a significant positive correlation between distractibility, impulsivity and hyperactivity. Impulsivity also seems to be indirectly related to activity level.

Many researchers have commented on the quality of activity in children whose behavior is characterized by overactivity. Impulsivity seems to be the chief characteristic of the type of activity exhibited by the hyperactive youngster. With respect to their cognitive abilities, there seems to be little direct relationship between verbal ability and impulsivity. However, impulsivity does appear to be related to at least one other form of cognitive style. Impulsive children tend to be field dependent. That is, they show little ability to structure and analyze their visual perceptions. Although the impulsive child's level of intellectual functioning is as likely to be average or above as the intellectual level of the reflective child, the impulsive child is most likely to show a lag in academic achievements. Impulsivity seems to differentially affect the performances of males and females on standardized tasks. Impulsive males seem to do better on tasks that require them to respond in a more reflective manner. Females on the other hand tend to do better on similar tasks when the instructions require them to be somewhat more impulsive. The overall findings in this area seem to indicate that a relationship between impulsivity and gender does exist. It appears that females tend to be more reflective while males are apt to be more impulsive. The exact cause of this relationship is unknown. At this point these differential effects seem to be related to differences in early childhood socialization between males and females. Generally speaking, there does appear to be an inverse relationship between increases in age and impulsivity. It appears that as age increases, impulsivity decreases. There appear to be critical stages in the development of cognitive response strategies during which impulsivity gives way to a more reflective cognitive style. Children who do not effectively progress through these stages seem to maintain an impulsive cognitive style long after many of the other primary characteristics of hyperactivity have dissipated. Perhaps one of the most impressive aspects of this characteristic of the hyperactive child is the fact that impulsivity remains so stable over such long periods of time and has such far-reaching effects on the entire spectrum of the child's academic activities. While there has been some support in literature for viewing impulsivity as a psychosocial phenomenon, research on the relationship between the cognitive styles of impulsive children and the styles of their parents indicate that these variables are independent of one another.

Treatment of impulsivity has a positive affect in decreasing impulsivity while facilitating a reflective cognitive style. However, chemotherapy alone does not teach the child to develop new and more effective response strategies. The research in this area has been particularly encouraging with respect to the discovery of which response strategies seem to be most effective. Generally speaking, a response strategy which teaches the impulsive child to identify the differences rather than the similarities between the elements of his visual field are most effective.

Behavior modification has shown itself to be quite effective in modifying impulsive cognitive style. Several studies on the effects of delay training indicated that cognitive tempo is relatively easily modified through the use of standard reinforcement techniques. Perhaps most encouraging in this particular area is the knowledge that fixed interval and limited hold schedules of reinforcement are capable of producing significant pauses in responding between the onset of the discriminative stimulus and the emission of the responses. To date, little research has been published on the effects of positive reinforcement on impulsive cognitive style. The few studies that have been published suggest that the introduction of a tangible positive reinforcer may serve to be disruptive to the learning process of the impulsive responder. Impulsive children receiving reflective training tended to become fixated on the presence of the reinforcer to the point that they became overly distractible. Much work needs to be done in this area in order to control for such variables. A most productive form of behavior modification in altering impulsive cognitive style has been that of social modeling. This method brings about behavioral change by having the impulsive child observe a reflective model who is reinforced for his long response latencies and closer scrutiny in evaluating response alternatives. Training in cover self-guiding speech has proven to be an invaluable addition to the list of treatment approaches. This approach teaches the child to use his inner speech as a means of controlling his overt behavioral responses. In effect this technique uses self-reinforcement, social modeling and other covert conditioning procedures such as covert sensitization and thought stopping to alter the impulsive cognitive style.

An effective training program is one which brings all of these elements together. Such a program offers response latency training. In addition, effective training includes the development of problem-solving strategies and the use of covert self-instruction. It appears that the most effective social modeling procedure is one that involves the use of a change model in which verbal and behavioral explanations of reflective cognitive style are demonstrated and the child is instructed in covert self-guiding speech. All of these procedures could be easily integrated into a classroom program by either having a classroom teacher act as a social model to her students or by developing more rigorous training programs in which impulsive students were paired with reflective peers who served as problem-solving models. The fact that cognitive tempo and impulsive problem-solving strategy show rather permanent changes with only a minimum amount of intervention time is encouraging.

REFERENCES

Ault, R. L., Crawford, D. E., and Jeffery, W. G.: Visual scanning strategies of reflective, impulsive, fast-accurate and slow-inaccurate children on the Matching Familiar Figures Test. *Child Development,* 43:1412-1417, 1972.

Ault, R. L.: Problems-solving strategies of reflective, impulsive, fast-accurate and slow-inaccurate children. *Child Development, 44*:259-266, 1973.
Bem, S.: Verbal self-control: the establishment of effective self-instruction. *Journal of Experimental Psychology, 74*:485-491, 1967.
Bem, S.: The role of comprehension in children's problem solving. *Developmental Psychology, 2*:351-358, 1970.
Campbell, S. B., Douglas, V. I., and Morgenstern, G.: Cognitive styles in hyperactive children and the effect of methylphenidate. *Journal of Child Psychology and Psychiatry, 12*:55-67, 1971.
Campbell, S. B.: Mother-child interaction in reflective, impulsive and hyperactive children. *Developmental Psychology, 8*:341-349, 1973a.
Campbell, S. B.: Cognitive styles in reflective, impulsive and hyperactive boys and their mothers. *Perceptual and Motor Skills, 36*:747-752, 1973b.
Campbell, S. B.: Mother-child interaction in reflective, impulsive, and hyperactive children. *Developmental Psychology, 8*:341-349, 1973c.
Campbell, S. B.: Cognitive styles and behavior problems of clinic boys: a comparison of epileptic, hyperactive, learning-disabled, and normal groups. *American Journal of Abnormal Child Psychology*, in press, 1975a.
Campbell, S. B.: Mother-child interaction: a comparison of hyperactive, learning disabled ,and normal boys. *American Journal of Orthopsychiatry*, in press, 1975b.
Cohen, S. A.: *A Study of Impulsivity in Low Achieving and High Achieving Boys from Lower Income Homes.* New York, Columbia University, 1969.
Conners, C. K., and Rothschild, G.: Drugs and learning in children. In *Learning Disorders,* Vol. 3, Seattle, Special Guild Publications, 1968.
Debus, R. L.: Effects of brief observation of model behavior on conceptual tempo of compulsive children. *Developmental Psychology, 2*:22-32, 1968.
Diamond, S., Bolvin, R. S., and Diamond, F.: *Inhibition and Choice.* New York, HarRow, 1963.
Douglas, V. I.: Stop, look and listen: the problem of sustained attention and impulse control in hyperactive and normal children. *Canadian Journal of Behavioral Science, 4*:259-281, 1972.
Douglas, V. I.: "Sustained attention and impulse control: implications for the handicapped child." U.S. Department of Health, Education and Welfare, Office of Publications, Office of Education, Psychology and the Handicapped Child, 1974.
Freidberg, V., Douglas, V. I., and Weiss, G.: The effects of chlorpromazine on concept learning in hyperactive children under two conditions of reinforcement. *Psychopharmacologia, 13*:200-310, 1968.
Gardner, J., Percy, L. M., and Lawson, T.: Sex differences in behavioral impulsivity, intellectual impulsivity, and attainment in young children. *Journal of Child Psychology and Psychiatry, 12*:261-271, 1971.

Gibson, A. J., and Gibson, J.: Perceptual learning: differentiation or enrichment? *Psychological Review, 62*:32-41, 1955.

Harrisoin, A., and Nadelman, L.: Conceptual tempo and inhibition of movements in black preschool children. *Child Development, 43*:657-668, 1972.

Hirschfield, T. P.: Response set in impulsive children. *Journal of Genetic Psychology, 107*:117-126, 1965.

Kagan, J., Rosman, B. L., Day, D., Albert, J., and Phillips, W.: Information processing in the child: significance of analytic and reflective attitudes. *Psychological Monographs, 78*, (Whole No. 578), 1964.

Kagan, J.: Individual differences in the resolution of response uncertainty. *Journal of Personality and Social Psychology, 2*:154-160, 1965a.

Kagan, J.: Reflection-impulsivity and reading ability in primary school children. *Child Development, 36*:609-628, 1965b.

Kagan, J.: Impulsive and reflective children: significance of conceptual tempo. In Krumboltz, J. D. (Ed.): *Learning and the Educational Process*. Chicago, Rand McNally, 1965c.

Kagan, J.: Modify ability of impulsive tempo. *Journal of Educational Psychology, 57*:359-365, 1966a.

Kagan, J.: Developmental studies in reflection and analysis. In Kidd, A. H., and Rivoiri, J. H. (Eds.): *Perceptual and Conceptual Development in Children*. New York, International University Press, 1966b.

Kagan, J.: Reflection-impulsivity: a generality in dynamics of conceptual tempo. *Journal of Abnormal Psychology, 71*:17-24, 1966c.

Kagan, J.: *Change and Continuity in Infancy*. New York, Wiley, 1971.

Kagan, J., Pearson, L., and Welch, L.: Conceptual impulsivity and inductive reasoning. *Child Development, 37*:588-594, 1966.

Klein, W. L.: *An investigation of the spontaneous speech of children during problem solving*. Unpublished doctoral dissertation, University of Rochester, 1963.

Knights, R. M., and Hinton, G.: The effects of methylphenidate (Ritalin) on motor skills and behavior of children with learning problems. *Journal of Nervous and Mental Diseases, 148*:643-653, 1969.

Kohlberg, L., Yaeger,, J., and Hjertholm, E.: Private speech: four studies in a review of theories. *Child Development, 39*:691-736, 1968.

Lowrey, P. W., and Ross, L. E.: *Severely retarded children as impulsive responders: improved performance with response delay*. Personal Communication, 1975.

Lovaas, O. I.: Properties of words: the control of operant responding by rate and content of verbal operants. *Child Development, 35*:245-256, 1964.

Luria, A. R.: The directive function of speech in development. *Word, 15*:341-352, 1959.

Luria, A. R.: *The Role of Speech in the Regulation of Normal and Abnormal Behavior.* New York, Liveright, 1961.

Maccoby, E. E.: *The Development of Sex Differences.* London, Travistoc, 1967.

Meichenbaum, D. H., and Goodman, J.: The developmental control of operant motor responding by verbal operants. *Journal of Experimental Child Psychology,* 7:553-565, 1969a.

Meichenbaum, D. H., and Godman, J.: Reflection-impulsivity and verbal control of motor behavior. *Child Development,* 40:785-797, 1969b.

Meichenbaum, D. H., and Goodman, J.: Training impulsive children to talk to themselves: a means of developing self-control. *Journal of Abnormal Psychology,* 77:115-126, 1971a.

Meichenbaum, D. H.: *The nature and modification of impulsive children: training impulsive children to talk to themselves.* Paper presented at the Proceedings of the Society for Research in Child Development Conference, Minneapolis, 1971b.

Meichenbaum, D.: Self-instructional training: a cognitive prosthesis for the aged. *Human Development,* 17:273-280, 1974.

Meichenbaum, D.: Self-instructional methods: In Kanfer, F., and Goldstein, A. (Eds.): *Helping People Change.* New York, Pergamon, 1975a.

Meichenbaum, D.: Toward a cognitive theory of self-control. In Schwartz, G., and Shapiro, D. (Eds.): *Consciousness in Self-regulation: Advances in Research.* New York, Plenum Pr, Plenum Pub., 1975b.

Meichenbaum, D.: *Cognitive factors as determinants of learning disabilities: a cognitive functional approach.* Paper presented at NATO Conference on the neuropsychology of learning disabilities. Korsor, Denmark, 1975c.

Mercurio, S. J.: *A teacher observation rating scale for impulsive behavior.* Unpublished master's thesis, State University College at Fredonia, New York, 1975.

Messer, S.: Reflection-impulsivity: stability and school failure. *Journal of Educational Psychology,* 61:487-490, 1970.

Mosher, S. A., and Hornsby, J. R.: On asking questions. In Bruner, J. S., Olver, R. R., and Greenfield, P.: (Eds.): *Studies in Cognitive Growth.* New York, Wiley, 1966.

Murray, H. A.: *Explorations of Personality.* New York, Oxford UP, 1938.

Odom, R. D., McIntyre, C. W., and Neale, G. S.: The influence of cognitive style on perceptual learning. *Child Development,* 42:883-891, 1971.

Parton and Newhall, N.: Social development of preschool children. In Barekr, R., Kounen, J., and Wright, H. (Eds.): *Child Behavior and Development.* New York, McGraw, 1943.

Ridberg, E. H., Parke, R. D., and Hetherington, E. N.: Modification of impulsive and reflective cognitive styles through observation of film mediated models. *Developmental Psychology,* 5:369-377, 1971.

Schwebel, A.: Effects of impulsivity on performance of verbal tasks in middle- and lower-class children. *American Journal of Orthopsychiatry,* 36:13-21, 1966.

Schwebel, A. I., and Bernstein, A. J.: The effects of impulsivity on the performance of lower-class children on four WISC subtests. *American Journal of Orthopsychiatry,* 40:629-636, 1970.

Segel, A., Babich, J., and Kirasic, K.: Visual recognition memory in reflective and impulsive children. *Memory and Cognition,* 2:379-384, 1974.

Shelley, E. M., and Riester, K.: Syndrome of minimal brain dysfunction in young adults. *Diseases of the Nervous System,* 33:335-338, 1972.

Seigel, I. E., Jarman, P., and Hanesian, H.: *Styles of categorization and their preceptual, intellectual and personality correlates in young children.* Unpublished paper cited in Maccoby, E. E.: *The Development of Sex Differences.* London, Travistoc, 1967.

Solley, C. M., and Murphy, G.: *Development of the Perceptual World.* New York, Basic, 1960.

Sprague, R. L., Barnes, K. R., and Werry, J. S.: Methylphenidate and thioridazine: learning, reaction time, activity, and classroom behavior in disturbed children. *American Journal of Orthopsychiatry,* 40:615, 1970.

Sutton-Smith, E.: A scale to identify impulsive behavior in children. *Journal of Genetic Psychology,* 95:211-216, 1959.

Sutton-Smith, B., and Rosenberg, B. G.: Impulsivity and sex preference. *Journal of Genetic Psychology,* 98:187-192, 1961.

Sutton-Smith, V., Crandall, V. J., and Roberts, J. N.: *Achievement and Strategic Competence.* 1964. Unpublished paper cited in Maccoby, E. E.: *The Development of Sex Differences.* London, Travistoc, 1967.

Vygotsky, L. S.: *Thought and Language.* New York, Wiley, 1962.

Wechsler, D.: *Wechsler Intelligence Scale for Children Manual.* New York, Psychological Corporation, 1949.

Weiner, A., and Berzonsky, M.: Development of selective attention in reflective and impulsive children. *Memory and Cognition,* 46:545-549, 1975.

Welch, L.: *A naturalistic study of free play behavior of reflective and impulsive four year olds.* Paper presented at the meeting of the Society for Research in Child Development. Philadelphia (Paper available from University of Chicago), 1973.

Werry, A. A., Weiss, G., Douglas, V. I., and Martin, J.: Studies on the hyperactive child. III. The effect of chlorpromazine upon behavior and learning. *Journal of American Academy of Child Psychiatry,* 5:292-312, 1966.

Witkin, H. A.: Differences in the ease of perception of embeded figures. *Journal of Personality, 19*:1-15, 1950.

Yando, R. M., and Kagan, J.: The effects of teacher tempo on the child. *Child Development, 71*:21-24, 1968.

Zelniker, T., Jeffrey, W. E., Ault, R., and Parsons, J.: Analysis and modification of search strategies of impulsive and reflective children on the Matching Familiar Figures Test. *Child Development, 43*:321-355, 1972.

Zelniker, T., and Oppenheimer, L.: Modification of information processing of impulsive children. *Child Development, 44*:445-450, 1973.

AUTHOR INDEX

A

Abramson, A., 70
Adametz, J. L., 40, 67, 81, 112
Alabiso, F. P., 31, 58, 67, 121, 129, 131, 138, 143, 157, 169, 173, 175, 229, 242
Albert J., 214, 243, 247, 308
Alexander, D. F., 70
Alexandris, A. R., 40, 67
Allen, F., 56, 67
Allen, K. H., 96, 99, 112
Allen, R., 70
Allport, F., 120, 175
Amassian, B. B., 40, 67, 81, 112
Amerongen, F. S., 40, 68, 81, 113
Anderson, D. B., 57, 67, 96, 112
Anderson, W. M., 34, 67
Annesley, F. R., 231, 242
Ault, R. L., 272, 286, 288, 306, 307, 311

B

Babich, J., 262, 310
Backus, R., 114, 146, 148, 177
Backus, J. T., 79, 117
Baer, R., 96, 99, 112
Bailer, R., 86, 115
Barekr, R., 309
Barnes, K. R., 51, 71, 280, 310
Barr, E., 70
Baumeister, A., 75, 80, 84, 112
Beck, A. T., 44, 67
Becker, W. B., 57, 69, 97, 115
Bekhterev, V. K., 119, 175
Bell, G., 86, 116
Bell, R. T., 92, 112
Bem, S., 248, 256, 307
Benson, C., 235, 243
Bentzen, F. P., 68, 242

Berkson, G., 91, 112
Berlyne, D. A., 127, 175
Bernstein, A. J., 277, 283, 310
Berzonsky, M., 262, 310
Bestor, S. L., 125, 175
Bianchi, L. T., 43, 67
Bijou, S. L., 170, 175
Bindra, D., 77, 112
Blatt, B. I., 154, 176
Bloom, I., 223, 242
Blough, D. D., 112
Boldruy, B. D., 70
Bolvin, R. S., 245, 307
Booksen, B. N., 112
Braddard, G. S., 52, 67
Bradley, C. E., 62, 67
Brickner, R. E., 43, 67
Broadbent, D. E., 131, 132, 175
Brooks, D. T., 154, 175
Broverman, D. N., 215, 242
Broverman, I. K., 242
Brown, D. C., 156, 176
Brown, L., 134, 159, 177
Brown, M. P., 122, 176
Brummet, H., 7, 31, 36, 50, 67
Bruner, J. S., 309
Buckley, N. S., 161, 166, 167, 179
Buckley, R. E., 43, 67
Bucy, P. A., 43, 69
Burks, H. P., 34, 48, 53, 67
Burnham, W. H., 120, 176
Bussaratid, S., 71

C

Camille, N., 82, 115
Campbell, S. B., 53, 67, 213, 215, 216, 242, 265, 273, 274, 275, 281, 307
Cantor, G. N., 78, 112
Cantwell, D., 44, 67

Carduc, W. A., 71
Carter, P., 227, 242
Casaer, P., 114
Castanera, T. J., 86, 112
Child, B., 114
Child, D., 146, 148, 177
Chung, R. M., 82, 113
Clarinda, M. K., 62, 71
Clarinda, N., 86, 116
Clarizio, H. F., 93, 94, 112, 229, 242
Clark, M., 235, 243
Clements, S. D., 5, 7
Cohen, L. A., 3, 31
Cohen, S. A., 267, 307
Cole, J. O., 52, 68
Connors, C. K., 48, 51, 52, 68, 85, 112, 280, 307
Connley, D. P., 53, 68
Conrad, W. G., 44, 68
Crandall, V. J., 310
Crawford, D. E., 306
Cromwell, R. L., 75, 80, 84, 86, 90, 113, 115, 128, 135, 176
Crosby, K. G., 154, 176
Cruickshank, W. T., 34, 61, 68, 227, 228, 242

D

Dahler, M. S., 139, 180
Daley, N. F., 109, 113
Daniels, G. T., 68, 105, 108, 113
Dashiell, J. N., 120, 176
Davenport, R. K., 91, 112
Davids, A., 85, 113
Day, D., 214, 243, 247, 308
DuBrose, S. G., 62, 68, 105, 108, 113
Debus, R. L., 295, 296, 299, 307
Denhoff, E., 38, 40, 42, 69
Denton, L., 68
Deutsch, D. R., 132, 176
Deutsch, J. N., 132, 176
Diamond, F., 245, 307
Diamond, S., 245, 307
DiVito, R. T., 40, 67, 81, 112
Doll, E. A., 3, 31
Douglas, V. I., 32, 52, 53, 67, 71, 72, 213, 216, 242, 262, 263, 265, 267, 271, 280, 289, 290, 307, 310
Duik, R. B., 44

E

Ebner, M. J., 94, 96, 113, 116
Egeth, E., 132, 176
Eisenberg, L., 51, 68
Ellis, N. R., 128, 134, 136, 176
Emmers, R., 82, 113

F

Farson, R., 108, 113
Faterson, H. S., 244
Fechner, E. T., 119, 176
Ferrier, D. L., 43, 68
Finley, K. H., 78, 117
Finnerty, R. J., 52, 68
Fisher, L. R., 129, 141, 142, 176
Foice, A., 78, 113
Forward, T. C., 54, 68
Foshee, J. G., 86, 90, 113, 128, 135, 176
Freeling, N. W., 45, 69
French, J. T., 40, 68, 81, 113
Friedberg, V., 307
Fullton, J. L., 43, 69

G

Gardner, J., 264, 268, 269, 270, 307
Gardner, W. I., 90, 91, 113, 128, 176
Gastaut, H. O., 43, 68, 90, 113
Geissler, L. R., 119, 120, 176, 178
Gellner, L., 77, 113
Gibbons, C., 68
Gibbs, E. L., 78, 113
Gibbs, F. A., 78, 113
Gibson, A. J., 286, 287, 308
Gibson, J., 286, 287, 308
Giles, D. I., 101, 118
Gilmer, B. S., 126, 178
Giradeau, F. L., 134, 176

Glavin, J. P., 231, 232, 242
Gofman, H., 4, 31, 228, 242
Goldstein, A., 309
Goltz, F., 82, 113
Goodenough, G. R., 244
Goodman, J., 248, 256, 258, 309
Gray, W. G., 154, 175
Greenfield, P., 309
Grindee, T. D., 96, 113, 114

H

Hanesian, H., 310
Haring, N. E., 229, 244
Harlow, H. F., 133, 176, 211, 242
Harris, S. A., 96, 99, 112
Harrisoin, A., 262, 270, 308
Harrison, S., 32, 116, 226, 243
Harter, S., 134, 159, 177
Hawkins, C. W., 128, 176
Hawkins, W. F., 75, 80, 84, 112
Hebb, D. O., 120, 177
Henke, L. R., 96, 99, 112
Henley, E. N., 101, 118
Hermelin, D. C., 129, 177
Hernandez-Peon, R., 40, 68, 81, 113, 114
Herring, A. T., 122, 177
Hetherington, E. N., 299 309
Hilgard, E. R., 78, 114
Hillcoat, B., 68
Hinton, G., 280, 308
Hirschfield, T. P., 246, 308
Hjertholm, E., 308
Hoernstein, S. R., 34, 62, 68
Hornsby, J. R., 271, 272, 309
Horowitz, I., 85, 114
House, B. A., 132, 133, 180
Hundert, J., 47, 68
Huntsman, N. J., 140, 177

I

Ingram, T. P., 35, 43, 69

J

Jacob, W. O., 56, 69
Jacobsen, C. C., 43, 69
Jacobsen, C. T., 43, 69
Jacobsen, E., 44, 69
James, W., 119, 177
Jarman, P., 310
Jeffery, W. G., 286, 306, 311
Jensen, A. L., 140, 141, 142, 177
Johnson, H. M., 120, 177
Johnson, N., 69, 85, 115
Jolles, I. L., 59, 69, 226, 243
Jones, C. C., 112
Jones, R. P., 128, 176
Jones, R. W., 61, 70

K

Kagan, J., 140, 177, 214, 216, 243, 247, 249, 250, 252, 253, 254, 255, 264, 265, 266, 271, 272, 273, 277 278, 282, 290, 291, 303, 308, 311
Kahn, F., 3, 31
Kaliski, L. E., 69, 225, 226, 243
Kalverboer, A. F., 87, 89, 114
Kanfer, F., 309
Kantwell, D. P., 69
Karp, S. A., 216, 243
Kaspar, J. C., 74, 77, 78, 79, 85, 90, 91, 114, 115, 116, 136, 144, 145, 146, 147, 148, 151, 153, 164, 174, 177, 179
Kassinove, H. O., 124, 177
Kaufman, M., 92, 115, 134, 177
Kennard, M. T., 43, 69
Kennedy, D. A., 154, 177
Kenny, T. J., 7, 31
Keogh, B. K., 58, 69
Kephart, N. C., 125, 179
Kimeldorf, D. J., 112
King, L. G., 101, 118
Kirasic, K., 262, 310
Kirk, S., 59, 69
Kirk, S. A., 205, 206, 209, 224, 240, 243
Kirk, W. D., 205, 206, 209, 243
Kissel, S., 45, 69
Klein, W. L., 248, 308
Kleitman, N., 82, 115
Klibern, L., 242

Knights, R. M., 280, 308
Knobel, M., 77, 115
Knowles, P. K., 155, 178
Koch, H. S., 122, 177
Koch, S., 176
Kohlberg, L., 247, 248, 257, 308
Konstadt, N., 216, 243
Koppitz, E. M., 198, 243
Korn, C. V., 108, 115
Koser, L. E., 57, 69, 97, 115
Koshaba, J. E., 146, 147, 151, 174, 177
Kothera, R., 235, 243
Kounen, J., 309
Kuhnke, E., 92, 115
Kulpe, O. A., 119, 178
Kulver, H., 43, 69

L

Laufer, M. W., 38, 40, 42, 69
Laviqueur, H., 32
Lawson, T., 264, 268, 307
LeCoultre, R., 114
Lehtinen, L., 59, 76, 117, 179, 222, 244
Lennox, M. A., 78, 115
Leontiev, A. N., 122, 123, 178
Levin, T. M., 43, 69
Levitt, H., 92, 115
Levy, S., 3, 31
Lewen, D., 32
Lewis, R., 73, 115
Lindsley, T. C., 81, 115
Lindy, J., 32, 116, 182, 183, 226, 243
Lipkin, M. P., 86, 116
Lipps, A. S., 119, 178
Livingston, R. F., 40, 81, 113
Lockey, A., 227, 242
Lott, I. T., 70
Lourie, R., 73, 115
Lovaas, O. I., 248, 308
Lowrey, P. W., 282, 308
Lundell, F. G., 40, 67
Luria, A R., 248, 258, 259, 308, 309

M

Maccoby, E. E., 268, 309, 310
Madsen, C. A., 57, 69, 97, 115

MaGoun, H. M., 40, 70,, 71, 80, 81, 113, 115
Marcus, R. J., 80, 82, 117, 118
Martin, G. L., 122, 160, 178
Martin, J. T., 72, 280, 310
Martinson, M. E., 62, 69, 229, 243
Mason, E., 77, 115
Mason, W. A., 81, 91, 112
Maynard, R. C., 49, 69
McCarthy, J. J., 205, 206, 209, 240, 243
McConnell, T., 86, 115
McDermott, J., 32, 72, 116, 226, 243
McIntyre, C. W., 286, 309
McKenzie, H. S., 235, 236, 243
McQueen, M. W., 154, 164, 178
Meichenbaum, D., 32, 248, 256, 257, 258, 259, 260, 262, 291, 292, 293, 301, 303, 309
Mendleson, W., 38, 69, 85, 115
Mentz, L. N., 120, 178
Mercurio, S. J., 246, 267, 309
Messer, S., 273, 309
Mettler, F. A., 117
Meyer, W. J., 159, 178
Miller, C. A., 78, 115
Millichap, J., 62, 70, 114, 146, 148, 177
Milner, B., 178
Minde, K., 4, 32, 45, 70, 71, 216, 242
Mitchell, J., 86, 116
Mollica, A. H., 40, 70, 81, 116
Morgan, C. T., 86, 115
Morgenstern, G., 53, 67, 213, 242, 268, 281, 307
Morrison, J. R., 43, 44, 70
Morrow, J. W., 154, 175
Moruzzi, G., 40, 70, 81, 115, 116
Mosher, S. A., 271, 272, 309
Moyer, K. G., 126, 178
Murphy, G., 286, 287, 310
Murray, H. A., 245, 303, 309
Murray, W., 242

N

Nadelman, L., 263, 270, 308
Naquet, R. P., 43, 68
Neale, G. S., 286, 309
Nelson, T. O., 156, 178

Nemeth, E., 32, 71
Newhall, N., 258, 309
Nixon, S. J., 96, 116
Noble, M. I., 35, 70

O

Obersteiner, H. B., 119, 178
O'Connor, N. ., 129, 177
Odom, R. D., 286, 309
O'Donnell, J. P., 141, 142, 178
Offenbach, S. I., 159, 178
Olver, R. R., 309
Oppenheimer, L., 287, 311
Osgood, C. E., 205, 240, 243
Ott, J., 93, 94, 116

P

Packard, R. F., 167, 168, 169, 178
Pager, E. K., 57, 69, 97, 115
Paley, E., 215, 216, 243
Palkes, H., 36, 70
Palkers, H., 32
Parke, R. D., 299, 309
Parsons, J., 286, 311
Patterson, G. R., 36, 61, 62 ,70, 85, 94, 95, 96, 116
Payne, R. S., 77, 116
Pearson, L., 282, 308
Penfield, W., 178
Percy, L. M., 264, 268, 307
Peterson, D. R., 243
Peterson, W. M., 134, 177
Phillips, W., 214, 243, 247, 308
Pihl, R. F., 61, 70, 96, 116
Pillsbury, W. C., 120, 178
Plum, G. E., 139, 179
Powers, R. P., 122, 160, 178
Pozmanski, E., 72
Prechtl, H. F., 114
Premack, D., 109, 116
Prior, M. W., 134, 176
Prutsman, T. D., 155, 178
Pryer, M. S., 136, 176

Q

Quast, W., 116
Quay, H. F., 154, 164, 178, 231, 232, 242, 243

R

Rapoport, J. L., 45, 52, 70
Ratzenburg, F. L., 68, 242
Reardon, D., 92, 116
Reeves, J. L., 131, 134, 135, 142, 158, 159, 173, 178
Reisman, K. M., 86, 116
Reynolds, N., 96, 99, 112
Rich, C. L., 78, 113
Ridberg, E. H., 299, 301, 309
Rie, H., 44, 70
Rieber, M., 92, 116
Riester, K., 271, 310
Roberts, J. N., 310
Rosenberg, B. G., 277, 310
Rosman, B. L., 214, 243, 247, 308
Ross, A. C., 137, 179, 229, 243
Ross, L. E., 282, 308
Rothschild, G., 280, 307

S

Safer, D., 49, 70
SantoStefano, S. P., 61, 70, 215, 216, 243
Scheibel, M. P., 40, 70, 81, 116
Schrager, J. M., 4, 32, 61, 73, 116, 182, 183, 243
Schrater, H. A., 124, 179
Schulman, J. L., 62, 71, 74, 76, 77, 86, 114, 116, 136, 146, 147, 148, 177, 179
Schwartz, G., 309
Schwebel, A. I., 246, 277, 283, 310
Sears, W. W., 92, 116
Secuda, L., 78, 117
Segel, A., 262, 310
Seigel, I. E., 268, 310
Shainman, L. D., 46, 56, 71, 224, 243

Shapiro, D., 309
Shatin, L., 92, 117
Shaw, D. T., 94, 116
Sheer, D. P., 46, 56, 71
Shelley, E. M., 271, 310
Sirvastava, R. K., 136, 137, 179
Skeffington, A. M., 203, 204, 240, 243
Skinner, B. F., 126, 179
Slaughter, F. E., 92, 117
Sly, W. S., 71
Smothergill, D., 140, 180
Smythe, J. R., 194, 143
Solley, C. M., 286, 287, 310
Solomon, C. I., 78, 117
Soltys, J. J., 52, 68
Son, C., 86, 115
Spearman, C., 185, 244
Sprague, R., 48, 51, 54, 71, 72, 154, 164, 178, 280, 310
Stayton, S. N., 61, 70
Stellar, P., 86, 115
Stevens, G. A., 79, 117
Stewart, M., 32, 35, 36, 69, 70, 71, 85, 115
Stover, C. E., 79, 117
Strauss, A. A., 3, 32, 33, 58, 59, 71, 76, 117, 125, 179, 222, 144
Strazel, T. K., 40, 70
Stumpf, T., 119, 179
Sullweld, F. R., 132, 179
Sully, P. N., 120, 179
Sutton-Smith, B., 268, 277, 310
Sykes, D., 52, 70, 71
Sykes, E., 32

T

Tannenhauser, M. M., 68, 242
Taylor, C. E., 40, 71
Thomas, D. H., 57, 69, 115
Thompson, I. J., 154, 177
Thompson, R. L., 97, 117
Thorne, F., 116, 179
Titchner, E. B., 120, 179
Tizard, B., 71, 86, 117, 129, 179
Touwen, B. P., 114
Turnure, A. E., 145, 146, 151, 179

U

Ullman, L. R., 244

V

Varenhorst, B. B., 108, 117
Vigouroux, R. N., 43, 68
Villa Blanca, J. R., 80, 82, 83, 117, 118
Vygotsky, L. S., 248, 256, 310

W

Wachtel, P. M., 139, 179
Walker, H. A., 161, 166, 167, 179
Walker, S., 80, 87, 118
Wang, G. H., 82, 113
Warren, R. J., 44, 71
Webb, G., 70
Wechsler, D., 184, 185, 244, 284, 310
Weiner, A., 262, 310
Weir, C., 68
Wehlen, R. I., 229, 244
Weiss, G., 32, 37, 48, 50, 52, 71, 72, 216, 242, 280, 307 310
Welch, L., 264, 282, 308, 310
Werner, H., 3, 32, 33, 58, 71
Werry, G. S., 7, 32, 35 51 61, 154, 164, 178, 229, 231, 242, 244, 310
White, S. H., 139, 179
Whittier, J. E., 61, 70
Wilson, P., 32, 116, 226, 243
Windle, W. D., 81, 118
Witkin, H. A., 214, 244, 274, 311
Wolf, M. M., 235, 243
Wolf, N. V., 101, 104, 118
Wolman, M. B., 77, 115
Woodburn, L. F., 81, 118
Woodrow, H .R., 120, 180
Wright, A. C., 139, 140, 180
Wright, H., 309
Wright, M. A., 61, 70
Wundt, W., 120, 180

Y

Yaeger, J., 308
Yando, R. M., 290, 291, 311
Yelon, S., 93, 94, 112, 229, 242

Z

Zapoorozhet, A. V., 77, 118
Zeaman, P. O., 132, 133, 180
Zelniker, T., 286, 287, 311
Zigler, E., 134, 159, 177
Zigler, E. F., 145, 146, 151, 179
Ziziemsky, D. D., 62, 72
Zrull, J. P., 44, 72

SUBJECT INDEX

A

Absenteeism, 183
Activity level, 7, 9, 73-118, 128, 132, 135, 148, 149, 268
  control of, 93-109
  definition of, 84
  and impulsivity, 263-264
  etiology of, 75-78
  measurement of, 83-87
  variables affecting, 87-93
Activity rating scales, 85-87
Actometer, 86
Adolescence, 37, 38, 39
Age
  and distractibility, 152, 153
  and impulsivity, 271-273
Amphetamines, 42, 47, 48, 49
Aphasia, 197
Apraxia, 209
Arithmatic reasoning, 185
Arousal, 132
Associative memory, 196
Attention, 8, 109, 119-122
  adult, 100
  auditory, 130
  and brain damage, 141
  case study of, 24-31
  definition of, 121
  concepts of, 122-144
  effects of environment upon, 122
  focus of, 138-143, 155-156, 171, 173
  and impulsivity, 262-263
  and modification of behavior, 153-162
  orders of, 123
  selective, 131-138, 156, 173
  span, 122-131, 154-155, 171, 173
  voluntary, 123
Auditory
  attention, 130
  distractibility, 150
  input-output systems, 203-209
  and short term memory, 196
  stimulation, 91-93, 125
Automatization, 215, 165
Autonomic nervous system, 220

B

Balistograph, 86
Baseline period, 102, 105, 170
Behavioral control of activity level, 93-109
Behavior modificaton, 57, 58, 61, 65, 95, 99-100, 101, 229, 235, 305
Behavior therapy, 292
Birth, 10, 16, 21, 26, 35, 45
Brain damage, 42-43, 135, 141, 148, 149, 150
  and focus of attention, 141
Brain dysfunction
  and distractibility, 152
Brain stem (*see* Reticular activity system), 39, 83

C

Cards test, 147, 150, 152, 153
Career choice, 38
Centering, 202
Central analyzing mechanism, 131
Cerebral cortex, 42, 63, 82, 184, 185, 193, 104, 218, 222
Change modeling, 296, 298
Chemotherapy (*see* Treatment), 47-54, 62, 64, 280-282
  and learning, 50-54
Chlorpromazine, 50

Classroom reinforcement strategies, 97-109; (see Reinforcement)
Clearness, 120
Clock test, 148
Closure, 207, 208
Cognitive abilities, 184-193
 and abstract reasoning, 185
 vocabulary, 186
Cognitive dysfunction, 8, 181, 244
 case of, 9-15
 definition, 181
 and educational programming, 239
 improved learning for children with, 227-228
 and impulsivity, 264-266
Cognitive response, 286
Cognitive styles, 213-229, 289, 303, 305
 automatization, 215
 field dependence and independence, 214
 and hyperactivity, 265
 measures of, 216-217
 reflection-impulsivity, 213-214
Cognitive tempo, 213, 252, 256, 260, 279, 283, 285, 287, 288, 301, 303, 305, 306
Comprehension, 185
Conceptual style test, 249
Constricted flexible control, 265
Convergent syndrome, 79
Covert sensitization, 292

D

Delay training, 282-285
Depression, 64
Design recall test, 249, 252
Destimulation, 59, 222
Development
 uneven, 60, 61
Developmental lag theory, 42, 52, 63, 64, 192
Dexedrine, 48, 49
Diagnosis, 5-6
Diencephalon, 34
Differential cue errors, 134, 212

Differential reinforcement, 104-107
Discrimination, 137, 139, 157
Distractibility, 160-161, 173, 174, 289, 290
 and age, 152, 153
 and brain dysfunction, 152
 concepts of, 144-153
 definition of, 121, 145
 and intelligence, 152
 measures of, 147-148
 reduction of, 227
 visual, 150
Drive theory, 78
Drugs (see Treatment and Chemotherapy), 47-54, 280-282
 side effects, 49
Dysfunctions
 learning arc, 218
 visual motor, 198-199

E

Educational programming, 58-62, 66, 93
 historical perspective, 222-229
Electrophysiological theory, 80-81
Embeded figures test, 274
Emotional conflicts, 35, 45
Encephalitic infection, 34
Endocrine glands, 45
Enuresis, 10, 26, 35
Environment
 and activity level, 87
 control of, 227-228
 engineer of, 231
 stimulation of, 87-91
Errors
 of commission, 254, 255, 265
 frequency of, 282
 response time, 289
Etiology
 of hyperactivity, 39-46
 of activity level, 75-78
Expressive process, 208
External stimuli, 125-127
Extinction, 94, 97, 99, 100, 101, 166, 168, 169, 285

F

Fidgetometer, 86
Fixed interval reinforcement (see Reinforcement)), 285
Frontal lobes, 83

G

Genetics
  and hyperactivity, 43-44

H

Habituation, 120
Haptic visual matching test, 252
Hippocampus fornix, 193
Homeostatic control, 79
Hyperactivity, 3-32
  causes of, 39-46
  definition of, 3-5, 79, 95
  evaluation of, 5-6
  genetic causes of, 43-44
  and high risk factors, 182-183
  psychogenic causes, 44-45
Hyperactive children
  and activity level, 73-118
  characteristics of, 6-8, 33-39
  and cognitive dysfunction, 181-244
  impulsivity in, 245-311
Hypothalamus, 40, 42, 193, 194

I

Individualization, 60, 224
Intelligence, 13, 36, 53, 54, 60, 128, 141, 142, 183, 261
  and distractibility, 152
  and impulsivity, 266-268
  tests of, 18, 22, 28, 184-185
Impulsivity, 8, 142, 214
  and activity level, 263, 264
  and age, 271-273
  and attention, 262-263
  case of, 20-24
  and chemotherapy, 280-282
  and cognitive dysfunction, 262-266
  description of, 245-249
  and intelligence, 266-268
  and modeling, 297
  and mother-child variables, 273-276
  nature of, 249-261
  and personality factors, 277-279
  physiological aspects, 245
  population characteristics, 266-279
  and reflectiveness, 246, 247, 248
  and sex, 268-271
  treatment of, 279-294
Impulsive tempo, 282

J

Jack-in-the-box test, 148

K

Kissel-Freeling Depression Scale, 45
Kinetometer, 86

L

Learning
  and chemotherapy, 50-54
Learning arc, 197, 198, 199, 205, 217-222
Learning discrimination, 132, 133
Learning set, 211-213
Learning theory, 56-58, 65, 93, 139, 154, 156, 175, 284, 291
Limit-setting, 19
Logical memory, 195, 220

M

Mainstreaming, 235
Maximum holding power, 126
Memory abilities, 193-211, 286
  definition of, 193, 194
  process of, 193-197
  recall, 193
  registration, 193
  retention, 193

Mental control, 194, 220
Mental retardation, 33, 59, 125, 128, 129, 130, 135, 136, 140, 141, 143, 146, 156, 159, 169, 185, 187, 188, 282
Methylphenidate (see Ritalin), 47, 281
Metropolitan Reading Readiness Test, 291
MFFT, 250, 251, 252, 253, 254, 258, 259, 262, 263, 265, 267, 269, 272, 273, 274, 280, 281, 283, 286, 287, 288, 289, 290, 291, 296, 297, 299, 300, 301
Minimal brain dysfunction, 5, 7, 87
Minimal cerebral dysfunction, 182
Modeling, 94, 295, 297
  social, 290-291
Money, 237
Mother-child variables
  and impulsivity, 273-276
Motivation, 191, 192, 255
Motor neuron theory, 75

N

Negative reinforcement, 94, 159
Neurons, 75
Neurophysiology, 74

O

Obstinant progression, 82
Operant conditioning, 65
  techniques, 57, 160
Overactivity
  case of, 15-20

P

Passivity, 268
Peabody Picture Vocabulary Test, 150
Peer reinforcement, 101, 107
Perseveration, 212, 213
Personality testing, 19
Phenothiazines, 49

Phenylketonuria, 152
Placebos, 48, 51, 281
Position preference, 133, 211
Positive reinforcemnt, 94, 97-99, 154, 156, 157, 159, 289-290, 305-306
Premack principle, 109
Primary reinforcement, 96, 136, 156, 165, 283
Problem solving, 185, 286, 288, 299-301, 306
Psychoanalytic theory, 55-56, 65
Psychogenics, 44-45
Psychological theories, 54-58
Psychostimulants, 47-49, 51, 52, 53
Puberty, 36

R

Rating scales, 85-87
Readiness tests, 183
Receptor-effector systems, 77, 184, 197-198
Reciprocal inhibition, 164-165
Reflectiveness, 250, 254, 255, 258, 259, 260
  and impulsivity, 246, 247, 248
Reinforcement, 57, 58, 62, 94, 96, 97, 99, 100, 101, 102, 103, 104, 105, 107, 108, 109, 110, 111, 134, 136, 139, 175, 284, 288
  of academic achievement, 235-239
  fixed schedules, 162
  limited hold schedule, 285
  positive, 289-290, 305-306
  primary, 96, 136, 156, 165, 283
  school and home, 235-239
  secondary, 96, 101, 165
  social, 158
  strategies of, 162-172, 231-239
  token, 157
  variable interval schedules, 163
  variable ratio schedule, 163
  verbal, 288
Remedial programs, 222, 225
Repetition, 192
Response delay, 282
Response errors, 133-134

Response latency, 250, 253, 282, 286, 287, 288, 291, 297, 298, 302, 306
training, 284
Response sets, 221
Response shifts, 211
Response shift errors, 134
Reticular activity system, 39-42
Reticular formation, 34, 63, 80, 81, 82
Ritalin, 49, 280

S

Secondary reinforcement, 96, 101
Selective attention
and activity level, 135, 136
definition, 132
process of, 131, 132
Self-concept, 14, 19, 23, 24, 29, 30, 37, 230
and impulsivity, 277
Self instructions, 302, 303
Self-reinforcement, 294
Self theory, 56, 65
Sequential memory, 194-195, 208
Set, 120
Sex
and impulsivity, 268-271
Sleep, 35
Social interactions, 186
Social modeling, 94, 290-291, 292, 296, 299, 300, 306
Social reinforcement, 107
Special education programs, 226
Stimulus control, 121, 126, 128
Stimulus intensity, 127
Stimulus perseveration, 133
Strategy training, 285-289
Synapse, 40, 41, 80, 81

T

Tactile systems, 209-211
Teacher attention, 97, 98, 99
Teacher
role of, 229-230, 231-235
Temporal lobe, 35, 42, 43
Tempo response, 80, 95
Thalamus, 40, 42, 82, 131, 132
Thought stopping, 292, 293
Time out room, 233
Token reinforcement, 101, 105, 235, 236, 237
Tones test, 148, 150, 153
Tranquilizing drugs, 44, 49-50, 51
Treatment approaches, 279-294
chemotherapy, 47-54
educational, 58-62
modes of, 46-62
psychological theories, 54-58
Twenty questions test, 288, 289

V

Verbal mediation, 256, 292, 293 301-303
Verbal skills, 185
Vestibular (*see* Vision systems), 202
Vision systems, 202-203
centering, 202
communications, 203
identification, 203
vestibular, 202
Visual-Motor
coordination, 187
errors, 200-201
system, 198-201
Visual reproduction memory, 196
Visual stimuli, 125, 127
Visual verbal systems, 201-203
Visualization, 218
Voluntary attention, 123

W

Wechsler intelligence scale, 252, 254, 266, 284, 294